Praise for
The Practice of
Embodying Emotions

"A grand accomplishment. A unique synthesis. With academic precision, and with a deep gift for reflection, Dr. Selvam takes us on a stunning journey, exploring the structure and function of emotion in the brain as well as the body, the role emotions play in health and dis-ease, and how the body can be used to create a greater capacity to regulate and tolerate emotions to improve cognitive, emotional, and behavioral outcomes in all therapies. *The Practice of Embodying Emotions* is a rich addition for all therapists, as well as a gift to laypersons wishing to contact their emotional intelligence and enrich their lives."

—PETER A LEVINE, PhD, developer of Somatic
Experiencing® and best-selling author of *Waking the
Tiger* and *In an Unspoken Voice*

"Our capacity to regulate our emotions is extremely important for healing our attachment wounds and for having healthy relationships. This book, which offers a simple and effective method for building in us a greater capacity to regulate our emotions through our body, is a must for all therapists who work with attachment and for those looking for a self-help approach to improve their relationships."

—DIANE POOLE HELLER, PhD, author of *Crash
Course* and *The Power of Attachment* and creator of DARe
(Dynamic Attachment Re-Patterning experience) Training

"Ripe for our times, this brilliant book sheds light on the vital importance of fully embodying emotions, whether painful, pleasurable, or in-between. With an abundance of research and empirical evidence, it makes the case that emotions have a stronger influence on cognition and behavior than the other way around. As a couples' therapist and a child advocate for mental health in our schools, I experienced this book as a joyous godsend. With the support of the compassionate presence of another, emotions can be felt and fully expanded within the body to make them allies rather than foes. Dr. Selvam generously provides details of his four-step approach to alleviate suffering and enhance pleasure through the vehicle of emotional embodiment."

—MAGGIE KLEIN, LMFT, Somatic Experiencing® faculty member, and author of *Brain-Changing Strategies to Trauma-Proof Our Schools*

"There are many things I like about this book. I like that it is not only about changing emotional reactions but also about changing cognition and behavior (for the better) through regulating emotions—and that it shows scientifically how cognition, emotion, and behavior are intimately related to each other in the brain as well as the body. I also like that it provides evidence that our cognition, emotion, and behavior are dependent on others as well as the broader environment. I like how the book alternates between theory and concrete examples and embodies the author's persistence and brilliance. I highly recommend it to all therapists and those who are serious about their personal and spiritual growth."

—LISBETH MARCHER, founder of the Bodynamic Somatic Developmental Psychology System, coauthor of *The Body Encyclopedia*, and former president of EABP (European Association for Body Psychotherapy)

"Raja Selvam's book is a revelation. Combining the findings of neuroscience, Western psychodynamic theories, and Western and Eastern insights into the mind-body relationship, he has created a powerful and transformative approach to the way we experience and work with emotion. His extensive work with traumatized individuals and groups has put this approach to the test, and the resulting techniques make an invaluable addition to all forms of psychotherapy. Every page of this book conveys depth, clarity, and substance."

—GLEN SLATER, PhD, cochair of the Jungian and
Archetypal Studies Program at Pacifica Graduate Institute

"This book is a must-read for anyone who is interested in understanding and working with the embodiment of emotions. It is the perfect combination of science, historical and cultural context, client case examples, and presentation of a well-articulated, innovative model. The reader is guided, eloquently and methodically, on an exploratory journey of interwoven threads of traditions, disciplines, and models for understanding emotion. That journey seamlessly leads into a clear and detailed description of Dr. Selvam's approach to working effectively with embodying emotions."

—KATHY L. KAIN, PhD, coauthor of *Nurturing Resilience*
and *The Tao of Trauma*

"Don't miss this book! A valuable guide for therapists and interested folks alike. Introducing new concepts, solid theory, and grounded practice for working to embody emotions in gentle and innovative ways. The concept of *sensorimotor emotions* is a unique and much-needed contribution to the field of human consciousness. Refreshing in its presentation, with clarity, guiding the reader along a path of discovery toward embracing their whole being."

—IAN MacNAUGHTON, MBA, PhD, psychotherapist
and author of *Body, Breath & Consciousness*

"Selvam's extraordinary book offers an in-depth explanation of how the human body is involved in generating, defending against, and later triggering traumatic emotional experiences—especially prelinguistic ones—and is therefore a vital source of understanding of the physiology of implicit trauma memories that dominate the work of those engaged in pre- and perinatal psychology. *The Practice of Embodying Emotions* is brilliant and humble, research based, and intuitive. It is a 'game changer' in the field of trauma therapy, and I personally rate it five out of five."

—WILLIAM R. EMERSON, PhD, psychologist, winner of US National Science Foundation Award for Significant Contributions to Psychology, and author of *Treatment of Birth Trauma in Infants and Children*

"This book unmasks what is most painful and hidden in our minds and bodies. It is gentle. It is compassionate. It helped me reduce my own fear and reclaim my body. One of its many compelling aspects is that it embraces all our experience: our traumas, anxieties, terror, joy, and on and on. Rather than discounting other approaches to therapy, it builds on them with honesty, wisdom, and self-awareness—ultimately offering me a logical and clear guide to my own healing. It is simply an amazing and superb book; it has deepened and broadened my life and sense of self."

—PAUL LIEBER, actor, poet, teacher at Loyola Marymount University and the American Musical and Dramatic Academy, and author of the poetry collections *Chemical Tendencies* and *Interrupted by the Sea*

"Raja Selvam's extensive work on embodying emotions and regulating them through the body is a wonderful addition to the field of trauma healing. The book also includes what I particularly cherish: an extensive cross-cultural awareness."

—GINA ROSS, MFCT, Somatic Experiencing® senior faculty, founder and president of the International Trauma Healing Institute, and author of several books on trauma including *Breaking News! The Media and The Trauma Vortex*

"As a trauma therapist and educator, I found *The Practice of Embodying Emotions* to be a deeply satisfying work. It offers a practical combination of well-thought-out theory and research and numerous case examples to demonstrate and clarify the concepts and the methods. Raja Selvam is clearly an exceptional clinician, and I particularly benefited from the experiential exercises provided in the latter chapters. This book is a must-read for therapists and will be profoundly relevant for the layperson committed to their own healing."

—ARIEL GIARRETTO, MS, LMFT, SEP, trauma therapist and educator

"Integral Somatic Psychology (ISP) on which this book is based is a breath of fresh air for the professional community and the general public. It weaves together current science, Eastern and Western philosophical traditions, the linear and nonlinear world of emotional experience, and takes us to the next level of healing. It is brilliantly written and offers a wealth of information for anybody who wishes to engage deeply with the complex arena of trauma work. I have already gained priceless insights into my traumatization, stemming from racism and being a Vietnam combat veteran. Especially now, in these troubled times, people can gain a deeper understanding of their own response to PTSD with the help of Integral Somatic Psychology."

—RALPH STEELE, MA, LMFT, SEP, ISPP, teacher of Embodying Emotions Through Somatic Meditation and author of *Tending the Fire*

"This wonderful book offers a deep yet simple practice that aims to increase our ability to withstand, process, and complete difficult psychological experiences. It is useful for psychotherapists of different modalities and specialists in other helping professions, as well as for everyone searching for ways to cope with emotional forces in everyday life without suffering from avoidance. The main idea of the approach is surprisingly simple: involve more of the body in the emotional experience by removing physiological defenses against emotions and stay with the emotional experience for a longer period. Expanding and sustaining emotional experience this way, in turn, has a positive effect on almost all human systems (cognitive, behavioral, relational, physical, energetic, and spiritual)."

—ELENA ROMANCHENKO, psychotherapist, psychologist, educator, and member of the European Association for Body Psychotherapy (EABP)

"Developing the capacity to competently deal with deep emotions is a critical element in accessing and resolving powerful responses that can have a major impact in our lives. In this wonderful book, Raja Selvam offers a roadmap for identifying, accessing, and processing both present-day and long-ago emotions that live in our bodies and unconscious processes across a lifetime, often arising unbidden to play their irresistible role in current relationships and circumstances. With practical suggestions and guidelines, he shows us the way to develop the skill and ability to meet and resolve distressing and previously overwhelming emotional experiences."

—NANCY J. NAPIER, MA, LMFT, psychotherapist specializing in trauma resolution, Somatic Experiencing® faculty member, and author of *Getting Through the Day*, *Recreating Your Self*, and *Sacred Practices for Conscious Living*

"Finally! We have been waiting for this book for years! In this ground-breaking work, Raja Selvam creates the long-overdue synthesis of psychotherapy, neuroscience, and quantum physics as well as of cognition, emotion, and behavior to provide a tool for working with emotions that will profoundly enrich and facilitate your therapeutic work, no matter what your specialty is. You and your clients will be grateful!"

—DR. ELISABETH PELLEGRINI, specialist in child and adolescent psychiatry, psychoanalyst, teacher at the Medical University of Vienna, the University of Vienna, and the Danube University in Krems, and a training analyst in the Vienna Circle for Psychoanalysis and Self-Psychology

"In this very approachable book, Dr. Selvam marries the science of embodied emotion with the practice of healing. Practicing therapists as well as lay people will benefit greatly from the specific prescriptions offered in the book. Particularly at this trying time in human history, Dr. Selvam's instructive book serves as a balm to our broken species, and as an instruction manual on how to recover from our collective traumas."

—AKSHAY R. RAO, PhD, General Mills chair in Marketing at the Carlson School of Management, University of Minnesota

The Practice *of* Embodying Emotions

The
Practice
of
Embodying
Emotions

A GUIDE FOR IMPROVING COGNITIVE,
EMOTIONAL, AND BEHAVIORAL OUTCOMES

Raja Selvam, PhD

North Atlantic Books
Huichin, unceded Ohlone land
aka Berkeley, California

Published by
North Atlantic Books
Huichin, unceded Ohlone land
aka Berkeley, California

Cover art © Nickolay Grigoriev/Shutterstock.com
Cover design by Mimi Bark
Book design by Happenstance Type-O-Rama

Printed in Canada

The Practice of Embodying Emotions: A Guide for Improving Cognitive, Emotional, and Behavioral Outcomes is sponsored and published by North Atlantic Books, an educational nonprofit based in the unceded Ohlone land Huichin (aka Berkeley, CA), that collaborates with partners to develop cross-cultural perspectives, nurture holistic views of art, science, the humanities, and healing, and seed personal and global transformation by publishing work on the relationship of body, spirit, and nature.

MEDICAL DISCLAIMER: The following information is intended for general information purposes only. Individuals should always see their health care provider before administering any suggestions made in this book. Any application of the material set forth in the following pages is at the reader's discretion and is his or her sole responsibility.

North Atlantic Books' publications are distributed to the US trade and internationally by Penguin Random House Publishers Services. For further information, visit our website at www.northatlanticbooks.com.

Library of Congress Cataloging-in-Publication Data

Names: Selvam, Raja, 1956– author.
Title: The Practice of Embodying Emotions : A Guide for Improving
   Cognitive, Emotional, and Behavioral Outcomes / Raja Selvam, PhD.
Description: Berkeley, CA : North Atlantic Books, [2022] | Includes
   bibliographical references and index.
Identifiers: LCCN 2021014095 (print) | LCCN 2021014096 (ebook) | ISBN
   9781623174774 (trade paperback) | ISBN 9781623174781 (epub)
Subjects: LCSH: Emotions. | Somesthesia. | Emotions and cognition. | Mind
   and body. | Psychotherapy.
Classification: LCC BF531 .S45 2021 (print) | LCC BF531 (ebook) | DDC
   152.4—dc23
LC record available at https://lccn.loc.gov/2021014095
LC ebook record available at https://lccn.loc.gov/2021014096

2 3 4 5 6 7 8 9 MARQUIS 27 26 25 24 23 22

This book includes recycled material and material from well-managed forests. North Atlantic Books is committed to the protection of our environment. We print on recycled paper whenever possible and partner with printers who strive to use environmentally responsible practices.

Contents

PART III PRACTICE: THE FOUR STEPS OF EMOTIONAL EMBODIMENT

Acknowledgments

My parents, Kannammal and Muthuswamy, made the life I have possible. Without their dedication to my growth throughout my life, it is hard to imagine how this book could be here. I therefore dedicate this book to them, in gratitude.

I express my gratitude to those on whose shoulders the practice of embodying emotion stands, many of whom are named in the introduction as important influences in my professional development.

Of thousands the world over to whom I am deeply indebted for this life of mine, some have engraved deeper imprints on my soul. Richard Auger, my Jungian analyst for over twenty-five years, has been more of a caring father than a therapist. Cécile Ziemons, my love, companion, wife, anchor, harbor, catalyst, and critic, and an award-winning writer, has been a constant support throughout the writing of this book. Cécile, I love you!

I am also grateful to my maternal uncle Jegadeesan, in whose love I found the support to live through early separations from my mother; my paternal uncle Ramaswamy, who admired and supported my interest in reading and predicted that I would write a book one day; Alice Matthews, my class teacher in the seventh grade, who gave me much-needed confidence through a timely reflection of my academic ability, in the English-language boarding school I joined in the sixth grade with hardly any knowledge of English; Mr. Murugesan, my headmaster in the Tamil-language village school, who helped me to prepare for boarding school during lunch breaks; and dear friend Ron Doctor, who has given me much personal and professional support over the years.

One of the blessings of this life of mine is the opportunity to interact on a deep level with people from so many different cultures on every continent, form close friendships, and realize how similar we all are as human beings. I would like to express my love and appreciation to all of them and thank them for letting me into their hearts and lives and making my life so rich.

I would also like to express my gratitude to my publisher, North Atlantic Books, a nonprofit organization that embodies sincerity, heart, and soul through every individual I have had the pleasure of working with there: Tim McKee, the publisher, who patiently worked with me to arrive at a contract and introduced me to my excellent developmental editor; Shayna Keyles, the acquisitions editor, who went beyond the call of duty to offer me valuable editing suggestions, chapter by chapter; Lisbeth White, my developmental editor, who not only made the book much better but also made me a much better writer in the process; Brent Winter, whose meticulous and informed copyediting made the book even better; and Trisha Peck, the production editor, for helping me move through the many complexities involved from manuscript submission to publication.

I would like to thank my colleague and friend Maggie Kline for taking the time to offer very valuable comments. And last, but not least, two special thanks are in order. Louise Peyrot, the manager of my organization Integral Somatic Psychology, LLC, single-handedly manages almost all organizational activities to give me the time to write. Louise, I cannot thank you enough for all that you do for me and the organization, with such professionalism, kindness, compassion, and spirit of service! And Robert Gussenhoven, who plays multiple roles for us, including business consulting and website design, with such ability and ease—I thank you also for taking care of the art in the book.

Introduction

What This Book Is About

This book is about emotion. The book is also about the body, in relation to emotion. Specifically, it is about how to build a greater capacity to tolerate emotion. Its aim is to scientifically establish that we can build a greater capacity for tolerating emotion—especially unpleasant emotion—by expanding the emotional experience to as much of the body as possible, and how that can improve not only emotional but also physical, energetic, cognitive, behavioral, relational, and even spiritual outcomes in all therapies.

This book also aims to offer concrete steps and tools for how one might go about "embodying emotion," or building a greater capacity for tolerating emotion through expansion of its experience to as much of the body as possible, to improve a range of outcomes. The book is for professionals in all therapeutic modalities who are looking for ways to improve outcomes in whatever work they do, as well as for those looking for self-help tools for managing turbulent emotions in daily life.

People seek help when they are feeling sufficiently bad about something that they cannot deal with by themselves. There is an emotional difficulty in the core of almost every problem that clients present to their therapists. There are many effective ways to resolve an emotional difficulty: through changing how we think about a situation (cognition), changing how we deal with a situation through expression or action (behavior), changing the state of the brain and body physiology through medication, or numerous other means such as exercise, nutrition, meditation, essential oils, bodywork, and even electric shock. Or we can stay with the emotional experience in whatever form it appears, for as long as is necessary, until it transforms—a common practice on many spiritual paths.

People come to us, their therapists, for help with their suffering. Why not reduce or simply take away their suffering through one of the above methods, without taking people deeper into their suffering to build a greater capacity for tolerating it by expanding the emotional experience to as much of the body as possible? The answer lies in the latest findings in neuroscience, which establish that all of our three important psychological functions—cognition, emotion, and behavior—depend not only on the brain but also on the body and its connection to the environment; and that inhibiting the involvement of the body in emotion compromises our cognition as well as our behavior relative to the situation that has to do with the emotion. These findings, in combination with the central thesis of this book—that involving more of the body in emotional experience can create a greater capacity to tolerate the emotion and stay with it for a longer period of time—offer the possibility of improved outcomes in cognition and behavior, even in therapies that focus primarily on cognitive or behavioral methods.

Emotion is a summary assessment of a situation's impact on a person's well-being. The brain that has a longer time to process an emotion—because it is more regulated from being more expanded through the body—has a greater chance of generating more functional cognitions and behaviors in relation to the situation. If I can tolerate my rage in a relationship setting, what I think and do in the situation is likely to be more regulated and relational. So, even therapies that focus on facilitating cognitive and behavioral change to bring about symptom relief can improve their outcomes by incorporating the practice of embodying emotion.

All of the usual methods for working with emotion—especially the strategy of staying with the awareness of the emotional experience until transformation occurs—do enable people to develop some capacity for tolerating emotion. However, the extent to which these methods can develop a capacity for tolerating emotions is limited because they either do not work with the body or, if they do work with the body, their focus is not on expanding the emotional experience to as much of the body as possible. Of all the methods, the strategy of staying with an emotional experience until transformation occurs is most likely to increase affect tolerance.

However, the transformation a person is working toward might take longer or not happen at all if they do not know that an emotional experience, especially a difficult one, potentially involves the entirety of the brain and body physiology. In addition, people need to know that one needs to work with physiological defenses against emotions to expand the emotional experience to as much of the body as possible. This will increase the capacity to tolerate it for a longer period and to fully grasp the impact that a situation is having on our well-being. There is also the risk of retraumatization in passively staying with an emotion wherever it appears, as opposed to actively working with the body to regulate the emotional experience by expanding it, thus reducing the likelihood of retraumatization.

For all of the above reasons, embodying emotion—expanding the emotional experience to as much of the body as possible, to acquire a greater capacity to tolerate it—offers the potential for improving various outcomes in combination with all therapies and all of the usual methods for working with emotions, including medication.

For those who are not working in the helping professions, the book has also been written to serve as a self-help guide for understanding and working with emotional difficulties, large and small. For those who intend to use the book for self-help, even if you are a therapist, please make sure to seek professional help in case you find yourself in a difficult place. Please remember that as far as emotions are concerned, sooner or later we always need the support of others to resolve things, no matter who we are.

I would like to briefly share with you my personal and professional journeys that led me to develop the work of emotional embodiment, with a nod to those who helped me along the way. Then I will present a chapter-by-chapter overview of the book, followed by suggestions for strategies you can use to get the most out of this book.

The Development of
Emotional Embodiment Work

In their insightful book *Faces in a Cloud: Intersubjectivity in Personality Theory*, intersubjective psychoanalysts Atwood and Stolorow make the case that the diverse psychological theories developed by psychologists Freud, Jung, and Reich were shaped by these thinkers' personal histories, needs, and personalities.[1] My Jungian analyst, Richard Auger, often observes that we teach what we need to learn. Looking back over my life and my choice of orientations in psychology, I find that my relationship with the work of emotional embodiment in Integral Somatic Psychology (ISP) is no exception. I developed ISP as a comprehensive psychological approach to the embodiment of all levels of the psyche, individual and collective, with emotional embodiment as its primary clinical strategy, to improve cognitive, emotional, and behavioral outcomes in all therapies.

I had a rough start in life. My mother and I nearly died during my birth. I got stuck in a birth canal too narrow for my head, with the umbilical cord wrapped tightly around my neck during a prolonged labor under the care of a very inexperienced midwife. It was a miracle that we both survived, as my paternal grandmother remembered it. The birth trauma brought me close to cerebral palsy; I learned this from the symptoms I experienced while processing the birth trauma in therapy and in a dream from that period. My mother and I became tightly bonded, I think in part because of this shared traumatic experience. The repeated and prolonged separations from my mother I experienced from between the age of ten months until I was five years old were probably all the more traumatic because of the birth trauma and the close bond between us. When you add the physical, verbal, and emotional abuse my father subjected me to, my history does add up to something! I once dreamed that I went into a room in a heavily guarded police station to find a filing cabinet full of folders containing descriptions of all the kinds of traumas I have experienced in my life.

I have always marveled at how people appear to choose professions that offer them the optimal setting and opportunity to not only be of service to others but also to heal themselves personally. I see this especially among therapists in their choice to become mental health professionals and in the therapeutic modalities they choose, both for training and for treatment. The same is true for me.

All the early traumas caused me to lose my connection to my emotions and my body, and I grew up as a brainy kid interested more in mathematics than music. Once when I went on a date with a girl who loved music, I proudly offered her a mathematical theory of music appreciation. I am sure you can imagine how that turned out! Therefore, it made sense that from the very beginning of my professional development in psychology, I was drawn to bodywork systems such as Postural Integration, yoga, and body psychotherapy systems such as Reichian Therapy, Bioenergetics, and Bodynamic Analysis. This is where I first learned about physiological defenses against emotions and other psychological experiences, and how to work with such defenses gently (and not so gently) to connect the head to the body and to access emotions to work with them, often cathartically or regressively.

Wilhelm Reich, a contemporary of Sigmund Freud, is considered to be the founder of the body psychotherapy tradition in the West. The system he developed is called Reichian Therapy. Body psychotherapy approaches such as Bioenergetic Analysis, with their origin in Reichian Therapy, are identified as neo-Reichian therapies. The field of body psychotherapy now consists of such neo-Reichian approaches as well as other modalities. In my opinion, Bodynamic Somatic Developmental Psychology, also known as Bodynamic Analysis, is the most sophisticated body psychotherapy system to date, with its empirically derived map of the psychological functions of the major voluntary muscles based on their psychomotor functions, and a complex character structure theory for seven stages of childhood development. This system is perhaps years ahead of its time, given how limited the orientation to the body still is in the larger field of psychology. I learned a great deal from teaching the Bodynamic Analysis psychology of muscles and character structure theory for a number of years. I cannot thank Lisbeth Marcher and her colleagues at the Bodynamic Institute enough for their contribution to my personal and professional development by offering me a detailed map of the emotional needs of the child in each state of its development.[2]

Many of the early traumas of my life involved so much stress and dysregulation in my body and brain that I suffered for a long time from symptoms of posttraumatic stress disorder (PTSD), such as sensitivity to noise, poor sleep, and extreme reactivity in relationships, without realizing they could be symptoms of PTSD. Traumatic stress, especially from early childhood, often involves high levels of stress, dysregulation, and reactivity in the autonomic nervous system and the viscera governed by it, and in the central nervous system areas of the brain and the spinal cord.

It helped me a great deal to train in a body-oriented trauma training called Somatic Experiencing (SE), which focuses on resolving trauma through autonomic regulation, and then teaching the approach all over the world on behalf of its founder, Dr. Peter Levine. These experiences were beneficial not only in healing my traumatic stress symptoms but also in providing me with a laboratory to develop my emotional embodiment work. Dr. Levine, whose book *Waking the Tiger: Healing Trauma* continues to be a bestseller in its category more than twenty years after its publication, is an exquisitely fine clinician with an incredible intelligence.[3] He is a master at downregulating highly aroused autonomic nervous systems that are often the cause of symptoms of traumatic stress. I owe so much personally and professionally to this exceptional individual and am very grateful for meeting him so early in my career in psychology.

My training in Biodynamic Craniosacral Therapy from Dr. Michael Shea helped me to understand how to work directly with stress and dysregulation in the central nervous system areas of the brain and spinal cord in others as well as myself.[4] The core areas of the brain and spinal cord are increasingly dysregulated with severe trauma, such as birth and early abandonment traumas, which I have in my own history. Biodynamic Craniosacral Therapy also taught me how to work with the body in its depth at the quantum or subatomic level, which can become increasingly dysregulated when the intensity of trauma worsens. This approach also taught me how to reconnect the body to collective healing energies in its environment, a connection that can be compromised in trauma to a greater or lesser extent depending on the severity of the trauma.

I experienced much difficulty in accessing my emotions and regulating them, and in sensing my body, both as an academic in business before I became interested in formal training in psychology and during my subsequent education and training to become a licensed clinical psychologist. This motivated me to study the findings of research on emotions and their physiology in depth, especially in affective neuroscience and body psychotherapy paradigms, to find clues for how to access and work better with emotions and the body, both for my clients and myself.

Body psychotherapies such as Reichian Therapy, Bioenergetics, and Bodynamic Analysis work with body defenses primarily in the muscular nervous system to access and express emotions. Of late, the focus of body psychotherapy has expanded to include the role of the autonomic nervous system. Somatic Experiencing, for example, focuses more on working with defenses and dysregulation in the autonomic nervous system to access and regulate emotions. The approaches based on meditative practices from the East, such as mindfulness-based stress reduction, deal with emotions through mindfulness practice. The intersubjective and Kleinian psychoanalytic approaches and the analytical psychology of Jung work with emotions primarily through cognition. The cognitive behavioral approaches regulate emotions through cognition and behavior. And the fine work done by bodywork and energy work approaches regulates emotions by regulating the body or energy respectively. These are all either evidence-based or time-and-market-tested methods that are effective in helping clients with a variety of clinical problems. However, I found them lacking somehow, or time-consuming, or incomplete in their approach to working with emotions, at least for some of my clients—especially for myself!

More than one surprise emerged from my in-depth study of the physiology of emotions in affective neuroscience, especially in an area called embodied cognition. One of these surprises was recognizing that our understanding of the physiology of emotion and of the physiology of cognition has been going through paradigm shifts in the last twenty years, turning earlier findings on their heads. It was also surprising to see that so little of what we understand about the physiology of emotion and of cognition has been integrated into the practice of psychology, even in body psychotherapy systems. In addition, I noticed that most of the research on emotion is focused on a limited number of primary emotions, such as anger and sadness, and neglects the larger number of always-present emotions that I started to refer to as sensorimotor emotions—emotions such as just feeling good or bad about a situation one finds oneself in. Finally, the more recent findings in affective neuroscience in newer research paradigms of embodied and embedded cognition, and embodied and enactive emotion, provide substantial theoretical and empirical evidence for the effectiveness of emotional embodiment work in improving cognitive, affective, and behavioral outcomes across therapeutic modalities, which I had been finding empirically for some time.

No work stands solely on its own feet. It always stands on a pyramid of shoulders that reaches far below into the past. I have many to thank for my education about the interrelated physiology of emotion, cognition, and behavior. I will, however, limit my thanks to those close to the top of this pyramid of accumulated wisdom. I learned that the body as well as the brain are involved in emotion from neuroscientist Antonio Damasio (in whose lineage Bud Craig has been making outstanding contributions of late) and from neuroscientist and psychoneuroimmunologist Candace Pert.[5,6,7]

The work of a number of brilliant minds taught me that emotion, cognition, and behavior are functions of not only the brain but also the body and the environment; that cognition, emotion, and behavior are fundamentally inseparable in the physiology of the brain and the body; that embodying emotion can improve cognition and behavior; and that emotion is dynamic and predictive. Those brilliant minds belong to Eugene Gendlin[8] from the University of Chicago, Marc Johnson[9] at the University of Oregon, Lisa Feldman Barrett[10] at Northeastern University, Sian

Beilock at Barnard College,[11] Giovanna Colombetti[12] at the University of Exeter in the United Kingdom, Evan Thompson[13] at the University of British Columbia in Vancouver, Paula Niedenthal[14] at the University of Wisconsin at Madison, and Rebekka Hufendiek[15] at the University of Basel in Switzerland.

Any effective work with emotion requires an understanding of the psychological defenses against intolerable or unacceptable emotions, as well as adequate outside support for emotional experiences. I was fortunate enough to learn how to work with psychological defenses against emotions and to support emotions in not just one but a number of psychological modalities: the humanistic psychology of Carl Rogers, the gestalt therapy of Fritz Perls, Heinz Kohut's self psychology, Melanie Klein's object relations, and the intersubjective psychoanalysis of Robert Stolorow.

I grew up in India and moved to the United States for higher education at the age of twenty-six. I grew up in a family in which dreams were seen as meaningful messages from the collective. In my culture, one's quantum energy body is real, and an individual's experience is deeply embedded in and shaped by the collective. Therefore, it was natural that I would be drawn to Jungian psychology from almost the beginning of my study of psychology because of its expansive view of the human psyche. It was also natural that I would eventually be drawn back to an Eastern psychology that proposes an even more expansive view of the psyche: Advaita Vedanta, a school of Hindu philosophy. In addition to incorporating all levels of the psyche from Jungian psychology, Advaita Vedanta theorizes that the individual is ultimately inseparable from and identical with the collective.

In order to work with emotions, which are the most difficult of our experiences, it makes sense that one needs to work with all levels of the psyche—physical, energetic, and collective—that bear upon them. Jungian psychology, Advaita Vedanta,[16] yoga, Randolph Stone's Polarity Therapy,[17] and Biodynamic Craniosacral Therapy[18] gave me the necessary understanding and tools to begin to work with all levels of the psyche in relation to emotions. Developing a greater capacity for opposites in experience, or building affect tolerance, is emphasized in intersubjective psychoanalysis for psychological health, in Jungian psychology for individuation, and in Advaita Vedanta for enlightenment. Seeing the importance that these diverse systems placed on affect tolerance was an early inspiration in the development of emotional embodiment work as a core clinical strategy in the larger framework of ISP, my comprehensive approach to the psyche.

When I set out twenty years ago to develop the approach of embodying emotion—focused on developing a greater capacity to tolerate emotional experiences—as a therapeutic tool, I did not have the benefit of all the scientific evidence available today for why that makes sense. During that time, there has been a virtual revolution in our understanding of the role of the body in both emotion and cognition. When I began, I was inspired to develop this work on the basis of two simple ideas: that developing a capacity for tolerating emotion is a good thing, based on my study of intersubjective psychoanalysis, Jungian psychology, and Advaita Vedanta; and that the entire brain and body physiology could perhaps be used to make the experience of emotion more tolerable. I developed the second idea after learning from my initial study of the physiology of emotions (especially from neurologist Antonio Damasio and molecular scientist Candace Pert) that the bulk, if not the entirety, of brain and body physiology can be involved in the generation of emotional experiences. I also learned from several body psychotherapy approaches that various physiological defenses against intolerable experiences could form in both the brain and the body to reduce suffering.

From observing emotional experiences in myself and my clients, it became clear that an experience of an emotion such as fear could occur in different body locations in different people, and in different locations in the same person on different occasions: sometimes in the chest, other times in the legs, the belly, the head, or the brain. For example, when I once asked a client where she was experiencing her fear, she first reported it as an experience only in her brain. When I asked her to touch the back of her neck, where muscles can often form a defense against an experience from the head extending to the body (and vice versa), she was surprised to experience fear all over her body not much later.

These observations, in combination with my observation that my clients and I often struggled to resolve difficult emotions that showed up in only very few places in our brain and body physiology, led me to wonder if processing the energy of a difficult emotion in more places in the brain and body physiology—processing in a bigger container, so to speak—would somehow make it more bearable to stay with, process, and complete the emotions. As I would later explain to my clients, to motivate them to embody difficult emotional experiences: just as a bag can be carried more easily with two hands than with one, it is easier to tolerate an emotion when it is carried by more parts of the body.

Thus, emotional embodiment work has been critical to my professional and personal growth. I am extremely pleased by this confluence, which continues to evolve from new clinical experiences and emerging streams of knowledge. Emotional embodiment has certainly benefited me, my clients, and my students, and in turn their clients. In writing this book, I am so looking forward to sharing this work with as many people as possible—mental health professionals as well as laypeople—all over the world.

Outline of the Book

The book is organized in three sections: an overview of this field (part I, "Overview," chapters 1–4), an exploration of the theories underlying it (part II, "Theory," chapters 5–9), and details regarding the practice of embodying emotion (part III, "Practice: The Four Steps of Emotional Embodiment," chapters 10–14).

Chapters 1–4 in part I offer a more substantive introduction to the work. They offer an introduction to the theory, the basic concepts, the practice of embodying emotion, and its benefits, with illustrative clinical examples in a variety of clinical contexts, and with clients with varying levels of affect tolerance or capacity for tolerating emotional experiences. Chapter 1 focuses on clients with high affect tolerance, with high levels of emotion and emotional intensity, wide and deep expansion of emotion in the body, and long cycles of emotional processing. Chapter

2 focuses on work with clients at the other end of the spectrum of affect tolerance, with low levels of emotion and emotional intensity, narrow and superficial expansion of emotion in the body, and short cycles of emotional processing. Chapter 3 presents clinical examples highlighting benefits that are possible through embodying emotion, such as improvements in cognitive, emotional, behavioral, physical, energetic, and spiritual outcomes. This chapter also presents a clinical example of emotional embodiment in long-term work and the possible limitations of the method. Chapter 4 focuses on clinical examples of emotional embodiment work in the treatment of severe traumas that involve considerable dysregulation of the brain and body physiology. I hope that after reading part I, readers will have a decent grasp of the approach so they can begin the practice of embodying emotions with themselves and others.

Part II, the theory section (chapters 5–9), presents the hard scientific evidence on which the practice of embodying emotion is based. Chapter 5 offers a detailed treatment of the physiology of emotion and establishes that the generation and experience of emotion can involve the entirety of one's brain and body physiology. Chapter 6 presents emerging evidence on how cognition, emotion, and behavior are dependent not just on the brain but also on the body and the environment; how inseparable the three are as they arise in the physiology of the brain as well as the body; and the implications of these findings for the work of emotional embodiment. Chapter 7 presents a framework of seven physiological dynamics through which emotions are generated and defended against in the brain and body physiology—dynamics that can be observed and manipulated in embodying emotion. Chapter 8, on affect tolerance, develops the book's central thesis—that expanding an emotional experience in the physiology can increase a person's capacity to tolerate the experience—based on the findings presented in chapters 5, 6, and 7 and on a simple model of physiological regulation. Chapter 9 discusses different kinds of emotions, including always-present and often-overlooked sensorimotor emotions such as simply feeling good or bad, to create a bigger range of emotional experience to embody from the first session with a client.

Part III, consisting of chapters 10–14, is focused on the nuts and bolts of the practice of embodying emotion. Chapter 10, "The Situation," discusses how to identify and process a situation so it can lead to an emotional response to work with. Chapter 11, "The Emotion," offers different ways of working with psychological and innate defenses against emotions to access emotions, as well as ways to support emotional experiences in oneself and others. Chapter 12, "The Expansion," looks at how to approach and work with physiological defenses against emotions, and ways to work with different parts of the brain and body physiology to expand an emotional experience in a regulated manner to as much of the body as possible. Chapter 13, "The Integration," covers the optional step of integration. This chapter discusses how certain resources—such as physiological energetic improvements, collective energies, and cognitive and behavioral shifts that can be expected to arise automatically in the process of embodying emotion—can be used to make emotional experiences more stable, contained, and tolerable, and to expedite symptom resolution. Chapter 14, "Interpersonal Resonance," presents evidence on how human beings have the innate capacity to exchange information directly with each other through short-range bioelectric and biomagnetic energies and long-range quantum energies. The chapter also discusses how to use interpersonal resonance to understand and support emotional states in others.

The last chapter, titled "Conclusion: The Future," discusses an interesting topic for neurological research in relation to emotional embodiment and the possible new dimensions that the practice of embodying emotion could add, such as the subtle or quantum level as well as the collective level of the psyche, to further improve outcomes in all therapies.

For the reader who is short on time or has little patience with theory, I would recommend that you start with part I, skip part II, go straight to part III, and then return to part II to learn more about the theoretical underpinnings of the practice of embodying emotion. For everyone, I highly recommend that you start the practice of embodying emotion with yourself and others as soon as you start reading this book. We are generating emotions all the time, and difficult emotional experiences, big and small, are a daily occurrence. So what are you waiting for? If you are reluctant to start to expand an unpleasant emotional experience in your body, start with a pleasant experience as a trial run.

As a medium for communicating how to go about the practice of embodying emotion, a book containing words and pictures is limited at best. To overcome this limitation, we have set up free secure online access to videos of complete demonstration sessions of emotional embodiment work, as well as shorter illustrative videos of the steps involved in the practice of embodying emotion. To gain access to this free online resource, please visit www.integralsomaticpsychology.com, then click "Books," then "Embodying Emotion," and then "Resources" in successive dropdown menus, and register.

PART I

OVERVIEW

The four chapters in this section present an overview of the theories, concepts, methods, and benefits of the practice of embodying emotion, in the context of a variety of treatment examples and their outcomes.

1

The Beginning

Chapter summary: an overview of concepts, methods, and outcomes in the context of treatment examples involving higher levels of emotional intensity, from earlier phases of development of the practice of embodying emotion.

To develop an understanding of emotional embodiment work, let's begin with real-life examples. This chapter and the next will present clinical examples of emotional embodiment, touch upon some key concepts that underlie the approach, and give the reader a feel for how the work developed over time. I will not be discussing in depth the specific skills for embodying emotion in the chapters in this section. A detailed treatment of the skills involved can be found in part III.

I first noticed the effectiveness of emotional embodiment treatments when working with clients experiencing high levels of emotion, and these are the case studies presented in this chapter. In the next chapter, I present examples of treatments working with clients involving lower levels of emotion, through which I learned the breadth and versatility of the effectiveness of emotional embodiment. The names and locations of some individuals have been changed to honor their requests for anonymity.

Petra, the Voice, and the Panic Attacks

Petra started having panic attacks at the age of seven. As she remembered it, she was playing in her room by herself when she heard a voice speak to her from her lower right abdomen: "Petra, it is time for you to die!" This was the start of fourteen years of suffering that involved panic attacks, depression, difficulty in school, and stress in low-paying jobs after high school. Petra went to work, came home, ate, and slept up to twelve hours a day. She did not want her parents to leave the house when she was at home because she did not feel safe. When I saw her for the first time, I was in the Netherlands facilitating a six-day training. At the end of the first day, her uncle, who was an assistant at the training, asked me to see Petra to determine if I could be of any help.

What I remember particularly about that first meeting was how dispirited her parents appeared to be. It made sense that they were not hopeful. Petra was their only child, and they had done everything they could think of to help her: medical doctors, psychiatrists, and psychoanalysts. At the age of twenty-one, Petra had already been through two psychoanalytic treatments and was on multiple medications. When I told her I could see her twice at the most during my short stay in her country and that she might have to do follow-up work with someone I referred her to, Petra was very clear with me that she did not want to do more psychotherapy. Instead of insisting that she should agree to see another therapist to ensure she was adequately cared for after the work we did together, I told her that she had a much better chance of improving if she did the things I taught her during our sessions.

The work I and others had done in Indian fishing villages among the survivors of the 2004 tsunami had taught me that clients could be active participants in their own healing.[1] Over a period of two years after that devastating natural disaster, I led five international teams of therapists to the state of Tamil Nadu to offer treatments, education, and training for the survivors and those involved in their recovery. Follow-up surveys from one of our trips to India found that respondents who practiced skills they had learned during treatment sessions were much more likely to report a greater reduction in their symptoms.

Petra's uncle had told me that she had had two surgeries soon after she was born in order to correct a life-threatening congenital defect in her large intestine—the same location where the voice announcing her time of death appeared to come from. I was curious about how that area might be involved in the formation of her panic attacks. I knew from my own experience and the experience of those I have treated that symptoms often involve dysfunctional patterns in parts of the body that have been most traumatized. An example from my own life: because I nearly died during my own birth because I was stuck for a long time in a birth canal too small for my head, whenever my degree of physical or emotional stress increases beyond a certain extent, the right side of my head has a tendency to become constricted and uncomfortable. This symptom is less evident now than it used to be, but it still makes its presence felt to this day.

I told Petra it was possible that unresolved traumatic patterns from her lifesaving surgeries might have something to do with her panic attacks. She was not surprised; one of her two psychoanalysts had made that connection already. I told her it is not unusual for energy to concentrate in an area of the body that has experienced trauma and to increase in intensity until it reaches an upper limit and triggers a symptom such as a panic attack, to reduce the intensity and bring about relief. The level of intensity at which the symptom forms is also referred to as the symptom threshold. I then suggested the following, both as a treatment and as a self-help protocol: whenever she felt stress in her life, no matter the cause, she should learn and practice ways to distribute the stress in her body so that it did not build and concentrate in the lower right abdominal area beyond the symptom threshold, which could trigger the voice and an ensuing panic attack.

To start, we chose to practice how she could cope with her work situation, as her boss was often a source of stress. I asked her to imagine a difficult interaction with her boss and then to notice the buildup of constriction, arousal, stress, and discomfort in her lower right abdominal area. I guided her to work with the physiological defenses in her abdomen and legs to redistribute the unpleasant arousal, stress, and discomfort she felt in her abdomen to adjacent areas of the legs using simple tools of awareness, intention, movement, and self-touch. I invited her to notice how this helped ease the intensity of the unpleasantness in the abdominal area, and how that area eventually settled. All of this did not take very long. I asked her to practice what we had done during the session on a daily basis whenever she felt that she was getting stressed, regardless of the cause, and to come back in five days, on the last day of my training. During the treatment, I found Petra receptive enough to my suggestions; but I also found her somewhat skeptical, which was understandable, given how long she had suffered without relief.

When Petra came back five days later, I noticed a change in her. She appeared to be in a better mood. I asked her whether she had been able to practice what she had learned in the previous session, and what changes, if any, she had observed in herself since. She said she did "the exercise" regularly, and her mother had observed that her energy had somehow changed for the better. What she told me next, however, surprised me. Petra had suffered from severe constipation all her life and was able to eliminate only once or twice a week, with a great deal of difficulty. Since our session, however, she was greatly relieved to be able to have an easy and regular bowel movement every morning. The "exercise" seemed to have really worked, she said, adding that she did it as often as she could. She now really believed in "the method" and was looking forward to learning more about it.

The method I taught her, on the basis of what I had observed had worked well for her during the first session, was simply this: Whenever she felt stress building up in her abdomen, she should move her legs to relieve any constriction in them. Then she should place one hand on her abdomen and the other on first one leg and then the other, to draw the energy down and distribute it more evenly between her abdomen and her legs, and then observe the changes that occur in her body, especially for the better. For example, the high level of arousal might automatically come down, and the body might feel better overall.

Years later, such quick changes in long-term, persistent, and serious symptoms in some clients no longer surprise me as much as they did when I saw Petra, even for symptoms such as asthma, migraine, and chronic pain, when they are psychophysiological in origin. People can form serious psychophysiological symptoms, such as chronic fatigue, at low levels of emotional stress. Psychophysiological (formerly called "psychosomatic") symptoms are physical symptoms that are caused or exacerbated by psychological conditions. (This book uses the term "psychophysiological symptoms" instead of "psychosomatic symptoms" because the latter has acquired a negative meaning of being only in one's head.) Teaching people how to experience emotional stress in a more distributed and regulated way within the larger container or space of the body can achieve a number of beneficial outcomes:

- It can create a greater capacity for emotional suffering, which helps by increasing the threshold or level of tolerance at which symptoms form.

- It can decrease the level of stress and dysregulation and increase the level of self-regulation throughout the organism.

- It can increase the body's connection to the environment, improving the possibility of interactive regulation.

- It can resolve symptoms more quickly and shorten the treatment period.

- It can make a person's overall system more resilient, so that symptoms do not form as easily in the face of stressors; and if symptoms do form, they can resolve more quickly.

Back then, knowing less than I do now, I could not rule out the possibility that Petra's constipation cure was just a "transference cure"—a sudden cure that can happen because the client idealizes the therapist or the method—which does not always last. Putting those thoughts aside, during my second session with Petra I turned my focus to the work she and I could do before I left the country the following day. It seemed as though she had come prepared to jump in with both feet and do a lot, encouraged by what she had been able to achieve in just a week. As soon as we started to process a stressful situation in her life, she reported a more coherent emotion of fear emerging in the chest area. Emotions in the body often emerge first in the chest area. That she could sense it there right away was a good sign that she had developed a greater capacity to not shut her body down in the face of the difficult emotion of fear. It is not unusual for people to continue to heal on their own and develop greater capacity for emotions once they learn how to use more of the body to process them.

Emotion can be thought of as an assessment of how a situation affects or impacts the well-being of the whole body.[2] This implies that the more the impact is distributed throughout the body, the easier it is to tolerate it subjectively. We have a tendency to use physical and energy defenses, such as constriction, to limit emotions to a few places in the body as a way of coping with them. All of us have a tendency to resort to this strategy for relief quite often, in a misguided attempt to reduce our necessary suffering. It is all too understandable, given our shared aversion to unpleasant experiences. Physical and energy defenses against emotions such as constriction, low arousal, or numbing can disrupt the various flows (blood, nervous system, lymphatic, interstitial or intercelluar fluid, and electromagnetic and quantum energy) that are vital for brain and body regulation and physical and psychological well-being. In this context, I use the phrase "expanding the body" to mean working to undo such physical and energy defenses to improve all of these vital flows from one part of the body to another, to help distribute the emotional experiences to more places in the body to make it more bearable, and to improve the level of regulation throughout the brain and the body to resolve psychophysiological symptoms.

As I taught Petra how to "expand" her body in order to expand the emotion of fear, and to stay with it and tolerate the sensations in more places in her body, the level of fear as well as the psychophysiological arousal became extremely high—so high that I wondered if I had helped Petra to open up too much too fast. This made me very concerned that she might decompensate or fall apart during or after the session.

We hung in there—Petra and I and her uncle, who was observing the session—for a long period of time, as the fear turned into terror, a response clearly disproportionate to the situation we had started with. I got Petra to split her attention between what she was experiencing inside her body and what she was noticing in her surroundings, to reduce the subjective intensity of her suffering. I had her make statements such as "My body is afraid; I am not" to introduce mindfulness. I interpreted the fear for her as possibly the fear of dying after her birth from the congenital defect and from the surgeries, so as to provide a meaningful frame to contain the fear. This anchored the context that it was not a fear of an unknown in the present, which would be harder to contain, but a fear response to something in the past.

Most importantly, I remained focused on working with the physiological and psychological defenses against her terror so she could expand her body in as regulated a manner as possible, in order to distribute the emotion to as much of her body as possible (the rest of the chest, the abdomen, the arms, the legs, the head, the neck, the spine, the brain, the front, and the back). This was intended to manage but not eliminate the states of physiological stress and dysregulation that are inherent in the generation and experience of unpleasant emotions such as fear. The purpose of all this was to have Petra experience the emotion as being as regulated and tolerable as possible.

The notion that the body is involved in emotions might sound strange to those who have been taught that only the brain is involved in emotional experience. The idea that the entire body can be involved in an emotional experience might sound odd even to those who do not dispute the body's role in emotion. As we will see later in this book, cutting-edge research on emotions has established that the experience of emotion depends not only on the brain but also on the entire body and its environment.[3,4,5] Once we accept the idea that the entire body can be involved in the experience of an emotion, it is easy to imagine how using more of the body to process an emotion might be to one's advantage, even though the scientific explanation might be indeed complex (as we will see in part II).

It was indeed a difficult and lengthy session for everyone involved, with a great deal of uncertainty about whether it would be helpful or harmful to Petra. I did not then have the confidence I have now that this method could or would work. In a way, I had no choice. The intense suffering was there all of a sudden, and I had to support her in managing it somehow to avoid another panic attack. Back then, I only had theoretical assurance: from neuroscience, that emotions could potentially involve the whole body; from intersubjective psychoanalysis, that healing involved greater affect tolerance; from cognitive behavioral therapy, that healing sometimes involved prolonged exposure to intense suffering; from Jungian psychology, that healing involved the development of a greater capacity to tolerate opposites; and from Eastern psychology, that the capacity to tolerate opposites in the body is a prerequisite for enlightenment, the highest possible spiritual achievement for the human psyche. Looking back, one could say I was being shown through treatments such as Petra's that increasing the capacity for necessary suffering in a regulated manner, by using as much of the body container as possible, can help resolve psychophysiological symptoms in a surprisingly efficient manner.

The length of the cycle, with fear and then terror, was nearly forty minutes; but Petra eventually settled. Exhausted yet relieved, I educated Petra about the additional things we had done during the second session to manage her fear, stress, and dysregulation, and I encouraged her to continue to practice these techniques to manage stress or other feelings as they came up, as often as possible. I referred Petra to a local colleague just in case she needed help, and I also asked her to keep me informed of her progress through her uncle. Probably shaken by the session, Petra took the colleague's contact information, although I learned later that she never used it. I left the country the following morning, and I might have said a prayer or two before leaving! Just in case you do not know this, there is evidence for the effectiveness of prayer, even in the treatment of cancer.[6] Researchers have observed higher rates of remission among cancer patients who had others praying for them than among control group members who were not prayed for.

Three months later, Petra's uncle emailed me with very good news about her that he wanted to share with me over the phone. Extremely curious and much relieved, I called him as soon as I could. What he had to tell me was very good news indeed: Petra no longer had any panic attacks, a symptom that had persisted for fourteen years. She had been using the skills she learned during our sessions to prevent an attack from occurring if she sensed that she was on the verge of one. She was feeling much better and more positive about her life. She was no longer sleeping as much and had even started jogging with her father. I told him I was so glad we were able to help a young woman move forward in her life.

The next time I saw Petra for a session was six months later, when I was back in the Netherlands to teach the second and final part of the training. It was late November, and the spirit of Christmas was already palpable. I saw her only once during this trip. The session was mostly about catching up and reinforcing the skills she had learned during the earlier sessions. She had made significant changes in her life: she had quit her old job and had found a new one that she liked more, she still was no longer having panic attacks, and she was working with her psychiatrist to get off all her medications by the end of February. Her psychiatrist, intrigued by her progress, wanted to know what "exercises" I had taught her that worked so well. At the end of the session, Petra wanted me to tell her story to others—and even gave permission to use her name in the telling—so others could benefit from "the method" as well. I was very touched by the sincerity, gratitude, and generosity of this remarkable young woman.

The next and the last time I spoke with Petra was in the spring of the following year. She had reached out to me through her uncle because she was having a difficult time. Her grandfather had just died. I was in the United States, so we talked on the phone. By then, Petra was off all her medications and was still free of the panic attacks. She was in general feeling much better. What had been difficult for her was the loss of her grandfather, who had always been a special person in her life. I told her that such a loss is indeed a painful experience. It takes time to heal and come to terms with that kind of experience, and we need the support of others to get through it. However, she could use the skills she had learned to cope with fear to cope with her sadness as well. We then worked on how to undo the physiological defenses, such as constriction, that easily form against unpleasant emotions such as sadness. We also practiced ways to redistribute the sadness from her chest area to the rest of her body in a regulated manner, using again the simple tools of awareness, intention, movement, self-touch, and expression. This time, she learned more consciously how working to more fully embody an unpleasant emotion such as sadness in a regulated manner made it more bearable to be with it for a longer period of time. We sat with the shared sadness for a while.

I was about to end the session to prepare for my next appointment when Petra asked if I had the time to help her with another thing that had been of concern to her. She said she used to be depressed, but now she often had so much energy that she did not know what to do with it—a level of energy she had formerly only experienced during panic attacks. I explained to her that when the body is no longer symptomatic and shut down in defense against unbearable experiences such as emotions, its energy is free and available for constructive and life-enhancing purposes. I asked her if she could think of anything she could use her extra energy to accomplish in her life. Petra responded that it was interesting that I should ask her that, because she had been thinking about going back to the university to get a degree. I encouraged her to do it. I even pushed her a bit by sharing with her that old symptoms could come back if she did not use the newfound energy constructively.

That phone session was the last time Petra and I worked together. I write "Petra and I worked together" instead of "I worked with Petra" because I believe that much of her progress had to do with her willingness to learn and to use more of her body as a container to deal with overwhelming experiences of emotion, and the stress and dysregulation that accompanied them. Like a proud parent, I have been tracking the strides that she continues to make in her life, through my contact with her uncle: She has a boyfriend. She has graduated from college. She has a new job. She has an apartment of her own. She and her boyfriend are now living together. And the last thing I heard, years ago, was that Petra and her boyfriend were on a long motorcycle journey through an Asian country. I am curious if that country is India, where I am originally from. One of these days, I intend to find out.

Connie, the Electrocution, and the Migraines

Connie, a woman in her midforties, had suffered from migraines for as long as she could remember. They occurred once or even twice a week. When they did, they were sometimes so intense that she had to lie down in a dark room to lessen their severity. Connie was a psychotherapist and a participant in a training I taught in Denmark. I heard from the team of assistant trainers that Connie found it difficult to stop crying during practice sessions with other training participants, leaving those who were trying to help her feeling helpless and puzzled, or she would come down with a migraine after the practice session. I did not have much history about Connie on the voluntary information and consent form she had submitted to be considered for a demonstration, but what I heard about her made me wonder if I could help her in some way.

During training, I usually do a demonstration of some aspect of the work with one of the participants in front of the class. I answer questions about what I did during the demonstration, and then I have the participants practice the demonstrated aspect in dyads or triads, under the supervision of an assistant trainer. I got the opportunity to work with Connie in a demonstration on the second or third day of the six-day training.

Even before we began, I knew that nothing would be accomplished if she just cried, and I made it clear to her and the class that this behavior had to be contained for any progress to be made. Although crying can often be therapeutic, it can also at times be a quick way to get relief or an indication of being stuck in a cycle of helplessness. It can rid the client of the suffering that is driving a symptom, but without providing the client or the therapist an opportunity to examine the suffering for the clues it might contain for the cure. In Connie's case, helpless crying appeared to have become a habitual response in therapy whenever any suffering was touched upon. It turned out that Connie had also done some therapy in which she had been encouraged to express her emotions strongly.

Getting Connie to contain her crying was indeed challenging. I introduced interventions such as asking her to open her eyes and not keep them closed, and guiding her to pay more attention to what was happening outside around her than to what was happening inside her body, in order to reduce the intensity of her suffering. I also insisted that she verbalize her inner experience as often as possible to maintain her ability to think and speak, which can often be lost in states of extreme emotional overwhelm. These helped her manage her crying and emotional overwhelm to some extent.

Between bouts of crying, with much guidance and reassurance, she was able to identify, tolerate, and express the suffering in her body in terms of the most basic sensorimotor emotions, such as feeling too bad or awful or intolerable. This was as opposed to noticing one unpleasant body sensation or another and reacting to unpleasant sensations negatively and helplessly after unsuccessfully trying to change them through different strategies, such as looking for pleasant sensations to counter them. These ways of tracking and reacting to what is happening in the body can be counterproductive and can be common among those who experience hypochondria or who suffer from severe symptoms such as chronic pain, and even among people who have learned to track their body sensations in great detail to regulate themselves in therapeutic or meditative modalities.

Interoception—becoming aware of events in the body by tracking body sensations—is an effective evidence-based tool for regulating not only the brain and the body, but also all psychological experiences that form within them. The use of interoception in psychology as a way to bring the body into treatment is becoming widespread. This is a significant and welcome development for the field of psychology, much of which has remained disembodied for a long time. However, as mentioned above, it also carries the risk of being misused to eliminate and avoid uncomfortable but meaningful psychological experiences.[7]

Basic sensorimotor emotions, such as feeling good or bad or pleasant or unpleasant, are always there in every moment of our lives, either as emotional experiences in themselves or as foundational layers of more complex emotional experiences such as sadness or happiness. The general lack of understanding in therapy and in life that experiences such as feeling good and bad or pleasant and unpleasant qualify as emotions—because they are meaningful psychophysiological reactions to situations—is based on a narrow academic definition of emotion as consisting of a limited number of primary emotions, such as happiness, sadness, fear, anger, disgust, and surprise, and their combinations. According to this theory, all emotional experiences other than primary emotions are secondary or complex emotions that are combinations of these primary emotions, just as all colors in nature are understood to arise from combinations of a limited number of primary colors.

This conceptualization of emotional experience often leads to the erroneous conclusion that many people have no emotions when they do not express primary emotions or their combinations. This limits the understanding and recognition of emotions and the work done with emotions across therapeutic modalities. Broadening the understanding of emotions to include the basic sensorimotor emotions such feeling bad or good can help all therapeutic modalities (including those that are already body-oriented) to contact, validate, support, develop, and differentiate their clients' emotional lives more effectively.

While working with the basic sensorimotor emotions, such as feeling bad, awful, or unpleasant, Connie was able to distribute her energy downward away from her head and toward her feet. The energy in her body had the habit of rushing towards her head and concentrating there, fueling her compulsion to cry for relief. When the brain is not able to cope with what is happening in the body, it too can become overwhelmed and symptomatic. Migraines, if they are psychophysiological in origin, often have such a pattern of top-heavy concentration of energy.

As things slowed down and stabilized, and Connie was able to notice, expand, and tolerate the basic sensorimotor emotion of not feeling good in her body, it became more possible to work with the primary emotion of fear that was there right from the beginning of the session. I have often observed this in myself as well as my clients. When basic sensorimotor emotions such as feeling bad or awful in relation to a situation are experienced and tolerated, it becomes more possible to differentiate other higher-order sensorimotor emotions, such as the painful emptiness in the complex emotion of loneliness, as well as primary emotions such as fear.

As for Connie's fear, it did not matter whether it was her fear of the suffering in her body or her fear of something outside. Because it was there, stronger and more differentiated than before, it made sense to expand the fear to as much of the body as possible. We will see later that there is neuroscientific evidence that expanding an emotion in the body can help improve the cognition of it.[8] That is, expanding an emotion in the body can help us understand our emotions better—what they are and where they come from. Between bouts of crying that decreased in frequency as the session progressed, Connie was able to embody her deep fear of whatever it was she was afraid of.

When Connie was in a relatively settled state toward the end of the session, I remarked to her that it appeared she was trying to cope with whatever she was coping with all by herself. Usually, at the end of a session I would feel as a clinician that my body had participated and worked somehow, especially if the session had been difficult. However, as difficult as the session with Connie had been, I felt that my body had not been taxed by the work at all. I was curious enough about this observation that I shared it with Connie and the class. When she started to cry again upon hearing this, I started to criticize myself for having made a bad intervention when things were finally settling, and I set about correcting it. Connie reassured me that she was okay, and she shared with us more of her story that, if I had known it earlier, would have probably made me far more cautious in the work I did with her, especially because I was still learning and developing my methods through the challenges that cases like Connie's presented.

When Connie was a year and a half old, a critical time for a child's brain development and attachment learning, she put her fingers in an unprotected electrical outlet and was badly electrocuted. She spent months in the burn unit of a hospital recovering from her wounds. As advised by the hospital staff, her parents did not visit her often. When they did, they often only saw her from behind a one-way mirror. To hear that history helped to make sense of many things: the migraine, a symptom that often forms when the central nervous system is overwhelmed; the rush of energy toward the head; the overwhelming helplessness and crying; the lack of trust in any help from outside, especially during difficult times; and the repeated experience of people letting her down during practice sessions.

Studies from multiple disciplines show that our bodies are constantly communicating with each other, regulating or dysregulating each other, through the measurable frequencies of the electromagnetic spectrum.[9] This process, which I call "interpersonal resonance" or simply resonance, is a valuable source of information about what is happening in others as well as a powerful tool for regulating others, despite the confounding complexities of possible transference and countertransference—the reactions of clients and therapists to each other that might have nothing to do with the other. Resonance is an ability we are born with, and it grows with the development of our physiology throughout our lives. Imagine Connie as a year-and-a-half-old child, with the medical staff peeling off her burnt skin or scabs, cleaning her wounds, and applying painful medications to help her heal in the absence of the reassuring presence of her parents, for months on end. One can appreciate why her body would shut down to interpersonal resonance and form an implicit distrust in its place. No wonder my body had felt barely used or taxed from the work I did with Connie.

In the days that followed, I heard that Connie was having a better time during practice sessions and was working with a great deal of sadness about her childhood, without crying as often, and allowing others to support her more than in the past. I thought these were good signs. From what I had already been observing in my clients and myself, when people are able to embody an emotion and tolerate it, they are often more able to work with other emotions in relation to the situation more fluidly. Their cognitions and behaviors often change for the better, not only in relation to the past, but also the present.

We will see later that there is growing evidence in neuroscience that it is emotion that drives cognition and behavior in every moment of our lives, as opposed to the conventional wisdom that cognition always precedes emotion, and emotion in turn drives behavior. Thus, it is common for dysregulation in emotion to lead to dysregulation or dysfunction in cognition and behavior. Therefore, tapping into the entire range of emotions, including the always present and often overlooked sensorimotor emotions, and regulating them by creating a greater capacity for experiencing and tolerating them, offers a better chance of improving not only emotions but also cognition and behavior—even among those who have poor access to primary emotions such as sadness and happiness.

Recently, when I was doing an online introduction to my system of Integral Somatic Psychology, I shared the case of Connie as anonymously as possible to give the audience an idea of the possible outcomes of the approach. At that moment I received a text message: it was from Connie, saying "I am here." Pleasantly surprised, I greeted her and asked how she was doing. Her response: "I am fine. And I am still without migraines. Thank you!"

Looking back, I realize that Petra and Connie were not the only ones who benefited from their treatments, because I gained a tremendous amount from working with them. Such cases were pivotal in reinforcing my emerging understanding that embodiment of emotions, especially unpleasant ones, in the larger container of the body in a regulated manner could be an efficient method not only for working with emotions and changing them, but also for working with and changing cognition and behavior in all therapeutic modalities. However, it has taken me some time to refine the method; test its effectiveness in diverse cases, clinical settings, and cultures; and accumulate the scientific reasons for the method's effectiveness. In addition, one reason why it has taken me this long to write this book is because the scientific findings that validate emotional embodiment as a potentially effective therapeutic method are from emerging and rather exciting paradigms in neuroscience and body psychotherapy.

That is what this book is all about: presenting a method of embodying and regulating a broader range of emotions to create a greater capacity for them, so as to improve diverse outcomes and reduce treatment periods in all therapy modalities; and providing the scientific basis for the method in emerging paradigms in neuroscience and body psychotherapy.

The work with Petra and Connie involved high levels of emotions at high levels of intensity (or subjective difficulty) for long periods of time, as well as deep and wide expansion of emotion in the body. These sessions made me wonder whether intense, prolonged, deep, and extensive embodiment of high-level emotion was always necessary for an expedient cure. Research on exposure therapy in the cognitive behavioral therapy paradigm has shown that it works best to resolve symptoms when the experience is intense and the exposure to the disturbing stimulus is prolonged.[10] Exposure therapy is an evidence-based therapy for posttraumatic stress disorder that research has found to be more effective than systematic desensitization, another evidence-based cognitive behavioral therapy modality for treating posttraumatic stress disorder. Systematic desensitization exposes clients to scenarios of increasing emotional level and intensity, and then it uses a relaxation protocol to calm clients after each encounter with the traumatic experience at increasing levels of intensity.

Exposure therapy suffers from a high dropout rate among clients and reluctance among therapists to practice it because they find its intensity too much for their clients or themselves. So I thought I had found a way to help therapists do exposure therapy with greater ease and regulation for both clients and therapists by using a larger and regulated body container to make the emotional intensity more manageable and tolerable to be with for a longer period of time.

However, as I continued to do emotional embodiment work with clients and teach it to therapists in different parts of the world, I discovered something else that made its applicability and usefulness more universal and versatile. Through my experiences with my clients and through the experiences of other therapists with theirs, I learned that emotional embodiment does not always have to involve high levels of emotion, be intense or prolonged, or have extremely wide or deep expansion in the body for it to be effective in improving outcomes in different therapy modalities. What appeared to matter more is a person's capacity for emotional experience in the body. It appeared that people often form serious psychophysiological symptoms, such as cardiovascular and respiratory illness, even at low levels of capacity for emotion in the body.

All of this made me curious, so I went back to look for clues in the literature on emotions and their physiology, especially in new and emerging research paradigms such as embodied cognition and enactive emotion in neuroscience, which I refer to broadly as the science of embodied cognition, emotion, and behavior. I found a number of new findings that, in combination with older findings on cognition, emotion, and behavior in neuroscience and body psychotherapy, helped to explain why emotional embodiment as I had conceived and refined it would work even at lower levels of emotion and intensity, and when emotional embodiment is less deep, wide, or prolonged.

Before we look at the method and its basis in science in a systematic and detailed manner in part II, let us look at a few other examples of successful emotional embodiment treatment that vary in the level, intensity, and duration of the emotional experience, and in the depth and width of its expansion in the body. These examples will also introduce us to other concepts in emotional embodiment work.

2

Variations in Emotional Embodiment Work

Chapter summary: an overview of concepts, methods, and outcomes in the context of treatment examples involving lower levels of emotional intensity, from later phases of development of the practice of embodying emotion, and in the context of long-term treatment.

Emotion: Level, Intensity, Depth, Width, and Duration

Embodiment of an emotion can be defined as the ability to expand the emotional experience to as much of the body as possible, in such a way that the person's ability to tolerate the emotional experience and stay with it is increased. When Integral Somatic Psychology (ISP) practitioners work with our clients or ourselves to embody an emotion, we expand the body in a regulated manner to manage any extreme physiological dysregulation and stress from the emotional experience that can lead to psychophysiological symptoms. At the same time we also expand the emotional experience to as much of the body as possible, to access the emotional information more fully. We try to stay with the emotional experience for as long as possible, to create a greater capacity to tolerate the emotions so they do not get acted out in dysfunctional thought or behavior. This also helps to give the brain adequate time to process the information in the emotional experience for optimal cognitive, emotional, and behavioral implications. In pursuing this strategy, we are informed by the emerging science of embodied cognition, emotion, and behavior that expansion of the emotion to as much of the body as possible will make it not only more tolerable to be with but will also improve what we think and do in the situation that is causing the emotional difficulty.

For a quick and simple example of what we do during a piece of emotional embodiment work, let us go to an Indian fishing village on the coast of the southern state of Tamil Nadu, where I took an international team of therapists for the first time to treat the survivors of the 2004 Indian Ocean tsunami. At the end of a sweltering summer day, as the sun was mercifully setting and we were packing up to leave, a twelve-year-old boy sought our help for relief from a symptom: his heartbeat became disturbingly high and irregular every time he thought another tsunami could come.

We worked with him by having him notice that he was afraid and that the fear was concentrated in his chest. We also had him notice how his chest was constricted as though it was trying to squeeze the fear out of the body. We helped him to expand his chest by having him breathe against the physical constriction and by supporting his chest with the touch of his own palm, with the intention to expand it. We kept the emotion of fear alive by talking about how afraid he might have been of dying during the tsunami and how everyone, including adults, feels such fear during a threat to one's life. We helped him to expand the fear from the heart to as much of the chest as possible by asking him to try to do it intentionally and by suggesting that he follow the spreading of the fear as the chest expanded with his breath and his touch. We repeated this process to help him expand his constricted arms by having him move his arms, and then we helped him expand the fear into his arms as well.

At the end of this really short intervention, he said he felt calmer, even though he still felt the fear in his chest and his arms. When we asked him if he was surprised that he did not have the disturbing heart-beat symptom, he said yes. We recommended that every time he got afraid that another tsunami could come, he should do exactly what we had done during the session. We also educated him that he might find the fear spreading to more places in the body beyond the chest and arms, and that it would be a good thing if that were to happen. In two follow-up research visits that took place three months and a year later, the boy gladly reported to our researcher that he no longer suffered from his frightening symptom.

When we go about the process of emotional embodiment, we might well find that experiences of emotional embodiment vary considerably, not only across individuals but also across time or situations for the same person. We have found that experiences of emotional embodiment can differ in terms of the level of the emotion, the intensity of the emotional experience, the width and the depth of the emotional experience in the body, and the duration of a cycle of emotional experience. Let us look at each of these variables in turn.

The level of emotion a person is generating and experiencing in the brain or body physiology can be high or low. But what is the level of an emotion? We often observe in ourselves or others that sometimes there is a lot of emotion, and at other times there is only a little bit of emotion. The level of emotion does not have to do with the level of energy or arousal. This is because some emotions, such as anxiety, are high-arousal emotions, physiologically speaking; other emotions, such as despair, are low-arousal emotions. A person might therefore report the level of anxiety as higher at higher levels of arousal, whereas a person experiencing despair might report the level of despair as increasing as the level of arousal decreases. The level of emotion is a subjective rating by the experiencer that is relative to the person's past experiences of the emotion. It is an answer to the question: are you experiencing more or less of the emotion than before?

Can outside observers assess another person's level of emotion as higher or lower than before? This is possible to some extent; it depends on how well the observer knows the person's experience. It also depends on how well the person expresses the emotion verbally and nonverbally, and on how well the observer can resonate with the person's experience. Interpersonal resonance—nonverbal communication between two bodies through electromagnetic and quantum mechanical means—plays an important role in how we communicate and regulate emotional experiences in each other (this topic is the subject of chapter 14). Assessing another person's level of emotion would also depend on the observer's capacity to tolerate the emotional experience. In any case, an observer's assessment of another person's level of emotion is subjective.

The experience of an emotion might also vary in its intensity from low to high. Intensity is defined here as the subjective psychophysiological difficulty a person has in tolerating and being with an emotion. We use the term "psychophysiological" because the difficulty in tolerating an emotion has both a psychological component and a physiological component. We know this from our experiences during physical exercises such as running. When we start to find an exercise strenuous, the more we tell ourselves it is difficult, the more physically difficult it becomes. We often say that an emotional experience is too intense when it is subjectively difficult for us to tolerate. Our assessment of how intense an emotion is does not have to do with what others on the outside might think about it, even though we might be influenced by our parents to find even low levels of emotion to be too intense. As with the level of an emotion, the assessment of the intensity of an emotion—whether by the person experiencing it or by a person observing it—has to be subjective as well.

What is the relationship between the level of an emotion and its intensity? It is reasonable to expect that a person would find the intensity of emotional experience to increase as its level increases. However, the extent to which the intensity of an emotional experience increases with its level might vary across individuals. Even though some people might consider a given level of emotion or level of intensity to be low, another person might find those levels to be unbearable. That is, a person might acknowledge that the level of an emotion is low and still find it unbearable, or a person might acknowledge that the level of an emotion is high and still find it quite bearable.

The level of emotion is only one of many factors that determine the intensity of an emotional experience. A level of emotion too intense for one person might not be as intense for another person due to many other factors, including thoughts and behaviors. A person who thinks it is bad to feel sad will find sadness more intense—at any level of sadness—than another person who does not have such a negative psychological evaluation attached to it. A person who is able to express an emotion is more likely to find an emotion less intense at any level of that emotion than another person who has difficulty expressing it. The physical fitness of a person might also have a bearing on the ability to tolerate emotional experiences. The more fit a person is, the more tolerable the emotional experience could be at any level of the emotion. Emotion can be thought of as an assessment of the impact of a situation on a person's brain and body physiology. Therefore, we can expect an unfavorable situation to have more adverse impact on a physiology that is less healthy to begin with.

As with the level of an emotional experience, the intensity of an emotional experience in a person can also be assessed by others to some extent, but the same caveats apply. It will also be a subjective assessment, and our ability to make that assessment will depend on a number of factors, such as how well we know the other person's emotional experiences.

People do appear to have the ability to differentiate between the level of an emotion and the difficulty with experiencing the emotion. We can infer this when they say they felt a lot of anxiety but they were okay with it or could tolerate it, or when they say they could not even tolerate a little bit of the anxiety they felt. The two variables are obviously related because they have at least one factor in common: the state of the body. The higher the level of emotion, the more change in the body one might expect. The greater the intensity, the more stress and dysregulation one might also expect in the body, because the level of stress and dysregulation is perhaps the most important factor making any body experience (including emotion) tolerable or intolerable.

Of these two variables—intensity and level—one can think of intensity as being more subjective than level, because level might have more of a physical basis than intensity. As subjective as these variables are, they can nevertheless be useful for regulating ourselves and others emotionally. We can learn to track emotional experiences along these two related dimensions in ourselves and others, so that we know when to ease up on or increase one or the other when we are working with others or ourselves.

When we are working toward embodying an emotion, the key variable we need to keep track of is the intensity of the emotion. That is, we need to stay in touch with the subjective difficulty experienced in tolerating and staying with the emotion without developing serious psychophysiological symptoms (such as the irregular heartbeat experienced by the boy in the Indian fishing village after the tsunami) and without losing connection to the emotion altogether, through defenses such as numbing and dissociation.

There are a number of ways to manage the intensity so it stays within a bearable range. One way is to manage the level of the emotion, because the level of emotion is one contributor to a person's inability to tolerate it. We can manage the level of emotion by reducing the support we are providing it with our awareness. For example, we can put only half of our attention on the emotion inside our body and devote the other half of our attention to what we are aware of outside the body. When we do this for a while, this tends to reduce the level of emotion because what we do not pay attention to within ourselves tends to diminish.

We can also manage the level of emotion by not thinking about the situation or aspects of the situation that are triggering the emotional response, or we can think about other aspects of the situation that are less evocative of the emotion. We can also help regulate the emotional experience in the body by switching our awareness to the purely physical level. Tracking body sensations usually regulates the body back to normalcy by setting up a feedback loop between the brain and the body.

Specifically, we can notice how our body and energy are doing better as a result of the hard work we have done to build more capacity for an emotion in the body.

In addition to managing intensity of emotion by managing level of emotion, we can also manage intensity by managing the other variables of emotional embodiment sessions: the width and the depth of body expansion involved, and the duration of the cycles of emotional processing. Let us now examine these variables and how they can be used to regulate the emotional experience.

The expansion of emotional experience in the body can be superficial or deep. For example, it can be superficial in the chest and involve only the musculature, or it can be deep in the chest and involve the lungs and the heart. The expansion can be wide and involve many areas or the entire body, or it can be narrow and involve only a few areas. An emotion such as grief might be present only in the chest, or it could include the face as well, or it could be felt throughout the body.

The length of time a person is able to stay with an emotion and process it can also vary considerably. Sometimes a person can stay with emotions only for short periods of time; sometimes people are capable of much longer cycles. This again can vary over time or across situations for the same individual.

Case Study: Working with Borderline Emotional States

Let us look briefly at how we might use the variables of width, depth, and duration to manage intensity to regulate an emotional experience and keep it from becoming unproductive. If a person has a very low capacity for tolerating an emotional experience, we might use very short cycles of emotional processing. That is exactly what I did when I worked with someone I was cautioned not to work with because she had been diagnosed with borderline personality disorder. People who have this disorder have an extremely limited capacity for emotional suffering. They tend to cope with it by either becoming extremely reactive to the world or by coming down with severe psychophysiological symptoms.

We can all think of situations in which we might have these "borderline" tendencies ourselves, so it is well worth knowing how we could build more capacity for such emotional experiences in the future by manipulating the duration of each cycle of emotion during our work.

The young woman I worked with in this case wanted to work on the distrust she felt, especially toward men. In our work together, I had her recall an experience she'd had with a man that she believed had added to her distrust. But she could not feel the distrust in her body. I had her notice where her body felt bad in recalling the situation. She could feel it in the chest, but only for a few seconds. She then looked at me as though she was asking me what was next. I had her recall the details of the situation again and had her notice where her body felt bad for another short cycle of less than a minute. Feeling bad in relation to a situation is a meaningful physical reaction and therefore an emotion—and feeling bad is present as a layer of every unpleasant emotional experience. Feeling bad is what we might call a basic sensorimotor emotion, a bodily state that is a meaningful reaction to a situation. Basic sensorimotor emotions do not appear on the lists of primary and secondary emotions that we learn in psychology courses. When we cannot tolerate a familiar emotion such as sadness or fear, first contacting and developing a capacity for how bad we feel can often help in making the sadness or fear more tolerable and conscious.

In order to expand the emotional experience of feeling bad in the chest, I had her make a sound to express how bad it felt in her chest. Verbal expression expands the emotion to the structures in the throat and the face involved in the expression, and it can help in expanding the emotional experience to other parts of the body. This is because verbal expression is almost always accompanied by nonverbal expression in the body. A cycle ended when she could no longer be with the emotion and her awareness turned to the outside. In successive cycles, each of which lasted around a minute, she was able to expand her experience only a little bit, mostly in the chest area. Her emotional experience had neither depth in any place nor width involving many places in the body. That is, it was shallow and narrow in the body.

We agreed in our assessment that the level of emotion itself was low. However, as we methodically went about this process in very short cycles, important changes started to occur. The sadness started to show, instead of her habitual angry outburst, and it became tolerable. This validated the implications of scientific research showing that unconscious cognitions, emotions, and behaviors will become increasingly conscious, optimal, and regulated with growth in the capacity for embodied suffering (the subject of chapters 6 and 8). As the session progressed, the cycles got longer, but not by much; the longest cycle of staying with an emotion and trying to expand it in the body might have been about two to three minutes. But the duration of the cycles proved to be adequate for her to make the changes we were able to observe after the session. That evening, a member of the training team observed her grieving what she had lost in her life by distrusting others. In the training days that followed, we saw her processing her vulnerabilities with greater ability during practice sessions with fellow trainees, instead of her habitual conflict with them about not receiving adequate support from them.

In this example, the cycles ended because the client ended them on her own when she could no longer tolerate being with her emotional experience in the body. There are other ways to control the length of a cycle of emotional processing. We can simply suggest shifting the awareness from the emotional experience to something else: the inside of the body, such as body sensations or how the body might be feeling better from the hard work with the emotion; outside of the body, to aspects of the present environment; or the mind, to reflect on cognitions and behaviors that might have changed from the work with the emotion. This last strategy is especially useful after a very long cycle or the last cycle in the session. We can also end the cycle by reducing the support we are providing the person for the emotion and/or shifting focus away from the situation that is triggering the emotional response.

When we sense that an emotional experience is getting too intense to handle, we can also use expansion strategies to help manage the intensity to keep it tolerable without breaking the cycle. In general, the longer we stay in one place in the body, such as the chest, the deeper the emotional experience will go into the area, and the more intense the emotional experience will tend to get. So if we find ourselves in a situation where we need to manage the intensity to make the emotional experience more tolerable, we could expand to other places in the same area; for example, to the sides and the back of the chest, beginning from the front, where the emotion is initially located. We could also expand to other places in the body, such as from the chest to the arms. That is precisely what we did with the boy in the Indian fishing village. We helped him to expand his fear that another tsunami could come from the chest to more places in the chest and then to the arms, in two relatively short cycles.

Why does an emotional reaction become more tolerable when more parts of the body are recruited to share the experience? An emotion is as an assessment of the impact of a situation on the whole body, so it is harder to tolerate the experience if we confine the energy of the impact to one place. Spreading the impact out over more areas of the body makes it easier to tolerate. Still, there are times when we have to stay in one place and go deeper into the physiology there for the healing to occur, and we will discuss those cases later. In this chapter, we are looking at cases where such deep work in one place is not necessary.

The two treatments we saw in chapter 1 involved emotions that had high levels, high intensity or difficulty for the subjects, deeper and wider expansion of emotion in the body, longer cycles, and faster outcomes. I presented them first because it is through such highly intense emotional cases I started to appreciate the effectiveness of embodying emotions. However, the norm for emotional embodiment work is to see steady benefits from a slower process over a longer period of time. Although there are some advantages to embodying high levels of emotions intensely, deeply, widely, and at length, emotional embodiment work can improve cognitive, emotional, and behavioral outcomes in all therapy modalities, no matter how emotions differ with respect to any of these variables. I learned these important lessons through cases such as the ones presented next in this chapter.

In terms of the dimensions that differentiate emotional embodiment sessions from each other, the two short cases presented below could be considered to be at the opposite end of the spectrum from the cases we have already discussed. We have already seen one example of this earlier in this chapter, in my work with a borderline client. Together, these cases illustrate the benefit of emotional embodiment work, even when the level and intensity of emotion are low, or its expansion in the body is superficial or narrow, or the duration of the cycles is short—a more likely scenario in therapy as well as in life.

Sally, Sadness, and Asthma

During the ISP professional trainings and workshops I teach, I demonstrate the different aspects of the work of emotional embodiment with training participants. In a training I was teaching in France, Sally approached me for a demonstration session. Sally suffered from asthma and wondered if we could work with it. Asthma, like many diseases, can have multiple causes, from genetic predisposition to hormonal fluctuations to allergies. It can also be psychophysiological in origin, as a consequence of defenses against emotional suffering that manifest in the physiology of breathing, especially in the lungs.

The most common physiological defense against emotional pain is holding back in the breathing muscles, such as the diaphragm and the intercostals, and in organs such as the lungs. When we are at rest, we do not need a great deal of oxygen, and the level of functioning of the lungs is lowered to the minimum through the autonomic nervous system. When the same mechanism is used to reduce breathing to lower the level and intensity of an emotional experience, breath can be inhibited to a greater degree than during rest, leading to bronchial symptoms such as asthma, especially in people who have prior genetic, hormonal, and allergenic dispositions for the symptom's formation.

In addition to asthma, which Sally treated with an inhaler when necessary, she said her other primary symptom was difficulty in bonding with and relating to others. The autonomic nervous system and the organs it governs, which include the heart and lungs, are important in emotional experiences in general, and in emotional experiences involved in bonding

45

with and relating to others in particular.[1] So it made sense to work with a situation in Sally's life that had to do with a disappointing relationship.

Even though Sally had been prone to asthma attacks since her childhood, the more recent and intense outbreak of it had been triggered by a breakup with a man she said she had loved more than any other in her life. It was not easy for Sally to track in her body how bad it felt and how sad it was that the relationship did not work out. Her physiological and psychological defenses appeared to be strong enough to keep the level and the intensity of emotion low and its presence in the body superficial and narrow, limited to the throat and the eyes. Sally had difficulty sensing and expanding the sadness, and she said she could barely feel it in her body or in her awareness. She needed a lot of psychological support from the outside, specifically from me and the group, to access her sadness and to stay with it, albeit for only a brief time each cycle. This indicated that she had not been given much support for her emotional experiences while growing up.

We supported her in experiencing as much emotion as possible in relation to the situation, and we suggested that she could use awareness, intention, breath, movement, expression, and self-touch as tools when she was on her own. We managed to expand the low level of sadness in her throat and her eyes to the rest of the face and to the chest, but only superficially and for very short periods of time before it disappeared. It was, therefore, more than a pleasant surprise to hear from Sally many months later that she no longer suffered from asthma since the session.

How can such apparently uneventful pieces of short-term embodiment work lead to the resolution of major long-term symptoms? The increasing tendency in the general population to form psychophysiological symptoms at rather low levels of emotional suffering—or, in other words, at low levels of emotion and intensity—offers one clue. Using emotional embodiment work to obtain even a small increase in the threshold of emotional suffering at which symptoms form could account for the outcomes observed in cases such as Sally's.

Sally exhibited a low threshold for emotional suffering in the body as demonstrated by her high resistance to sensing the presence of sadness in her body and by her finding the limited experience of sadness in her body to be not intense (subjectively difficult) at all. Therefore, increasing Sally's capacity for emotional suffering in the body just a little bit, by working with both her psychological and her physiological defenses, led to the surprising shift in her asthma symptoms.

Sabine, Crying, and Migraines

Sabine, another student I taught, suffered from migraines. Three months after a difficult interaction with her boss, the migraines started to occur more often, and she started having flashbacks of her boss's angry and disapproving face when the symptom appeared. The difficult interaction involved Sabine yelling at her boss when she got an unfair evaluation from him, and she thought of that as a good thing because when she was a child she could never speak up and defend herself to her abusive stepmother. Sabine reported suffering a lot in her childhood relationship with her stepmother, who punished her harshly and arbitrarily, both emotionally and physically. When I worked with Sabine during a demonstration in front of her class, I noticed that it was hard for her to access her vulnerability, both in relation to the incident with her boss and in relation to an incident when her stepmother slapped her for rearranging flowers in a vase.

Sabine showed a great deal of resistance to experiencing her vulnerability. Resistance to the experience of emotions can be either innate or psychological. Our brain innately resists unpleasant experiences because they imply states of stress and dysregulation in the body, which are associated with reduction in one's physical health and well-being. On the other hand, pleasant emotional experiences imply states of reduced stress and increased regulation in the body, which are associated with improvements in health and well-being. Freud called this innate tendency to seek pleasure and avoid pain the pleasure principle. Because the generation of unpleasant emotions involves increases in the level of stress and dysregulation in the physiology of the brain and the body, we all have an innate resistance to them. There can also be resistance to pleasant emotions because the brain also innately resists the unfamiliar, so both pleasant and unpleasant emotions can run into innate resistance if they are unfamiliar.

Psychological resistance to emotional experience can have many sources. Families and cultures have a strong influence on which emotions are allowed and how they can be expressed. Concepts of the role of emotion in life and attitudes toward emotion vary by culture, and they can also vary across therapeutic modalities. The influence of the conventional wisdom that emotions always lead to irrationality in cognition and behavior can be seen not only in the general population but also in some therapeutic modalities.

Such biases against emotion are under increasing challenge by science. Recent research in neuroscience shows that cognition, emotion, and behavior are more inseparable in the physiology of the brain[2] and the body[3] than previously believed. Research has also found that emotion influences all aspects of cognition and behavior in every moment of our lives, just as cognition and behavior are known to affect our emotional states. In addition, emotion appears to drive cognition and behavior more than cognition and behavior drive emotion, because all aspects of our cognition that precede behavior, including attention, are influenced by our emotional state.[4] The presence of emotion and its embodiment have been found to improve cognition, emotion, and behavior, and the absence of emotion impairs them.[5] Emotion—an assessment of the impact of a situation on a person's well-being—potentially involves the entirety of the brain and body physiology.[6,7] We will see in chapters 6 and 8 how these findings imply that embodying emotion, or expansion of emotional experience in the body, can improve not only emotion but also cognition and behavior. Unfortunately, these findings have not yet made their way into public life or therapy modalities to a great extent, a gap this book is intended to bridge.

Improving the work we do with emotions in ourselves and our clients requires an understanding of facts about emotions such as these, which are important but not widely known. Therefore, it is always good to educate clients about the important role emotions play in our lives and about the physiology of emotions. It is important to acknowledge the innate and psychological resistance to experiencing our emotions so we can work with the resistances to overcome them. Discussing how emotion, cognition, and behavior are intricately bound together in the brain and the body, and how the body is involved in cognition, emotion, and behavior, allows clients to understand how we might compromise not only our emotions, but also our cognition and behavior, when we shut the body down to avoid emotions that feel unbearable.

Sabine, as a trainee, already knew about the important role of emotions in life and in therapy. Regardless, in her process we often had to work with considerable resistance against emotions, and we provided strong psychological support for her emotions. It turned out that for her to access, stay with, and make sense of her emotions, what she needed most during the session was the validation and support she got externally, from me and the class. This made a lot of sense given Sabine's history. Research shows that a child's ability to generate, access, and express emotions depends a great deal on the modeling and support provided by their primary caregivers.[8] Sabine did not appear to have had a great deal of support for her emotions growing up, something she confirmed herself.

Using the images of her disapproving boss from her migraine-related flashbacks and of the stepmother during the flower vase episode from her childhood, I had her track and expand in her body the unpleasantness she experienced in those situations. We began at the sensorimotor emotional experience of unpleasantness because she could not find any primary or secondary emotions other than anger, which appeared to be her habitual defensive reaction to such situations as an adult. The level of the emotion of unpleasantness and of the reported difficulty in experiencing it (intensity) were both low, the expansion of emotion in the body was narrow and superficial, and the cycle was short; but it was enough to allow us to begin reorganizing the body somewhat. We had her redistribute the energy concentrated in her head downward toward her legs—a good direction when one is working with energetically top-heavy symptoms, such as migraine.

Toward the end of the session, when I asked Sabine what other feelings she could imagine herself having in those situations, she seemed to very briefly and lightly touch upon more differentiated emotions related to vulnerability, such as sadness, fear, helplessness, and loneliness. However, when I asked her where she was sensing those emotions in her body, Sabine quickly replied that she sensed them everywhere. To me, this seemed to be an improbably huge step compared to how limited her embodiment of unpleasantness had been, even though I knew that creating a capacity for such basic sensorimotor emotions can often lead to more differentiated and complex sensorimotor or primary and secondary emotions in clients. It is possible that Sabine merely recalled the memory of such emotions experienced in the body at some point in her past.

My skepticism of her self-report that she was feeling these emotions at all, let alone all over the body, also had to do with my observation in Sabine of a strong tendency to not appear as if she was failing or lacking in her process. As I ended the session, I thought it was possible that she had sensed them for a fleeting second in her brain or a part of her body and made the rest of it up.

Given the low level and intensity of Sabine's rather short-lived emotional experiences, the superficiality and narrowness of their expansion in the body, and her tendency to perform that made me doubt some of her statements about her inner experiences, I did not think much change would come from that session and thought rather poorly of the work we had done together. And I had another reason to be disappointed with how the session went: no matter how much experience I have as a therapist, my ego always appears to get the better of me when it comes to demonstrations I do in front of groups, because of the tendency to equate intense and dramatic pieces of work with good work. That way the ego can remain appeased and secure.

I didn't learn about the outcome of the session with Sabine until almost a year later, during the very last module of the training. When she went home after our work together, she started to cry. What she had experienced as a gentle drizzle of tears during some of her practice sessions prior to the demonstration session became a torrent. She cried all night long, interrupted only by fits of sleep. If I had found out the next day that she had cried all night long, I would have been concerned that she had fallen apart as a result of the session. But here is the thing: she has not had a single migraine since! Somehow the behavior of expressing her emotions through crying eliminated a severe symptom. All this came from an otherwise "unremarkable" piece of emotional embodiment work that I had so badly underestimated. I was once again pleasantly surprised to be reminded that it was not what happens and how it happens during the session that really matters. What really matters is what the outcomes are for the client in the long run.

Outcomes depend strongly on the level of suffering at which a client's psychophysiological symptoms develop, i.e., their symptom threshold. Because people with a low threshold for suffering tend to form symptoms at low levels of emotion and intensity, they can very well have "miraculous" cures resulting from small pieces of emotional embodiment work that increase their capacity for suffering only marginally. On the other hand, among people with a great deal of capacity for suffering, in whom symptoms form at higher levels of emotion and intensity because of their higher thresholds for emotional pain, emotional embodiment work might be characterized by high levels of emotion and intensity, deeper and wider expansion, and longer cycles of embodiment. Please remember that emotional intensity refers to how difficult a person finds an emotional experience to be psychophysiologically, regardless of whether the level of emotion is high or low.

Affect Tolerance, Symptom Threshold, Level of Body Expansion, and Formation of Psychophysiological Symptoms

We will now look at some core ideas in embodiment work in relation to building capacity for emotional experiences. This will involve examining the relationships between level of emotion, level of intensity, symptom threshold, and level of body expansion. In general, when more of the body is open and available to participate in an emotion, lower levels of intensity or psychophysiological difficulty are experienced. When more parts of the body participate in an emotional experience, the intensity or psychophysiological difficulty will be less in every part that is involved than when fewer parts of the body are involved. Also, when more parts of the body are involved in an emotional experience, it is possible to experience a higher level of emotion even with a lower level of intensity or subjective difficulty.

With Petra and Connie, we were able to work through their psychological and physiological defenses relatively easily to expand their body to access higher levels of emotions at higher levels of intensity, and to expand the emotions widely and deeply in the body while staying with them for longer periods. With Sally and Sabine, their stronger psychological and physiological defenses would only allow us to access relatively lower levels of emotions at lower levels of intensity, and to expand the body and the emotions only to a limited extent for shorter periods of time. They also had surprisingly quick symptom relief, underscoring the point that what matters is not how much emotion, intensity or psychophysiological difficulty, expansion of body and emotion, and duration of emotion were present in the treatment; what matters is whether the client was able to work with levels of emotion and intensity just beyond their threshold or emotional capacity for suffering without forming symptoms.

The symptom threshold is the level of suffering—which is the combination of level of emotion and intensity of emotion—beyond which a person forms a psychophysiological symptom. Symptoms could be cognitive, emotional, behavioral, physical, energetic, relational, or spiritual. These symptoms form when the threshold for suffering is exceeded in a part of the body including the brain. When this happens, the body shuts down or becomes dysfunctional, which further increases the level of stress and dysregulation in the body. This in turn further increases the person's difficulty with tolerating emotions. A psychophysiological symptom and the suffering it causes can be thought of as an unconscious compromise that a person's psyche makes to cope with unbearable suffering. This might very well be the best one could have done in a past situation, given one's history and one's resources at the time. However, when these reaction patterns become habitual responses to other situations in the future, they can exact a high price upon a person's well-being.

Psychophysiological symptoms constitute a dilemma. If the defenses were not there, the person would suffer from a lower level of functioning in the world and a higher level of stress and dysregulation. But if the defenses remain in place and become habitual, they contribute to the person's ongoing suffering in different ways: lower functioning in the world from some symptoms, high levels of stress and dysregulation, and low threshold for the emotions defended against. The symptom threshold can be thought of as a person's edge. In order to help clients heal, we need to be willing to help them work past their edge, or the boundary of their capacity, in such a way that symptoms do not form while their emotional capacity is expanded. This is possible when support for emotions is combined with the use of a more expanded, regulated body container. Therapists and clients need to understand that both support for emotions and work with the body are necessary for optimal outcomes, so that there is as little resistance as possible in the client as well as the therapist to do what is necessary to challenge the status quo.

Please note that a number of factors, including a person's physical, social, and cultural environment, might determine how much of the body can be expanded, how much emotion can be generated, and how much a person can tolerate emotional experiences without forming symptoms. For instance, we often find that we have shorter fuses when we are with our parents than with our friends; or a person might have greater capacity for one emotion, such as anger, than for another emotion, such as sadness. So it is important not to think of an individual's capacity for emotion or affect tolerance as fixed, as though it were independent of the environment or attitudes towards particular emotions.

Of all the factors that determine a person's ability for tolerating emotions, two stand out: the attitudes we have toward our emotions that make it possible to experience, express, tolerate, and stay with them; and the support we have from others for our emotions. Within relationships, the affect tolerance of either person is a function of the relationship.

Psychiatrist Daniel Siegel states that when two people come together, they form a synergistic supersystem wherein the capacity of the dyad is greater than the sum of the capacities of the two people forming it.[9] So in addition to the expansion of the body container, inner attitudes and support from others have a bearing on the affect tolerance profile of an individual in a given situation.

Through treatments such as Sally's and Sabine's, I learned that low-level, low-intensity, short-duration emotional embodiment work with narrow and superficial body expansion can be just as effective as high-level, high-intensity, long-duration emotional embodiment work with deeper and wider body expansion, which we saw in the treatments of Petra and Connie. This realization marked the second and the more subtle phase of my learning about the power and versatility of emotional embodiment. In a way, it made sense that I learned in the order I did. We tend to give more importance and significance to more dramatic events in which a lot happens. In the belief that such events are necessary to bring about change, we might push ourselves or our clients past thresholds for suffering, which can be counterproductive. Either we can end up being retraumatized with worse symptoms, or we can shut down because of psychological and physiological defenses that arise to defend us against suffering.

As I started to realize the importance of low-level, low-intensity, short-duration emotional embodiment work and began highlighting it in my trainings, other therapists I have trained in the method started telling me about its effectiveness in similar cases. This also made sense. I had biased the therapists I trained with my own bias toward high-level, high-intensity, long-duration emotional embodiment work, a bias I had developed from learning first about its effectiveness through intense treatments such as Petra's and Connie's. In trying to replicate that type of treatment as a formula, I had developed such a strong filter that it could only be broken through equally quick and dramatic outcomes from low-level and low-intensity treatments such as Sally's and Sabine's at the other end of the spectrum.

There is a growing tendency, in life as well as in therapy, to regulate emotions away rather than deal with them because of the suffering they bring. As a consequence, thresholds for emotional suffering in the population are getting lower. This has been an important factor in the formation of increasingly more serious psychophysiological symptoms in our times, as evidenced by increasing levels of addiction in the population. Recent studies show that as many as one-fourth to one-third of medical symptoms that motivate people to seek the help of medical professionals are psychophysiological.[10,11] This means therapists are going to be working more with clients characterized by a low threshold for emotional suffering. Therefore, the effectiveness of emotional embodiment even at low levels of emotion and emotional intensity makes it applicable not only for the minority who have a high capacity for emotion and its intensity, but also for the majority who do not.

Emotional Embodiment Work in Long-Term Treatment

All the cases we have seen so far have demonstrated the power of emotional embodiment in short-term work. But most therapeutic work takes place over the long term. The science of embodied cognition, emotion, and behavior and the empirical evidence from ISP therapists all over the world who integrate it as a complementary modality offer the possibility of reduction in the time it takes therapists in any modality to help their clients in long-term treatment to resolve their symptoms. One of the benefits of emotional embodiment work could be the reduction in the length of long-term treatment in different therapeutic modalities. Below I present a case from my practice that needed long-term treatment. I invite you to guess how long it would take a case like this to resolve symptoms; at the end of the story, compare your guess to the actual length of time it took.

Steven and His Flying Phobia: A Long-Term Treatment

Steven came to me for help in my private practice with a couple of symptoms. For one thing, he had developed a flying phobia causing him to have anxiety attacks when he flew. Because he was a musician who often had to fly to gigs out of town, it was very inconvenient that he could not fly without suffering an anxiety attack or being heavily medicated. His other symptom was that he could not sleep in a horizontal position. He could only sleep in a reclining position, as in an economy-class seat on a plane. Steven shared with me that he had developed both symptoms after the death of his mother, with whom he had had a difficult childhood.

We worked with the two symptoms and the loss of his mother, progressively taking care to ensure that the emotions involved in each step were not so overwhelming they would worsen the symptoms. In relation to his flying phobia, I had him at first just imagine a sequence of events in which he planned a trip that involved flying, taking time to embody emotions in each step. In relation to the sleeping difficulty, I had him attempt to sleep in my office with the lights dimmed. At first he was situated at the angle he was used to, and then we progressively reclined him in steps toward the horizontal position in a reclining chair. We tried to expand and embody the discomfort, the feeling of the lack of safety, the fear, the anxiety, and other emotions that arose in each step along the way in a series of sessions. We also tried to expand and embody the emotions that arose as we explored the significance of the loss of his mother as well as Steven's childhood memories of her.

In the end, it took about six months of steady work before both symptoms resolved, allowing Steven to fly without an anxiety attack and sleep in a horizontal position. There is an interesting story around the resolution of Steven's panic attack symptom. Steven did not fly much during the treatment; he took a break from work because he was going through so much. When he did start flying again toward the end of the treatment period, he actually had a panic attack on his first outbound flight. But he did not have any panic attacks after that. It is possible that when we work with emotions at a level of intensity close to the threshold when a symptom is triggered, the client may come down with a symptom. I have now made it routine to inform those whom I work with of this possibility so they do not have a strong negative reaction to it that derails the treatment.

3

The Contribution of Emotional Embodiment to Working with Individual, Collective, and Intergenerational Traumas

Chapter summary: an overview of concepts, methods, and outcomes in the practice of embodying emotion, in the context of treatment examples involving individual, collective, and intergenerational traumas.

Trauma and Emotional Embodiment Work

Emotional difficulties are universal and commonplace. So are low thresholds for suffering and the formation of psychophysiological symptoms—even serious ones—due to unprocessed emotions, even from ordinary life events. Traumas are generally understood as extraordinarily difficult life experiences with the potential to cause serious harm to the organism. In situations such as war or repeated physical abuse, the threat to the life of the organism is literal. The levels of stress and dysregulation endured are so high that, if left unresolved, they could be the basis of serious psychophysiological symptoms, including death. Those who are diagnosed with PTSD are understood to have suffered from such traumas and to have high levels of stress and dysregulation in their physiology.

It has also frequently been observed that there are many events, such as emotional neglect or emotional abuse, that are not physical threats to a person's life but that can nevertheless stress and dysregulate the physiology to the same extent as severe life-threatening events. This fact has necessitated consideration of broadening the definition of trauma in the *Diagnostic and Statistical Manual* to include things such as emotional neglect and emotional abuse. Therefore, the extent of stress and dysregulation left in the person's brain and body physiology after the experience can be used as a conceptual yardstick to assess how much the experience traumatized the person. The high level of stress and dysregulation in the physiology of traumatized people suggests that therapies that deal with trauma could be more effective if they also incorporated interventions for directly working with the physiology to manage the level of stress and dysregulation in it.[1]

Psychiatrist Bessel van der Kolk has been emphasizing the need to work with the body in any treatment of PTSD, and van der Kolk's claims are backed by evidence. This is demonstrated by the effectiveness of the psychopharmacological approach of psychiatry, and in body-oriented trauma modalities such as Somatic Experiencing[2] and mindfulness-based stress reduction.[3] However, body-oriented trauma treatment methods that track body sensations share a weakness in that they can sometimes thwart emotion by tracking body sensation instead of emotion. This is especially a problem for clients who either do not have an adequate inner capacity for emotional experience or who have insufficient support from others for their emotional experiences.

If the body is regulated too much when working with unpleasant emotions, the emotions can disappear, as sometimes happens when a person is medicated excessively. The systematic expansion of the body and of emotion along optimal pathways in the body—as suggested by models of body and energy regulation and utilized in the emotional embodiment work in Integral Somatic Psychology (ISP)—ensures a balance between physiological regulation and emotional regulation. This ensures that excessive physiological regulation does not end up countering the meaningful emotional experiences involved. As opposed to approaches in which physiological regulation and emotional regulation are performed in alternating order, the possibility of tending to both simultaneously offers the advantage of providing the client with maximum emotional support, without the distraction of going away from it to tend to the physiology, which could compromise the emotional experience.

The ability to work with both physiological and emotional regulation at the same time during emotional embodiment work gives this approach the flexibility to work with emotion from traumas, which is characterized by high levels of physiological stress and dysregulation, and with emotions from ordinary but difficult life experiences, which are characterized by lower levels of physiological stress and dysregulation. In fact, we will see later in the chapters on the physiology of emotion and sensorimotor emotions that states of stress and dysregulation can themselves at times be thought of as sensorimotor emotions, because they make sense as meaningful reactions of the organism to the traumatic event. For example, the shock a mother experiences on losing a child is a proportionate and meaningful physiological reaction to the event. It therefore qualifies meaningfully as an emotion. However, a word of caution is in order. There are times when the level of stress and dysregulation is so high, as when a person is about to faint or is completely dissociated, that it makes sense to focus on the physiology and bring the stress and dysregulation down to a manageable level to make the psychological experiences, including emotions, coherent enough before proceeding with the difficult work of emotional embodiment.

That said, the guideline to regulate the physiology when it is extremely dysregulated before working psychologically or embodying emotion has its exceptions, as can be seen in the following case.

Anita: A Woman Who Could Not
Sleep without the Lights on at Night

During a training I was doing in India, Anita approached me for help with a symptom that caused problems for both her and her husband: she could not sleep at night without the lights being on all night long. She said she did not exactly know how her symptom came about, but she had had it for a long time. I assumed fear must be driving the symptom, so in a demonstration session I had Anita close her eyes and imagine trying to sleep without the lights off, to trigger the fear so we could work with it through embodiment. Specifically, I had her notice how scary or unsafe she felt and where in her body she felt that way. Anita started to dissociate as soon as she started sensing the fear. She said her body started to feel numb and she felt she could very well be outside her body.

Usually at that point I would have had a client in this situation open her eyes and reorient to the present, rather than tracking the overwhelming fear and the situation triggering it, to make her feel more present, stable, and safe before going back in for another cycle of embodying the fear. For some reason, with Anita I chose not to do that at that moment. Instead, I continued to keep the situation and the emotion alive and stay with that part of her that could still feel the fear somehow. I kept asking her where she could feel the fear in her body, despite the counteracting numbness, by trying to get her to ignore the numbness as much as possible. When she said she could faintly feel the fear somewhere, I quickly asked her where *else* she could feel it going, hoping we could encourage as much superficial and wide expansion of the fear in as much of the body as possible, to keep the experience tolerable. As for working with the fear despite the strong pull toward dissociation, we can think of it as working with the fearful self in the dueling presence of the dissociating self, I explained to her and the class.

In a way, this is what exposure therapists might do when they expose their clients to a fearful stimulus in a prolonged manner—but with one difference. Exposure therapy is a variant of cognitive behavioral therapy, which is based on classical conditioning principles, and that school of therapy typically pays no attention to experiences in the black box of the body. By contrast, in my work we pay a great deal of attention to the experience and regulation of the body while attending to the emotion and the situation at the same time. The balance between attention to the body and its regulation and attention to the emotion and the situation varies on a case-by-case and trial-and-error basis. This variation involves managing variables such as level of emotion, its intensity or subjective difficulty, width and depth of body expansion, and the length of each cycle of emotional processing. In Anita's case, the balance was tilted so far in the direction of the emotion and the situation that at the end of the session she said she could hardly remember what she had experienced during the session, indicating the presence of a great deal of stress, dysregulation, and dissociation in the session.

I am sure you are as curious about the outcome as I was after the session ended, from which I emerged a bit numb and dissociated myself. Would she decompensate or fall apart later, especially that night? When she showed up for the following day of training, she said she had slept well the night before, although she did leave the lights on. She had traveled alone from the city where she lived to attend the training, and she was not ready to experiment with trying to sleep with the lights off without her husband sleeping next to her. At that point she shared with the group her idea that a sexual abuse trauma she had experienced repeatedly as a child might be related to her symptom—a significant cognitive insight. Anita used to be in the habit of getting up early in the morning, well before her parents, when it was still dark outside. The man who delivered milk to her house in the morning had repeatedly sexually abused her, and he threatened to harm her and her parents if she told anyone about the abuse. It made sense that such abuse could be related to her feeling unsafe in the darkness of the night. I thought at the time that if I had known she had suffered from such abuse as a child, I might not have been so brave as to work with her fear as much as I did, and to ignore the dissociation to the extent that I did.

I do not get to India often, once a year at the most. When I was in India a year later, I met Anita in another training, this time as an assistant.

She said she was so impressed by the work we had done together in our session, and by how she felt afterward, that she continued to get more sessions of emotional embodiment from the local trainer. She became so interested in emotional embodiment work that she became an assistant in the next training so she could learn more about it. And she no longer needed to keep the lights on at night to be able to sleep! It took Anita only five or six sessions with the local trainer to rid herself of her night-time symptom, demonstrating the potential of emotional embodiment work to hasten outcomes and shorten treatment times in all therapies and in daily life, even when severe trauma is involved.

When I wrote Anita to ask her permission to share her story in this book, she replied that in those five or six sessions she not only worked with her fear but also her shame in relation to the abuse, and she made deeper embodied connections between the abuse, her fear of darkness, and her symptoms. In conclusion, she wrote: "Today after seven years of my journey with Integral Somatic Psychology, I can say that not only did I overcome that symptom but also achieved many more milestones in my life. I have sweet harmony in my life, living successfully every day, and thanking you and the universe for allowing me to learn and practice ISP every day in my personal and professional life."

Sessions such as Anita's taught me that it is sometimes expedient to work with emotional embodiment when the body is in a state of extreme stress and dysregulation, even during dissociation, as long as there is enough of a witness in the person's awareness and enough of the capacity to suffer without the development of a major symptom. We cannot always know in advance whether a person has such capacity, so we must sometimes resort to trial and error.

There is also a theoretical reason for why we have to sometimes work this way in situations characterized by extreme stress, dysregulation, and even dissociation, when it is usually contraindicated: the dependence of the emotion on such an extreme state. Emotion is an assessment of the impact of the situation on a person's well-being. If the impact involves an extreme state of stress, dysregulation, and/or dissociation, then if we try to access the emotion when the body is regulated away from the underlying physiological and psychological states that generate the emotional experience, we run the risk of not being able to fully grasp the extent of the situation's impact—i.e., "the emotion."

As we have seen earlier, the level of stress and dysregulation involved in an emotional experience can be so great as to cause severe psycho-physiological pathologies. Even in such instances, one can imagine that the extreme method employed in Anita's session might apply. However, it is more likely that a more gradual approach might work better, with the capacity for difficult emotional experiences growing steadily, perhaps with shorter cycles and lower levels of emotion and intensity, and lower levels of stress and dysregulation in the body. In this way the client can move in small steps toward and beyond the level of stress and dysregulation at which symptoms form.

Such a gradual approach might be particularly suited to situations in which the level of stress and dysregulation in the person is so very high that no coherent psychological experience can be accessed, the person's capacity for suffering is very low, and the psychophysiological symptom's severity is extreme, such as migraine. The gradual approach might also be indicated when the person's capacity for suffering is not adequate to maintain a steady witness in relation to the overwhelming experience. The more capacity one has for an experience, the more tolerable the experience is, and the easier it is to remain a witness to it in a steady manner. However, a word of caution is in order: there is no need to approach every person gingerly, because people vary widely in these capacities, even when they have extensive trauma histories.

Psychopharmacology tends to diagnose all psychological problems as having to do with excess stress and dysregulation, and to treat it with medication. There are times when this diagnosis is appropriate and medication is necessary to regulate the physiology away from serious, debilitating psychological and psychophysiological problems and into a realm of coherent physiological and psychological experiences. In these instances, medication acts as a regulating stabilizer allowing healing to take place on one's own in one's social networks, with professional help if necessary.

The tendency to approach all psychological and psychophysiological problems as being caused by stress and dysregulation, and to regard reduction in stress and dysregulation as the key to all symptom resolution, can also be seen in some bodywork and body psychotherapy approaches, especially the more recent ones. Again, it might well be true in some instances that such caution is warranted. However, it bears repeating that excess reliance on such a clinical strategy, with a bias toward downregulation of stress and dysregulation in the body, runs the risk of avoiding significant psychological experiences of suffering for which greater capacity needs to be built. Approaches that constantly seek to reduce stress and dysregulation may miss the opportunity to ensure that clients have physiological and psychological resilience in the face of those emotional experiences in diverse situations that might trigger them, and may fail to give them the resilience that would allow them not to form symptoms or to resolve symptoms quickly when such emotional experiences come up in the future.

Intergenerational Traumas

It is well known that anxious parents tend to raise anxious children, and depressed parents, depressed children—even though some children might adopt the opposite position as a defense against the suffering caused by identifying with the parent.[4] However, when parents have not worked through their own traumas, such as physical and sexual abuse or significant losses, their reactions to the present tend to be colored by their experiences and reactions related to their unresolved traumas. This can mold the child's experiences and reactions throughout its development, going as far back as life in the womb.

This transfer of the effects of trauma from one generation to the next can happen in different ways. Our brains and bodies are known to communicate with and regulate each other by sharing internal states, experiences, and reactions (including physical and energetic defenses) with each other through measurable short-range energies of the electromagnetic spectrum.[5] We are particularly capable of tuning into the internal states of our parents this way because of the implicit, and even instinctual, trust we have in our parents as the best custodians of our survival and interests. We can also see these mechanisms as a nonverbal means through which parents inculcate their children with their worldview so as to maximize their well-being, in light of the parents' own experiences and expectations.

Another way this can happen is when parents become the perpetrators themselves, subjecting their children to the same traumas they were subjected to. Even though not all parents who were physically abused as children physically abuse their children in turn, we run into those who do. We even encounter such intergenerational abuse in instances where the parent is determined not to visit their own suffering upon their children and to break the cycle of violence across generations. Although conventional wisdom has it that abused children who have not worked through their abuse tend to become abusers themselves, a large longitudinal study has found that people abused as children are no more likely to become abusers than those who were not abused as children, which perhaps is a testament to the resilience of the human spirit.[6] Through observation and imitation of the parent, the child can also learn outmoded traumatized perceptions, such as the world appearing to be unsafe, and dysfunctional defenses such as fight or flight.

My father was easily slighted and reacted to perceived slights with anger. He projected his vulnerabilities, such as shame and hurt from his unresolved traumas, outward in order to rid himself of them. It is as though he used his anger as a missile to project his vulnerabilities onto the person he was angry at. I would, of course, have my own reactions of shame and hurt from being verbally, emotionally, and physically abused by my father. What I did not know then is that I was also taking in and identifying with my father's disowned vulnerabilities, in addition to experiencing my own reactions to his abuse.

A theory from Kleinian psychoanalysis called "projective identification," which is used to explain one method that parents use to regulate their children, can be helpful in understanding how children might end up absorbing their parents' vulnerabilities during abuse.[7] When a baby feels an anxiety that is too much to bear, it projects the anxiety onto the parent. The parent, who is uniquely equipped to regulate their child, "identifies" with the projection, making it their own. Then, in addition to soothing behaviors such as holding and rocking the child, the parent uses their more mature physiology to transform the projection of anxiety they have received. The parent then nonverbally projects the remaining traces of anxiety, along with calm, back to the child. The child identifies with such nonverbal help gratefully, just as a young bird would swallow the partially digested food that the mother bird places in its mouth. During abuse, the parents could project their vulnerabilities from being abused themselves into their children, who then identify with their parent's disowned vulnerabilities to maintain their connection with them.

The scientific evidence for the possibility of such nonverbal information exchanges between people through short-range electromagnetic energies emanating from the body, such as the electromagnetic energy field emanating from the heart that has been observed to travel several feet beyond the skin, provided a solid basis for my understanding of the process of projective identification. In projective identification, there is a willingness on the part of the receiver of the projection. In violent experiences such as physical abuse, in addition to identifying with the parents' projected vulnerabilities to maintain their connection with them, the child might simply be a victim of it, unable to prevent itself from taking in the strong energies directed at it.

My late father-in-law was all of five years old in World War II when the Germans and the Americans were fighting for territory in Belgium in what became known as the Battle of the Bulge. Caught between the two armies on a farm in Belgium, where his German father had sent his family to be safe from the intense Allied bombing unfolding toward the end of the war, he would hide under his bed, shaking in fear. As he grew up, he developed the habit of raging at whoever was around him when he became fearful. My wife internalized this pattern through observation and projective identification when she was a child. When she became an adult, if something on the road scared her while she was driving, she would sometimes curse and scream to get rid of her anxiety. Through my own reaction and projective identification, I would then experience a great deal of fear for a long time—the fear that a five-year old might have felt in the night under a bed on a Belgian farm some seventy years ago.

There are a number of ways to learn about our heritage of intergenerational traumas. One way, of course, is to get a detailed history of the traumas our family members went through. This might be easier said than done, as there can be a great deal of resistance to talking about one's traumas or seeing them as such. This was particularly true of Germans who were traumatized by the war, for many reasons, including the guilt of belonging to the country that initiated the war. So indirect methods such as the ones presented later might help people understand their inheritance of trauma.

One powerful way to get at the unresolved traumas our ancestors might have passed on to us is to imagine them in their habitual postures or reactions and try to use our own bodies to get a sense of what they might have been feeling inside of their bodies. Another way is to do a "family constellation" in therapy. Family constellation therapy was developed by Bert Hellinger in Germany to unearth and resolve intergenerational traumas that clients might be suffering from without knowing about them—traumas that their ancestors might have taken to their graves with them. In this modality, other people stand in for their ancestors in a family constellation and trust that the world-soul will guide the souls of the ancestors into the bodies of their stand-ins, to bring up and resolve the intergenerational traumas that continue to unconsciously affect the lives of the clients and their families. If you are skeptical of his method, which is quite popular in Germany, try doing a family constellation of your own with a therapist competent in this modality.

Intergenerational Collective Traumas

Working in Europe, especially in countries like Germany, one runs quickly into the ghosts of World War II. Intergenerational collective traumas—the effects that major collective traumas experienced by one generation have upon subsequent generations—continue to shape the emotional reactions of postwar generations. In the United States, we can see the effects of the intergenerational collective trauma of slavery in the African American population and the effects of the genocide of Native American populations in their descendants to this day. These inherited patterns, when unresolved, add to a person's reaction to current traumas and make it difficult to process the current traumas. The following treatment examples from Israel and Germany provide an idea of the efficacy of emotional embodiment work in cases where the weight of intergenerational collective traumas bears heavily on current traumas and symptoms.

Claudia's father was the mayor of a small town in Germany during the Third Reich. He and his family felt constantly endangered during the war due to his resistance to the Nazis. Claudia, born well after the war, inherited her father's social conscience and willingness to buck the system. Today she is passionately involved in efforts to protect the environment. She does whatever she can, personally and as a therapist, to help Jewish Israelis as well as Germans work through their intergenerational collective traumas from the war. She has been to Israel many times over the years as an assistant trainer in a trauma training program to help Israelis learn how to work with all kinds of traumas. I met her during one of the training sessions I taught there.

Claudia asked me for help with her symptoms of arrhythmia—sudden, scary irregularities in the heartbeat—and high blood pressure. The symptoms were sufficiently stressful that she was on beta blockers, a medication that can regulate both heartbeat and blood pressure. We did two sessions focused on her anxiety about things large and small in her life, to create greater capacity to embody and regulate the anxiety in the larger physical container of her body in order to help her resolve severe psychophysiological symptoms. The work was not easy, because of Claudia's tendency to regress to child states and cry helplessly. We had to constantly orient to the present to work as much as possible in her adult ego state.

As she developed her capacity to tolerate her anxiety—which clarified itself as the fear of dying, or worse, as the terror of being killed or annihilated by the world—Claudia told me how, for as far back as she could remember, her life had been ruled by a general sense of dread, anxiety, fear, and terror that something suddenly could happen to end her life. From time to time, depending on what was happening in her life, she would diagnose the fear as having to do with this or that in the world and try to deal with it in one way or the other, only for it to rear its ugly head again. Since she was a child, she had had a lot of psychotherapy in her life, which helped to manage this fear but not to resolve it to any degree of satisfaction.

The fear of being killed and the terror of being annihilated by the world are common themes we run into in the processing of life-threatening prenatal or perinatal trauma. Claudia once interviewed her mother to learn if she had had any significant prenatal or perinatal trauma, and it turned out that she had not. Still, I explained to her that babies could be traumatized even in the womb by the mother's unresolved traumas. Her parents, who went through the collective trauma of World War II while resisting the Nazis, could reasonably be expected to have unresolved activation, especially because postwar Germany had neither the time nor the resources to tend to its healing during the reconstruction of a country that had undergone incredible destruction.

It also made sense to Claudia that the collective war trauma carried by almost everyone around her might have continued to affect her as she was growing up in a number of ways. One of these avenues could be interpersonal resonance, the ability our brains and bodies have going back to the womb to exchange information with other brains and bodies nonverbally through the energies of the electromagnetic spectrum, such as electromagnetic energies emanating from the heart.[8] Another avenue of influence could be the ability we have to communicate with each other rapidly at the level of subatomic particles.[9]

When overwhelming emotional reactions and the defenses against them from inherited collective traumas such as war have not been worked through, it is harder to work with emotional reactions to current life difficulties and resolve symptoms that form from them. Exposure to intergenerational collective traumas such as World War II and the Holocaust can happen from childhood onward in all the ways such exposure can take place through the family as well as the community. These inherited collective traumas can make processing of emotional reactions to current traumas more difficult, because accessing difficult emotional reactions to current situations can quickly trigger the larger and more overwhelming emotional reactions to the intergenerational collective traumas, bringing them to the surface. It is as though the larger reactions to past events are just beneath the skin, and even a small scratch can trigger them, making healing the present as well as the past a tricky and difficult proposition. This is something I have observed not only in Israel and Europe in relation to World War II and the Holocaust, but also in Sri Lanka among the survivors of a thirty-year civil war, and in the United States in the African American population.

Therefore, when I saw Claudia on a subsequent trip to Israel, I was indeed surprised to hear that she no longer had any symptoms of arrhythmia and high blood pressure, and that her doctor was intrigued that her condition could change so much in such a short period, after just two sessions. I experienced a similar surprise when I worked with Silvia, an older German woman who was born closer to the war than Claudia and whose parents also experienced much hardship during World War II, including the trauma of displacement. After just a single session together, Silvia reported that she no longer had allergy symptoms, even though she continued to test positive for allergies.

In the session with Silvia, we focused on a great deal of fear she had in relation to a current situation in her life. Interestingly, when we spoke years later, she no longer remembered that we had worked with fear! What she remembered from the session were the significant and impressive changes in her energy during the session. This made sense. When the body has a greater capacity to be open and regulated during overwhelming experiences through emotional embodiment work, deeper healing energies often arise to resolve the symptoms. Paying attention to and supporting such energies are important parts of emotional embodiment work. Silvia, a psychologist by profession, had no doubt about how much her parents' and grandparents' traumatic experiences during the war and its aftermath continued to affect her.

For a therapeutic method to have validity, it has to be effective not only when its developer employs it, but also when those who have learned it have success in applying it. That is why I am always glad to hear of successful outcomes of treatments given by others. Short descriptions of two such treatments from Israel follow.

Sderot is an Israeli city close to the Gaza Strip. Rockets from the Gaza Strip fall regularly in the area. A man who lived in Sderot and who loved gardening could no longer spend time in his outdoor garden without having an anxiety attack. The panic attacks started happening after a rocket landed close to his house. I recommended to the therapist who was in one of my classes that she work with her client's fear and anxiety using the emotional embodiment technique, which at times I call the expansion technique, in order to develop a greater capacity in him to tolerate these emotions. A few months later, the therapist reported on the man's progress: "I worked with him only a few times. He is still afraid of the danger that rockets pose in the area, but he no longer has panic attacks when he goes out to enjoy working in his garden."

Areas adjacent to the Gaza Strip have recently been under a new threat: fires started by small incendiary balloons filled with hydrogen or helium and sent toward Israel. I heard from another therapist that a family she has been treating in that area is suffering from a great deal of anxiety, and the relaxation and discharge protocols she had taught family members to cope with anxiety were no longer working. She wanted to know if she could work with them by having them embody their anxiety. I replied through email that it was worth giving it a shot. When I was in Tel Aviv a month later, I asked the therapist about the family. Her response: "I only worked with the mother to begin with, because I was not sure whether the children could handle the intensity of staying with an emotion such as fear. When I spoke to the mother recently and asked her how she was doing, she said she was doing just fine. Whatever I had done with her had worked. Her children were, however, still not okay, so she wanted me to start treating the children just as I had treated her so effectively."

The outcomes for Claudia and Silvia from Germany, along with equally rapid and effective outcomes reported by Israeli practitioners, taught me that emotional embodiment work could be efficient in treating serious psychophysiological symptoms when the capacity to process emotion is quite limited by the baggage of intergenerational or contemporary collective trauma, which can make the symptom threshold for the suffering of new traumas low and the probability of regression, helplessness, and falling apart high. When major symptoms form at low levels of suffering, it is possible that increasing the capacity for suffering only a little bit could help resolve some symptoms quickly, even when intergenerational collective traumas are involved. This does not mean that all aspects of the trauma, past and present, have been worked through; but it does mean that people do not have to live with serious psychophysiological symptoms or work with all aspects of their traumas for long periods of time before getting relief from their symptoms. Thank God!

4

Diverse Benefits of Emotional Embodiment in Various Clinical Settings

Chapter summary: an overview of benefits of emotional embodiment that have been observed in different therapy modalities, and in different clinical contexts such as cognitive and behavioral therapies. The chapter also presents an overview of findings from both older and newer paradigms of research in neuroscience, cognitive psychology, body psychotherapy, and general psychology, which explain the observed range of benefits in diverse therapy settings.

Improvement in Diverse Outcomes from Emotional Embodiment Work in Different Therapy Modalities

Therapists trained in the emotional embodiment work of Integral Somatic Psychology (ISP) use it as a complementary modality to improve outcomes in whatever therapy modalities they happen to specialize in. Their professional backgrounds are diverse: they are psychoanalysts, psychiatrists, Jungian analysts, psychotherapists, social workers, cognitive behavioral therapists, counselors, body psychotherapists, psychologically oriented body workers, energy workers, educators, trainers, and teachers of meditation and spirituality. They work with different aspects of psychological experience as a means to help their clients.

In their work, some focus more on cognition, while others focus on factors such as emotion, behavior, brain, body, energy, and so on. Some work more with trauma, and others with ordinary but difficult life experiences and all kinds of symptoms. They are already trained in evidence-based therapies, do really good work, and help a lot of people. They are dedicated professionals continually training in new modalities to improve their practice. They recognize that the complex human psyche as it manifests in all individuals cannot be understood completely or treated effectively with one psychological theory or treatment approach. It is from such a diverse body of professionals that we continue to hear that integrating the emotional embodiment work of ISP into their practice as a complementary modality has helped them improve diverse outcomes and reduce treatment periods.

How does one explain the effectiveness of emotional embodiment work in improving outcomes across therapeutic modalities and in diverse domains such as cognition, emotion, behavior, body, energy, relationship, and spirituality? Let us look at how both older and newer findings in neuroscience, cognitive psychology, body psychotherapy, and general psychology could predict these outcomes, with examples from emotional embodiment work.

Emotional Outcomes

When emotions are more available to be experienced, we are able to appreciate more fully the significance of situations in our lives. When emotions become more bearable through their embodiment, we can imagine that we would live through and survive a difficult emotion, such as a broken heart, if it were to happen again. Then we do not have to shut the heart down, avoid relationships, or engage others halfheartedly. We can get to a place where we sense that our work with that emotion is resolved, to the extent that we can express it in statements such as "I am no longer as haunted by the loss." When the emotion is experienced as just a difficult state within the body, it is possible to become truly mindful of the emotion without the development of secondary unhelpful reactions to the emotional experience. This includes unhelpful cognitive conclusions, such as "I am not worthy of love," or self-destructive behavioral reactions, such as "I need to drink to get away from this pain."

Mindfulness has been found to be a key factor in affect regulation.[1] When one has a greater capacity for an emotion involved in a projection, such as when one believes that the distrust experienced in relation to the father is the distrust one is feeling toward the partner in the present, it becomes more possible to take back the projection. The following statement from a client demonstrates how this principle works: "Now that I can sense how deep the emotion of distrust is in my body, and that it is just an experience in my body, I can see that it is not my husband who is the cause of this distrust."

When emotions become more tolerable through the body container, we can stay with them longer and more deeply in order to differentiate them, which gives our emotional experience the "granularity" that research in cognitive psychology has shown to be a key characteristic of psychological health.[2] Emotional granularity refers to the ability to differentiate the emotional experiences of one's body through language, especially metaphor, and in particular through body metaphor. Being able to describe the impact of a loss only as good or bad would indicate a low level of emotional granularity. Being able to describe the impact of the same loss in terms such as "It was a blow to my heart" or "It is as though all the energy drained from my body in an instant" would indicate a higher level of emotional granularity.

Cognitive and Behavioral Outcomes

Emerging findings from the evidence-based paradigm of embodied cognition, emotion, and behavior in neuroscience inform us that cognition, emotion, and behavior are ultimately inseparable in the brain as well as in the body.[3] Additionally, cognition, emotion, and behavior are a function of both the brain and the body, and of the environment.[4] Therefore, when the brain and body shut down through physiological defenses to cope with intolerable emotions, the availability of the body and its connection to the environment are compromised, not only for the function of emotion but also for the functions of cognition and behavior. When our primary experiences of cognition, emotion, and behavior are compromised, so is every psychological experience, such as relationship or spirituality.

Research has shown that the presence of emotion strengthens a person's ability to generate relevant behavioral alternatives for a situation, as well as the person's ability to choose the best course of action in a situation given a number of alternatives. Conversely, the same research has shown that the absence of emotion impairs these functions.[5] Research has also shown that expanding emotions from the brain to the body improves cognition, both about the emotion and about its context.[6] What this means for psychotherapy is that embodying emotion can help us learn about the emotions we have and what they mean, not only in relation to the present but also in relation to our past. These are connections almost all therapies try to make in order to help clients make sense of and heal their current emotional difficulties.

Even though cognition and behavior have long been known to be involved in generating and altering emotional experiences, emotion is now known to be the primary force driving cognition and behavior in every moment of our lives (when emotion is broadly defined to include the basic sensorimotor emotions of feeling good or bad, and cognition is broadly defined to include attention, focus, and perception).[7] It is common for dysregulated emotions to lead to dysfunction in cognition and behavior. For example, I feel such unbearable worthlessness when she leaves me (emotion); I am so convinced that she is the cause of my worthlessness (cognition); I see no choice but to continue to beg her for her forgiveness (behavior).

When we can generate emotions and tolerate them for longer periods in the larger container of the body, we can regulate them better, giving our brains more time to process the cognitive and behavioral implications of the situation we find ourselves in so that our cognitive and behavioral responses to the situation are optimal. We can avoid blaming and acting out. For example, for someone who is in the habit of eating compulsively in the evenings to make themselves feel better, embodying the vague discomfort that triggers the compulsion would allow the person to develop a greater capacity to be with that feeling. The person might then be able to recognize the vague discomfort as loneliness, which might lead them to combat the loneliness by reaching out to a friend rather than to the food in the refrigerator. Also, when emotion is more available and embodied, we can offer the body adequate motivational emotional energy for carrying out the behavior necessary for dealing with the situation.

Examples of Improved Cognitive, Emotional, and Behavioral Outcomes from Emotional Embodiment Work

Discovering that a problem in the present has roots in the past, an act of cognition, is often therapeutic. Almost all psychotherapy modalities emphasize the importance of such insights in healing. At those points of healing, clients often say something like: "I knew that A was connected to B, but I did not know it as convincingly as I do now." This often happens more expediently during emotional embodiment work, two instances of which are presented below.

I met Kim, a mental health professional in her midfifties who has never been married, at a training I taught in China. She asked for help to get over a depression she had suffered from for about six months, ever since a man had walked out on her. The man was her high school sweetheart, the love of her life. He had a pattern of coming back to her from time to time only to abandon her again, either to return to a former lover or to form a relationship with a new woman. Kim could not let go of this man or engage another person in a relationship, so she never formed as deep an attachment to anyone else. In our session we worked with embodying the sensorimotor emotion of how bad the most recent betrayal felt in her body, and then the primary emotion of how sad it made her feel. The sadness was hard to contact, but it eventually surfaced when I had Kim imagine her boyfriend walking away from her into the horizon.

As we tried to stay with the sadness, Kim suddenly reported that she was beginning to feel fear. Interpreting the fear as possibly the fear of permanent loss, I encouraged Kim to stay with it and expand it in her body. She became terrified. Her body started to contort, and her arms and legs became twisted. The more she got into that state, the more terrified she became. She wanted to open her eyes and get out of the state her body was in. When I asked her whether her body has ever gotten into that state during a session before, she said, "Never."

As a body psychotherapist herself, Kim has had years of training and treatment in a trauma-focused body psychotherapy approach. Because certain emotional states can only be reached in certain body states, and regulating the body state toward normalcy could eliminate the emotional experience altogether, I encouraged Kim to stay with the terror—which appeared to be an affect state from early childhood, given the way her body was contorting—and expand the emotion to as much of the body as possible, especially by expressing emotion through vocalization. This technique can help expand the emotion in the body nonverbally, in addition to giving the client some relief. I told Kim it did not matter whether the terror was her terror of the contortions happening in the body or if it was an integral part of the emotional experience in the past situation.

At some point during her experience of terror, Kim remarked that she was born prematurely and was incubated for about a month. She also said she had been separated from her parents from time to time and that for much of her childhood her grandparents had cared for her. I sensed that she was making deeper connections to her past as a result of embodying and tolerating her terror and other feelings in that unusual body state, which can often be seen in physically disabled children. I interpreted her terror as the terror of dying, which is common to experiences of premature birth, incubation, and separation from the mother at birth. This terror is likely to have been reinforced every time she was separated from her parents and her grandparents in childhood, and by the repeated separations from her lover in adulthood.

When I thought she had been with the terror long enough, I stopped supporting that emotion and asked her to do the same. I then asked her to orient to the present, and I had her body slowly recover to a normal state. Toward the end of the session, Kim became quiet and reflective. She shared with us that she had had no idea until then that her long-standing difficulty of not letting go of her high school sweetheart might have anything to do with the threats to her existence around birth. In the days that followed, Kim continued to work with her fear, sadness, and anger on a deeper level in her practice sessions and in private sessions she received from the assistants during the training.

On the last day of the six-day training, Kim told the class she had never been able to remember a dream before, but that day she was surprised by having remembered a short dream from the night before. She had dreamed that her boyfriend appeared, and he wanted to say just one thing to her: "Congratulations!" Kim reported waking up feeling good, with a certain emotional conviction that she was finally over him. Now she felt she could move on and engage someone else in a relationship in a way she had not felt before. A year later when I was back in Hong Kong, I talked with Kim, and she shared with me that she had indeed moved on. She no longer felt that her relationship with her ex-boyfriend was hanging around her neck like a millstone. It hardly crossed her mind, and it caused no anguish, she said.

Another example of deepening insight resulting from emotional embodiment involved a man named Peter, who could not bear to live in the same house with his girlfriend and their two children. Peter volunteered to work with me in front of a class I was teaching in Switzerland. In addition to the house he shared with his girlfriend and children, Peter also had an apartment across the street, to which he retreated from time to time. This was becoming a real problem, not only financially but also relationally between him and his partner. In the session, I had Peter close his eyes, imagine living in the same house with his girlfriend, and sense how unpleasant, bad, or uncomfortable it would feel if he did not have his apartment across the street. I had Peter continue to sense the close presence of his girlfriend as we explored and embodied the unpleasantness, lack of safety, and fear he felt.

After a while, Peter started to sense his body as extremely small and vulnerable in relation to the larger body of his girlfriend. As I encouraged and helped him to embody the vulnerability and stay with it, Peter arrived at a new and significant insight having to do with his twin brother. When the twins were born, Peter was very small compared to his brother because his brother had flourished in the womb, and Peter had not. Peter had always known this about himself, but he had not understood how this fact was playing such an important role in his current life and intimate relationship until he embodied and tolerated the difficulty affectively during the session. I do not know whether Peter was able to change his living arrangement after the session, but his ability to tolerate the vulnerability of being close to his partner and what it brought up, and to make the significant connection between his past and present in that deeper state, is the kind of development I have often seen lead to real change in behavior in people.

Gaining an important and transformative insight is an act of cognition. How can emotional embodiment facilitate such an act? As we saw earlier, the new paradigm of embodied cognition in neuroscience has accumulated evidence showing that cognition is a function not only of the brain but also of the body and the environment. When a body is shut down, with its connection to the brain and the environment broken, that person's cognition is therefore compromised. Also, as we saw earlier, research on emotion has shown that embodying emotion improves cognition, and the lack of it compromises cognition.

Cognition can be defined narrowly or broadly. When defined broadly, acts of cognition involve awareness, attention, focus, perception, abstraction, association, evaluation, memory, imagination, and even language. Findings in embodied cognition research show that emotion affects every one of these cognitive processes, starting with the aspect of the environment one's awareness is directed to before perception begins.[8]

Therefore, it makes scientific sense that Kim and Peter were able to arrive at important and potentially transformative "embodied" insights during their sessions of emotional embodiment work, when they had access to their emotions in a regulated manner and their body was more available for cognition because it was not shut down to avoid unbearable emotion. In both cases, the increased ability they showed to process difficult emotional experiences and resolve them shows the efficiency of emotional embodiment work not only in resolving emotional problems but also in arriving at significant therapeutic cognitive insights. That Kim had moved on from being stuck in an on-and-off relationship of many years shows the effectiveness of this work in changing a long-term behavior.

Physical Outcomes

The Adverse Impact of Childhood Experiences study documents a correlation between adverse childhood experiences and physical health throughout one's life.[9] There is a strong correlation between psychophysiological symptoms on the one hand and the combination of adverse childhood experiences and low capacity for emotional experiences on the other.[10] A group of health care professionals in medicine and psychology founded an organization called the Psychophysiologic Disorder Association, which maintains an extensive bibliography of research articles on the relationship between adverse childhood experiences and physical symptoms such as chronic fatigue, fibromyalgia, and irritable bowel syndrome.[11] Most studies show that as many as one out three symptoms for which people seek medical help may be psychophysiological in origin.[12] Let us see how this might be happening to such a large extent, and how the work of emotional embodiment could be of help in alleviating it.

When the physiology of the brain and body shut down in defense to cope with painful or unacceptable emotional experiences, the physiology is often fragmented, and nervous system communication, blood circulation, lymphatic flows, interstitial (intercellular) flows, and electromagnetic and quantum energy flows between different parts of the physiology are compromised. The resulting decrease in the level of overall functioning and the increase in the level of stress and dysregulation throughout the organism constitute one possible basis of physical symptoms, ranging from minor symptoms such as headaches to major symptoms such as cardiovascular disease. Emotional embodiment work can reduce fragmentation and dysregulation of the body physiology and can efficiently contribute to the reduction of psychophysiological symptoms by increasing the body's capacity to tolerate intense emotional experience, as we saw in the examples of treatment in chapters 1 and 2.

Relationship Outcomes

When we shut our bodies down as our emotional experience becomes unbearable, our ability to process difficult emotional experiences—something we need to do to remain open and connected in relationships—is compromised. In this state, we are more likely to find that others are responsible for the problems we have with them, increasing our distrust in them. Our ability to communicate, regulate, be regulated, and exchange vital energies in relationships is also impaired, further eroding the quality of our relationships. Our attachment patterns in childhood can become reactivated and reinforced. When we shut ourselves down in important relationships in our immediate environment, we also compromise our connection to the collective body and psyche and their resources. Because emotional embodiment work creates a greater capacity for the intense emotional experiences that often characterize relationships, it can help us remain open and connected to significant others, heal wounds from old relationships, and transform our earliest and most entrenched attachment patterns, which often take the form of implicit emotional memories in the brain and the body.

Attachment theory has found affect regulation to be crucial in repairing attachment wounds.[13] Embodied attunement—the ability to sense emotional states in another's body within our own body—is the key to affect regulation.[14] When we are able to tolerate emotional states

82

in ourselves, we can remain open to sensing, tolerating, and regulating others through interpersonal resonance. Interpersonal resonance refers to the ability our bodies and brains have to sense and regulate the emotional or physical state of another person by sharing information with each other through energies of the electromagnetic spectrum when we are near each other,[15] and through quantum mechanical principles, such as quantum entanglement, even when we are at a great distance from each other.[16] Developing the capacity to tolerate difficult emotions in the body through emotional embodiment work can therefore be of great help to both clients and therapists engaged in attachment work.

People often seek therapy because bad experiences in past relationships are causing them to have relationship problems, hardship in current relationships, or difficulty in forming new relationships. We saw that pattern in the cases of Kim and Peter. Let us now discuss another example of treatment in which emotional embodiment work was of great help in expanding relationship capacity.

When Sonia's husband told her he had fallen in love with their secretary, she said she just accepted it and moved on. She was in another relationship when she attended a workshop I offered in Germany. The symptom she wanted help with was her inability to feel close to her new partner. No matter how hard she tried, she could not feel as loving toward him as she had felt toward her ex-husband. Sonia had worked on the end of her marriage in therapy, and she was therefore quite surprised how much energy, shock, and hurt there was behind her closed heart when we worked with it through awareness, intention, movement, self-touch, and expression.

In the session, we worked with the consequences of a broken heart—something to which we can all relate. When people have their hearts broken, the pain is so great that they sometimes end up in hospital emergency rooms, thinking they are having a heart attack. There is grief, hopelessness, despair, shame, guilt, and worthlessness. There is also the hurt, ache, and rawness of a wounded heart, and the stress, disorientation, and dysregulation that usually accompany loss of significant support in one's life. No wonder people shut their hearts and bodies down to cope with such awful experiences, with cognitive, emotional, and behavioral problems as a consequence.

Using the larger body container and the support of the group, we helped Sonia to expand and process her overwhelming emotions from the experience of betrayal that had shut her heart down. When I heard from Sonia many months later, she said she was so happy about the session and its effect on her relationship that she summed it up in one sentence: "That session alone was worth the price of the workshop!"

Spiritual Outcomes

At times, I hear from trainees and clients who tell me they're noticing improvement in their spiritual practice or that their spiritual practice appears to be getting deeper from emotional embodiment work. It is hard to know what they mean specifically by "improvement in spiritual practice" because there are so many spiritual practices and there is so much variation among different spiritual paths. Still, let us explore how emotional embodiment work could improve outcomes in any spiritual practice.

Spiritual growth can be defined broadly as improvement in the relationship between the individual and a greater power, called "God" in some religions. Spiritual growth can also be conceptualized nonreligiously as improvement in the connection between the individual and the whole. Quantum physics tells us that the individual is ultimately inseparable from the whole at the subatomic level. The ability to tolerate emotion at the individual level by making the body more available for interactions with the environment can improve the individual's connection to the collective level of our existence.

Jungian psychology—whose goal is individuation, or the development of a stable and healthy relationship between the individual ego and the collective self (which is defined as the totality of collective matter and psyche)—emphasizes that the basic requirement for individuation or personal growth is the ability to tolerate opposites at the level of the individual. Advaita Vedanta cites the same ability—the capacity to tolerate opposites in experience at the individual level—as a basic precondition or qualification for enlightenment, a state wherein the individual achieves a stable expanded awareness that the individual and the collective are one and the same. The Western alchemy tradition requires the ability to tolerate opposites as a basic prerequisite for transforming base metals (ordinary psychological experiences) into gold (extraordinary psychological transformation).

When we develop a greater capacity to tolerate opposites in emotional experience, such as hope and despair or love and hate, the individual body—and therefore the individual psyche—need not shut down in the face of seemingly unbearable or unacceptable emotional experiences. They can remain more open and connected to the collective body and psyche. Therefore, it makes sense that emotional embodiment work has been found to be helpful in improving outcomes in diverse spiritual practices that strive toward increasing the connection between the individual and the collective in whatever way it may be conceptualized. When awareness is not distracted by or concentrated in suffering at the individual level, it can soar to own the individual as well as the collective level as itself, which is another way of describing enlightenment.

Summary of Cases Presented in Part I

In the examples of emotional embodiment work presented in chapters 1, 2, 3, and 4, we worked with experiences ranging from extraordinary traumas, such as electrocution and premature birth, to ordinary but difficult life experiences of separation and loss of adult relationships. The levels of stress and dysregulation and the levels of emotion and its intensity varied from low to high, and the traumas ranged from purely physical to purely psychological. They involved shock (posttraumatic stress) traumas, developmental traumas, and developmental shock traumas, where shock trauma has developmental implications or developmental traumas have led to shock. Almost all the cases presented in these chapters had prior psychotherapeutic or psychopharmacological treatment. Almost all the cases had prior body psychotherapeutic treatment as well. These cases, their outcomes, and reports of similar outcomes by therapists from multiple countries with different orientations to therapy who have integrated emotional embodiment into their work show the versatility of emotional embodiment work as a complementary tool for improving diverse outcomes across a range of therapeutic modalities, including those already oriented to the body.

When Does Emotional Embodiment Not Work?

No method works for everyone, and no method works for the same person at all times. That is why there are many psychological methods, to meet the differing needs of individuals as well as changing needs of the same individual over time. A meta-analysis of research studies on the effectiveness of different therapies shows that, across all therapy modalities, 50 percent of clients reported measurable improvement in eight sessions, and 80 percent of clients reported measurable improvement in six months.[17] The ongoing viability of the various methods in the marketplace also indirectly attest to the efficacy of all therapy modalities. It appears that people stay with therapy modalities that work for them and leave those that do not, possibly explaining why studies among clients of different therapy modalities show that those modalities were more or less equally effective in meeting the needs of their clients.

There is also growing evidence that including the body in some way can improve the effectiveness of all therapies. That is probably why mental health professionals are repeatedly placing body-oriented courses and presentations at the top of their lists of things they would like to see more of in *Psychotherapy Networker* magazine (the magazine with the largest circulation among mental health professionals in the United States) and its conferences. That is also probably the reason for the steady increase in the offering of courses on body-oriented methods for continuing education of mental health professionals.

The aim of ISP is to increase the effectiveness of all therapy modalities, body-oriented or not, by involving the body in their work in a particular way. The primary clinical strategy used by ISP is emotional embodiment. This happens through the embodiment of a greater range of emotions, especially the often-overlooked but always present sensorimotor emotions, in as regulated a manner as possible, with simple tools that can be easily incorporated into the diverse therapy modalities out there. It is a complementary method for incorporation into all therapy modalities. It is best not to approach it as a therapy modality in itself, as that could severely limit its potential use and benefit when perceived as just one among many competing modalities. Because emotional embodiment work brings a broader understanding of emotions, and because it emphasizes educating clients about different kinds of emotions, it offers therapists a better chance of getting clients in all therapy modalities to sense and work with emotions in their body, to help resolve their symptoms efficiently.

All methods have limitations. So, despite the evidence that emotional embodiment is effective in improving outcomes in all kinds of therapies and all kinds of individuals in different clinical situations, an answer to the question of when it might be ineffective or contraindicated is very much in order. Emotional embodiment is unlikely to work when a person's emotional development is so lacking that they are not able to access and stay with emotions. It is also not likely to work when a person cannot sense their body, at least at the level of emotion, because emotional embodiment work requires the ability to sense emotion in the body. It is also not likely to work with people who easily decompensate when body awareness is brought to bear in relation to emotions. Emotional embodiment is not likely to work with those who lack enough of an observing ego for their experiences, nor with those at the extremes of the clinical spectrum, such as schizophrenia. Other limitations of the work will surely emerge as it is incorporated and tested in different therapeutic modalities for different ends.

However, a person's ability to sense one's body and emotions depends very much on the therapist's understanding of the different types of emotion and the role the body plays in emotional experience, and on the therapist's ability to educate, guide, and support clients to sense different types of emotions in their body. I often hear therapists say their clients cannot sense their body or get in touch with their emotion. Based on my experience, I think this often occurs because the therapist is working with either too narrow a definition of emotion or is not giving their clients adequate education about emotion, sufficient emotional support, or enough motivation to work with emotion.

Clients come to therapy not because they are feeling good but because they are feeling bad enough to do something about it. They have to feel bad enough in the body for them to come into therapy and spend hard-earned money to find relief. Now, feeling bad is an emotion—a basic sensorimotor emotion, or an aspect of the experience of any unpleasant primary emotion, such as sadness or fear. Feeling bad is something they could easily and readily sense in their body if their therapist guided them there. In my experience, clients are able to arrive at more differentiated emotional states when they first work with the basic sensorimotor affects, such as feeling bad or awful in the body, which are almost always available. This technique is effective because it is the "feeling bad" aspect of an emotion that often makes it intolerable. Asking clients what they sense in the body or what they feel and where they sense it in the body in the abstract is unlikely to motivate them enough to get there.

Clients also need to be educated about why it is important to sense something unpleasant in the body, and why it is helpful to expand the unpleasant emotional experience in the body. Most people seek treatment to rid themselves of their suffering. They will not be motivated to suffer any more than they already are if they do not get some simple explanation from the therapist that explains how what they are being asked to do is connected to the healing of their symptoms. For example, a therapist could say: "Just as it is easier and faster to carry a load with two arms than with one, it is easier and faster to process an emotion that is causing a symptom with more parts of the body than with one." Here is a more detailed example:

"When painful feelings become unbearable, we shut the body down to cope with it. Then, the body becomes more stressed and dysregulated, and its connections to the brain, other people, and the world at large are compromised. Psychophysiological symptoms form as a consequence.

When we expand the body by working with defenses against emotions to expand the painful emotions in the body, it can help the body to get regulated and remain open and connected to the brain as well as to other people and the environment. In that way, our symptoms can resolve. And we might even find that the pain of the emotion is bearable."

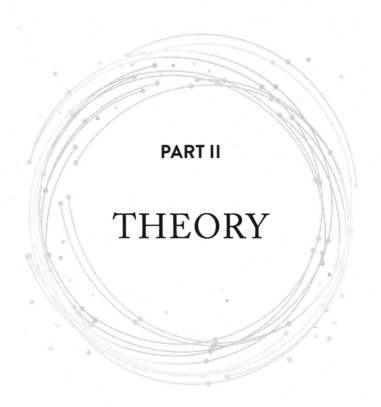

PART II

THEORY

In this part of the book, chapters 5–9 will present the scientific evidence for the practice of embodying emotion.

5

The Physiology of Emotion

Chapter summary: presents evidence from research on the physiology of emotion to elucidate all the ways in which emotions are generated in the brain and body physiology, and to establish that an emotion and its conscious experience can involve the entirety of the brain and body physiology.

As we saw in the examples in chapters 1, 2, 3, and 4, emotional embodiment involves the expansion and regulation of the body and the brain to expand and regulate the conscious experience of emotion in as much of the brain and body physiology as possible, to create a greater capacity to tolerate and stay with the emotional experience over a longer period of time. Two critical assumptions underlie this method:

- Emotion could involve the entirety of the brain and body physiology.

- It is possible to expand the conscious experience of emotion through both the brain and the body, even though it might not be necessary to involve all of the physiology to improve clinical outcomes in specific instances.

These assumptions might sound bold and even a bit crazy. After all, it is not at all our common experience that we experience emotions throughout our brain and body physiology. The question of whether there is adequate scientific evidence to support such assumptions comes up often and early among therapists in every country where I teach. Other questions also arise on a regular basis: What do emotions have to do with the body? Isn't emotion strictly a brain phenomenon?

Even after I have demonstrated that a difficult emotion, such as grief or fear, could be experienced consciously throughout the body and brain physiology, someone will invariably ask: Is that real, or is it caused by your suggestion? Or by the participant's need to perform in front of the group? These are very reasonable questions. I also ran into them in my own mind in the early stages of developing the work of emotional embodiment.

Why Emotions Are Not Commonly Experienced throughout the Brain and Body Physiology

We do not consciously experience emotions throughout the brain and body physiology on a daily basis. This is in part because we are limited by a lack of awareness that we bring to the experience of the body, in life and in therapy. It is also in part because, as we will see later, we defend against the greater involvement of the brain and body physiology in the generation and experience of emotions, through psychological as well as physiological defenses that eventually contribute to our pathologies. Despite the mounting scientific evidence of the role of the body in emotional and other psychological experiences, the research most therapists are exposed to in their training is focused more on the brain than on the body. The public at large is also exposed to the same media bias toward the brain when research on emotion is presented.

The most important reason why we do not consciously experience emotions all over the brain and body physiology is because it is not necessary to do so to live a healthy life. Emotions do not have to be always fully embodied or conscious experiences for them to play an important role in our lives. Just feeling a jolt of fear on the right side of my body when a car approaches dangerously close on the right might be enough to alert me to step aside, and I might not even consciously experience the fear before I move to protect myself. Therefore, it is important to remember that there is no lifestyle prescription whatsoever implied here. This book does not suggest that we ought to consciously experience every instance of emotion in every waking moment in as much of the brain and body physiology as possible. It does suggest that we use the potential we have for such complete emotional embodiment as the basis for developing a greater capacity for emotion as a therapeutic and self-help method, to resolve unresolved emotions and the difficulties they cause.

Emotions Are Complex

Emotion is a very complex phenomenon. There are many different theories about how the brain and the body are involved in generating and experiencing emotions, with differing perspectives on the importance of the brain versus the body. There are differing views on the extent to which emotions are innate dispositions endowed upon us by evolution, the extent to which cognitive appraisal is involved prior to emotional experience, and the extent to which emotions are constructed by our brains based on our body experience with the aid of language. There is contradictory evidence on whether different emotions have different distinct neural (brain) and body patterns. There are also different opinions on the function or purpose of emotion, e.g., for communicating our inner states to others, a quick assessment of how we are doing with respect to our homeostasis, energy management, survival, or some other purpose.

The more I study the research on emotions, the more I am convinced there is no one way in which emotions are generated and experienced in the brain and body physiology; rather, there are many ways. The debates in the field of research on emotions, especially the brain versus body debate, brings to mind the old Indian story about a group of blind men touching different parts of an elephant. The man who touched the trunk thought he was touching a thick snake, the one touching the tail thought it was a rope, the one touching the leg thought it was a tree trunk, and so on. Each man insisted that his own unique experience of the elephant was correct, and the others had to be in error. For those of you who wish to explore our present scientific understanding of emotion, I highly recommend two books: *The Nature of Emotion: Fundamental Questions* edited by Fox, Lapate, Shackman, and Davison (2018)[1] and *The Feeling Brain: The Biology and Psychology of Emotions* by Johnston and Olson (2015).[2]

Before we review and discuss the key findings on the physiology of emotions that are relevant to the work of emotional embodiment, let us get clear about the terminology we will use throughout the book. For the sake of simplicity, we will use the single term "emotion" to refer to the various terms such as affect, feeling, mood, and temperament that are used in the literature to differentiate states or types of emotion. For example, both mood and temperament can be thought of as persistent emotional states. Damasio defines a feeling as a conscious emotion, in which emotion comes first and feeling later, distinguishing emotion from affective experience.[3] Here, we will use conscious emotion and unconscious emotion as terms if we need to distinguish between conscious and unconscious emotional experience. A person might or might not be consciously aware of their envy when they make disparaging statements about a person they envy. The terms "experience of emotion" and "emotional experience" will refer to a conscious experience of emotion unless specified otherwise.

The James-Lange Theory: The Body Is Necessary for the Generation of Emotion

The earliest theory of emotion in the history of the physiology of emotion, the James-Lange theory, gave the body the primary role in generating emotion. American psychologist William James published his essay "What Is an Emotion?" in 1884.[4] A year later, Danish physician Carl Lange published his independent findings in an essay titled "On Emotions: A Psychophysiological Study."[5] The combined findings of these two pioneers came to be known as the James-Lange theory of emotion. This theory proposes that emotion is first generated in the body through changes in the voluntary muscles by the somatic nervous system; changes in the organs, glands, and blood vessels by the autonomic nervous system; and changes in the secretions of the glands of the endocrine system, such as the adrenal glands that empty products such as cortisol directly into the bloodstream.

When there is a significant change in a person's environment, the person has to do something with their body to cope with the change. If a hiker were to be suddenly confronted by a menacing bear, then the person has to generate a lot of energy through the autonomic nervous system and the endocrine system to fuel the voluntary muscular system to run from the bear or fight it. According to the James-Lange theory, the pattern of body sensations generated by these changes is what the brain becomes aware of as emotion. The brain was assumed to have the capacity to differentiate, recognize, and experience body sensations as different emotions. In our bear example, the person who runs will generate body sensations of fear, and the person who fights will generate body sensations of anger. One could presumably alternate between the two emotions in quick succession, generating both of them.

Please note that the James-Lange theory did not rule out a role for the brain in emotional experience. Emotions are ultimately experienced through the brain. What it implied was that the body is absolutely necessary for the generation of an emotional experience; that is, it cannot be generated in the physiology of the brain alone. The theory said the sensory and motor cortices of the brain, which belong to the external layer of the brain called the cortex, are the areas where the emotion generated in the body became conscious. The theory did not offer any insight on whether the brain was involved in any conscious or unconscious process other than the perception of the environment and the generation of automatic responses in the body, programmed by evolution, that became the basis of emotional experiences. The brain's ability to instantly recognize a pattern in the incoming information about the environment that triggers the instinctual response was implied. Please remember that this theory was formulated in the 1880s, when what we knew about the brain was quite limited.

The James-Lange theory was a paradigm shift in our understanding of emotion.[6] It not only put behavior ahead of emotion; it also made behavior the cause of emotion, at least to begin with. It challenged and still challenges our common experience of the order in which things unfold, which runs as follows: we perceive the world, evaluate it, have an emotional response on the basis of our evaluation, and then respond to the world with appropriate behavior to safeguard our well-being in the situation. To this day, this is the model that most of us use, in therapy and in life. However counterintuitive the model of behavior preceding emotion might appear, the accumulated evidence that this happens in most (if not all) instances is considerable. Please see the book *Feelings: The Perception of the Self* by Larry D. Baird (2007) for evidence from hundreds of studies in which behavior precedes and determines emotion.[7] For example, the work of Ekman and his colleagues shows that voluntary facial action generates emotion-specific nervous system activity.[8]

The Cannon-Bard Theory:
The Body Is Not Needed for the Generation of Emotion

The James-Lange theory was challenged in 1927 by James's former undergraduate student (and later his Harvard colleague) Walter Cannon, a neurologist who is often credited with the conceptualization of the "fight or flight" and "freeze" responses that are the staple of trauma therapy these days. Cannon is also known for the concept of homeostasis, which is the body's tendency to maintain optimal internal conditions in the face of widely fluctuating external conditions.[9] Cannon and his former student Philip Bard did not just say that emotion is generated in the brain and that behavior followed emotion; they declared that there is no way the body could be involved in the process of generating or regulating emotion.[10] What about the all-too-common experience of feeling gripping fear in the abdomen or the happy feeling of love in the chest? They are just sensations from the brain preparing the body to deal with the change in the environment triggering the emotion in the brain. Expressing emotion was seen as a means to return the organism to homeostasis or a balanced state of internal well-being.

The James-Lange theory located the conscious experience of emotion in the cortex, the outermost layer of the brain. The Cannon-Bard theory also identified the cortex as the place where emotion became conscious as an experience. It did not precisely locate any brain region where emotion is generated. However, it pointed to the subcortical or interior layer of the brain, especially the thalamus and the hypothalamus, as the location where emotional expression is initiated.

The James-Lange and Cannon-Bard theories are extremely important because almost all the subsequent orientations of emotion research were inspired by one or both of them. The Cannon-Bard theory shifted the focus of emotion research from the body to the brain for a very long time, until research on the brain itself started to point back to the importance of the body toward the end of the twentieth century. This turnaround has led to a renewed interest in the James-Lange theory, and the updating of it with new evidence from brain research. As for the Cannon-Bard theory, its influence on research on the role of the brain in emotion is also substantial. The subsequent discoveries relating to the role of subcortical brain structures in the generation and expression of emotion, as well as the role of cortical brain structures in regulating cognition and emotion and making them conscious, all have roots in the Cannon-Bard theory.

No theory, including the James-Lange theory, denies a role for the brain in emotional experience. The issue all along has been the extent to which the body plays a role in this experience. The neuroscientific evidence that has emerged since the second half of the twentieth century shows that body experience is involved in the generation and experience of emotion in the brain[11] and that the brain can generate emotional experiences without current input from the body by recalling past emotional experiences generated by past body experiences (to quickly predict possible emotional reactions to current situations).[12] This evidence poses the question of whether it is possible to generate and have experiences of emotion in the brain that do not involve the present or past experience of the body in any way. We will answer this question later in this chapter. For now, let us turn our focus to how modern brain research has made the body once again a key player in the generation and experience of emotion.

How Modern Neuroscience Put the Body Back at the Center of Emotional Experience

Recent neuroscience research returned the body to the center of emotional experience in a couple of ways. First, it countered the theoretical and empirical limitations of the research on the Cannon-Bard theory that led to the conclusion that the body is not involved in emotional experience. Second, it used painstaking neuroanatomical work to show how the brain gathers information from the body and uses it in the construction of emotion. Let us look at each of these streams of research in turn.

The body can be likened to an orchestra with a large number of instruments (or body systems) that can play a wide variety of melodies (or emotions) by creating complex arrays (patterns) of physiological changes. During Cannon's time, it was believed that the autonomic nervous system, and especially its sympathetic nervous system, behaved in the same way in all the areas controlled by it. We now know that the autonomic nervous system can vary its reactions from one part of the body to another.[13] For example, different people's bodies might all be involved in dealing with a shared situation (such as a common threat) but in different ways, with each of them generating similar but differing arrays of physiological changes, even when all of them are running away from the threat. Every person does not use the same muscles to the same degree in the act of running away from a threat. Similarly, when a given person faces multiple instances of a similar occasion, their body might not be involved in the same way each time, creating similar but varying arrays of physiological changes in response to the situation.

These similar but varying physiological responses to the same or similar situations can be likened to the similar but variable patterns we might observe in a kaleidoscope on successive turns of it. For a few turns at least, we can continue to see the original pattern, even though the elements get rearranged with every turn. Just as our brains can observe a common pattern among the variable patterns created by successive turns of a kaleidoscope, our brains are capable of recognizing a unique pattern of physiological changes for an emotion such as fear as a result of observing slightly different variations of it on different occasions. And just as our brains can observe, after many turns of the kaleidoscope, that the original pattern has been replaced by a new pattern, even though we might still observe some arrangements that are common to both patterns, our brains can also detect different patterns of physiological changes for different emotions in arrays of physiological changes that might have some (but not all) elements in common.

The brain is now recognized as having the ability to recognize such patterns in complex and overlapping information from a very early age.[14] The research that established the Cannon-Bard theory of emotion typically measured only a few changes, such as heart rate and breath rate, and concluded that the body cannot be the source of emotion if two distinct emotions such as fear and anger measured the same (either low or high) on both. In order to realistically study whether there are different physiological patterns for different emotions, such as happiness and sadness, later research usually involved the measurement of a greater number of physiological changes.

A study measuring heartbeat and skin conductance rate showed different patterns of physiological changes for different basic emotions, such as happiness, sadness, fear, and anger.[15] More recent studies took more differentiated measurements of changes in the autonomic nervous system itself, such as different styles or types of breathing as opposed to the simple breath rate.[16] Other research took more detailed measures of cardiovascular and respiratory responses such as properties of heart rate and its variability, changes in the respiratory period, and the interval between respiratory waves, and analyzed them by multivariate statistical methods.[17] Newer research has been more successful in providing evidence that the body could be involved in the generation of distinct emotional experiences through generating distinct patterns of sensations for different emotions.

Also, more recent studies based on self-reports of broad changes in parts of the body in the experience of all basic and some complex emotions have found different patterns of body changes for different basic emotions, such as happiness and sadness, and for complex emotions, such as anxiety and depression.[18,19] These cross-cultural studies involved a large number of subjects and employed multivariate statistical methods that allowed for variations across individuals to arrive at "a common pattern of body changes" that is distinct for each emotion.

We now turn to the other set of findings in neuroscience that restored the body to its important role in emotion.

How the Brain Gathers Information from the Body

We start with what we know now about how the brain receives and processes information from the body. From previous research we know that the brain constantly receives information through different body systems: the nerves, the blood, and extracellular fluid, the fluid that circulates between cells, bringing them nutrients and messages. Chemical messengers, such as peptides, which are capable of traveling between the brain and the body, are found in extracellular fluids of the brain and the body. The brain gathers a great deal of information about activity on different levels within each body system. For example, the brain gathers information about what is happening at the level of individual muscle cells in terms of chemistry, as well as at the level of an entire muscle in terms of tension or relaxation. The brain receives and processes information such as "signals related to pain states; body temperature; flush; itch; tickle; shudder; visceral and genital sensations; the state of the smooth musculature and other viscera; local pH; glucose; osmolality; presence of inflammatory agents; and so forth."[20]

The neural or brain image of such detailed information about the body is called a detailed "body map." We know the brain is capable of processing such detailed information to produce higher-order body maps through aggregation and abstraction. For example, the brain can be aware of individual sensations in different parts of an arm or of how the whole arm feels overall—"good" or "bad"—by collecting and inferring the meaning of individual sensations into an overall neural body map of the arm feeling good or bad. The overall sense of feeling good or bad is an example of a higher-order body map of the arm. The sensations from different components of the arm, such as the skin, the muscles, and the joints that contribute to this higher-order body map experience of feeling good or bad, are called lower-order body maps of sensations from the skin, the muscles, and the joints.

We also know the brain is capable of storing and recalling information about different parts of the body at different levels of aggregation and abstraction for prediction.[21] For example, if we want to predict and compare the emotional consequences of different behavioral responses to a current situation in order to choose the best way to respond to the situation, we can run such simulations in the brain by recalling similar experiences from the past.

How the Brain Generates Emotions from Body Experience

The brain generates and experiences emotions based more on the aggregate or abstract neural images it creates than on the detailed information it receives from the body.[22] What do we mean by an aggregate or abstract neural image? When we look at Georges Seurat's pointillist painting of a woman with an umbrella holding a child's hand on the bank of a river on a summer evening, consisting of thousands and thousands of colored dots, we are observing the image of the woman, the umbrella, the child, and the river at an aggregate or abstract level. However, when we move close enough to the painting, all we can see are the thousands and thousands of dots the images are made of. In the same way, we come to know that we are feeling good, bad, or neutral about a relationship by aggregating and abstracting a large number of microsensations from the body, which can be likened to the thousands and thousands of dots that make up Seurat's painting. The images of the woman, the umbrella, and the river are likened to the higher-order neural maps of the body in the brain, and the dots of paint that form those images can be likened to the lower-order neural maps of the body.

These higher-order body maps that give rise to the emotions of good, bad, or neutral might break down in terms of body changes that can vary considerably across individuals for a single emotion, and they can vary in the same person across different occasions.[23] One can be happy or sad in different ways on different occasions, depending on which body systems are involved and how they are involved. For example, an instance of sadness or happiness can involve one's heart and lungs to different degrees. It can involve the breath rate and the constriction or relaxation of the lung tissue. It can also involve the heart rate and the constriction or relaxation of the heart musculature, or it can involve both to different degrees. Such variability can also occur across individuals when they are all experiencing similar emotions (fear, horror, and sadness, for example) in a shared situation, such as watching the Challenger space shuttle explode and fall to the earth a few minutes after takeoff.

Likewise, the same orchestra can play the same melody with different combinations of instruments, and everyone who knows the melody can still recognize it. Even someone who does not know a melody can find the common melody after being exposed to a number of different renditions of it with different sets of musical instruments. In the same way, the brain is known to be capable from infancy of finding patterns in data and creating categories out of the patterns it observes.

How Emotions Are Constructed from Present as Well as Past Body Experience

So far, we have seen how the brain can generate emotion from current body experience. According to Damasio, the brain also has the ability to generate quick predictions of emotional reactions to familiar situations by recalling past body experiences without involving the body in the present.[24] This ability, which he calls "the as-if body loop," conserves energy and makes optimal use of past experience to respond to familiar situations. In Barrett's constructivist theory of emotions, such predictions are always involved in every emotional experience.[25] Every emotional experience is constructed by the brain as a combination of:

- predictions based on past experiences (about the situation, about how a person should optimally respond to it internally and externally to adjust one's energy and behavior to cope with the situation, and about the body changes that would be necessary to carry out the internal and external responses); and

- current information that is constantly coming in about the situation, how the person is responding internally and externally to it, and how it is affecting the body in the moment.

In case there is any disbelief that prediction is a component in emotional experiences, please note that there is now adequate evidence that prediction based on past experience is involved even in perception through the five senses.[26]

How Language Is Involved in the Construction of Emotional Experiences

In her book *How Emotions Are Made: The Secret Life of the Brain*, Lisa Feldman Barrett describes how language is involved in the construction of simple and complex emotional experiences.[27] From infancy, the brain is capable of recognizing patterns in inner and outer experience and attaching words to them. Every flying object might initially be called a "bird," a simple concept. Eventually, flying objects are differentiated into more complex concepts (e.g., "peacock," "robin," "passenger plane," "fighter plane") that are based on observations of features that distinguish them, even though they all fly. In the same way, a situation, as well as the emotional experience of it, can be described with simple emotion concepts such as "good," "bad," "painful," "pleasurable," "sad," or "happy"; or with more complex emotion concepts such as the "fear of failing to live up to one's father's expectations" and "fear of falling from a high place."

How Emotional Experiences Can Vary across Individuals, Families, and Cultures

Every instance of "fear of falling from a high place" is going to vary, from "fear of falling from a building" to "fear of falling from a tree" to "falling down while walking on posts on a fence in childhood," for example. Every instance of "falling from a building" or "falling from a tree" or "falling from a fence" will also vary, because our prediction, as well as our actual behavior, is never exactly the same in each of these situations. Two individuals exposed to the same situation, "the risk of falling from a high place," cannot be expected to have the same predicted or actual perception and evaluation of the situation, nor the same inner and outer behavioral responses initiated to cope with it, nor the same body changes that occur as a consequence. For example, faced with the same situation of falling from a fence, one person might predict worse consequences from the fall than another person, depending on their past experiences of such falls. One person might make further attempts to avert the fall, whereas another might take the fall for granted and prepare the body for the inevitable fall.

People can, however, communicate their diverse emotional experiences with simple emotion concepts in words such as "bad," "scary," and so on. In order to communicate their emotional experiences more accurately, they have to describe them with complex emotion concepts in phrases such as "fear of falling down while walking on posts on a fence in childhood." We can expect even greater variation in perception, evaluation, behavioral response, and consequent body changes involving "fear of failing to live up to one's father's expectations" across individuals, families, subcultures, and cultures.

"Fear of failing to live up to one's father's expectations" is a complex instance of emotion with much potential variation, especially across cultures, as the terms of relationship with one's father might vary. In more complex emotional experiences such as this, language plays a greater role in identifying and communicating one's emotional experiences to others. Those within the same culture and the same family system are more likely to be able to communicate and understand such complex emotional experiences in each other.

How We Communicate Our Emotional States to Each Other

We communicate emotional states verbally, through language with simple and complex emotion concepts, and nonverbally, through such features as facial and body expression, and tone of voice. When others receive such information from us, they can try to understand what we are going through by using their past experiences to simulate what they might feel in similar situations in their brains and bodies, or by mirroring our body and facial expressions and tone of voice. The research on "mirror neurons" focuses on identifying neurons in our brains that mimic the movements we see others make, in order to get at the inner experience of others.[28] As an example, I remember how good my body felt as I came out of an afternoon performance of a Cirque de Soleil show. It felt so good because my brain could, without moving, share the pleasure their bodies were experiencing as they executed such masterful routines.

All human beings share a common genetic heritage. Our brains and bodies are close to each other in their physical makeup. We might vary widely in terms of our psychological response to similar situations, but we share many common experiences: pain and pleasure, aversion and attraction, feeling good or bad, feeling regulated or dysregulated. These experiences might vary due to constitutional variations in people's physical makeup, but we have enough in common that we can understand each other when we use these simple words to communicate aspects of our emotional experience to each other.

Perhaps this is how the universal or basic emotions of sadness, happiness, fear, anger, disgust, and surprise evolved and became shared patterns of emotional experience. Perhaps the more frequent universal experiences of feeling good or bad can be called universal or basic sensorimotor emotions, which might be harder to express through facial expression than Darwin's list of universal basic emotions (happiness, sadness, fear, anger, surprise, and disgust). A sensorimotor emotion is a psychologically meaningful physiological state of the brain or the body that cannot be deconstructed into basic or complex emotions. Because basic sensorimotor emotions, like pain and pleasure, are always present either on their own or as part and parcel of all simple and complex emotions, we will see later how they can be useful in emotional embodiment work, especially with those who have difficulty in experiencing or differentiating their emotions.

Let's return to the earlier example of "fear of failing to live up to one's father's expectations" to examine how it might be communicated across individuals and cultures. It is a complex instance of emotion with much potential variation, even within the same person across all the situations in which it is evoked. This is even more true with regard to differences across cultures, which can affect the terms of how the relationship with one's father might vary. Therefore, perhaps there is a greater chance of communicating this emotion in terms of simple emotion concepts such as "bad" or "painful" or "sad," to at least get some essential aspect of the experience across. Such simple emotion concepts might well be the candidates for universal basic emotions that can be communicated across cultures, because all cultures appear to have words to describe otherwise complex and varied emotional experiences through simple and reductive emotion concepts.

However, such concepts might not quite capture the complex experience of "fear of failing to live up to one's father's expectations" across individuals and cultures. Those within the same culture and the same family system, who have shared lived experiences, are more likely to be able to communicate about and understand complex emotional experiences such as "fear of failing to live up to one's father's expectations" in each other. In more complex emotional experiences, language therefore plays a greater role in identifying and communicating one's emotional experiences to others.

How We Might Also Learn about Emotions from Each Other Directly through "Resonance"

The standard assumption is that we come to understand each other's emotional states and to empathize with each other by exchanging information about emotion through the five senses. This assumption, based in Western phenomenology, posits that the only way for individuals to gather information about the inner body and brain states of others is to use their external senses of sight, sound, smell, taste, and touch. This assumption strengthens the idea that it is not so easy for individuals to share their unique emotional experiences with each other.

Now, however, considerable research from multiple disciplines shows that our bodies and brains are capable of sending and receiving information through the measurable frequencies of the electromagnetic spectrum, the phenomenon we have already referred to as interpersonal resonance, or simply resonance.[29,30] Even though our unique bodies might still filter the information received through resonance, we can directly exchange information on emotions with each other in this manner. We can use resonance to learn about how others experience, understand, and label different emotions, which increases the likelihood that we have more shared brain and body patterns in the experience of different emotions than the constructive theory of emotion might lead us to believe.

The Hard Science That Reestablished the Role of the Body in Emotional Experience

The parts of the brain that have been identified as being involved with processing information from the body have now become collectively known as the "interoceptive network." Scientists such as Antonio Damasio and Bud Craig have identified several parts of the brain, especially the insular cortex, as constituting the interoceptive network. For example, Damasio identifies the sensory motor cortices (I and II), the insular cortex, the cingulate cortex, the thalamus, the hypothalamus, and the brain stem nuclei in the tegmentum as participating in the interoceptive network.[31] Many brain areas that have been identified as involved in processing emotion (in studies by leading researchers such as Walter Cannon, Philip Bard, James Papez, Paul McLean, and Joseph E. LeDoux) have also been found to be involved in processing body information. Important brain areas that constitute the interoceptive network, such as the anterior insular cortex, have been found to be the same brain areas that become active when people report that they are subjectively experiencing emotions.[32]

Now, the findings showing that brain areas that specialize in processing body information are also involved in processing emotion do not necessarily mean that one has to do with the other. Emotional experience need not necessarily depend on or derive from body experience; it could just be that those brain areas happen to have more than one function in common. Still, there is growing evidence showing how body states shape emotions.[33] There is also increasing evidence that our capacity for conscious emotional experience is highly correlated with our capacity for conscious body experience.[34] This also suggests that emotions are dependent on body states.

The senses of smell, taste, hearing, sight, and touch are called the external or exteroceptive senses. The sense through which we come to know what is happening in our body on the inside is called the internal or interoceptive sense. The brain's conscious and unconscious interoception of the body helps us perform a number of functions, including homeostasis, energy management, and survival.[35] It turns out that those of us who are better at interoception or body sensing—for example, those who can reliably estimate how many times their heart beats in a certain time period—also experience emotions more consciously and at higher levels of intensity than those who have a poorer interoceptive sense. (It also turns out that they have better cognitive functioning, and they spend less energy during strenuous exercise.)

The findings we have discussed in this chapter constitute a strong case for the potential involvement of the entire body in the generation and experience of emotion. To review, those findings are as follows:

- The brain processes information from all systems in the body gathered through different means.

- The areas of the brain that have been identified as having to do with the processing of body information are a subset of the areas of the brain that have been identified as having to do with the processing of emotion.

- The emotions are shaped by body states.

- The capacity for conscious emotional experience is dependent on the capacity for conscious body experience.

- Different emotions have different body patterns at the micro level (with measurements of cardiovascular and respiratory functions) and at the macro level (with measurement of different patterns of general activation in different parts of the body for different basic and complex emotions).

There is near unanimity among emotion researchers of all stripes that one of the important functions of emotion is the same as the primary goal of interoception: helping us with homeostasis, energy management, and survival. All other functions that are attributed to emotions— expressing emotions to let others know how we feel (which has to do with communication, attachment, and bonding), releasing inner tension and regulating ourselves through acts such as crying (related to healing), and guiding all aspects of cognition and behavior (providing energy and motivation for action)—can ultimately be reduced to the three fundamental functions of homeostasis, energy management, and survival. When I notice that I am feeling bad after separating from my wife, I cannot be doing well in terms of my homeostasis, energy management, or survival. When I enjoy being with my wife, that feeling moves my brain and body physiology in the direction of greater well-being.

Emotion and interoception thus share the same goals: homeostasis, energy management, and survival. Therefore, it makes sense that the information they use to achieve their common goals is the same— information on the body's condition—even though they might use different aggregates and abstractions of the same data. For instance, the sense of loss of balance that helps us prevent a fall and the unpleasant emotional experience of sinking and falling endlessly upon learning that a dear one has suddenly died in an accident have much in common in terms of physiological changes that give rise to them.

To summarize what we have learned so far from the overlapping bodies of research on interoception and emotion: the interoceptive sense and the interoceptive network gather information about the body and process in the brain to generate two types of information. One type of information is about body states (such as "fall in blood sugar level," "hunger," or feeling "good" or "bad") that are not commonly understood as emotions. Another type of information is about feeling "good" or "bad" or "sad" or "mad," states that are widely understood as emotions when feeling "good" or "bad" can be connected psychologically to situations we face. Both types of information are geared to help the organism with homeostasis, energy management, and survival in different ways. Emotional states, especially those that tell us how we are doing socially, can guide subsequent behavior toward improvements in our homeostatic condition, energy utilization, and survival. Information in the form of body states and emotional states is helpful to the organism, even when these states are not conscious experiences. However, conscious experiences of body states and emotional states confer additional advantages for homeostasis, energy management, and survival.

Can the Brain Generate Emotion on Its Own?

Because neurotransmitters such as dopamine and serotonin can induce and alter emotional states within the brain's physiology, it appears that the brain has the ability to generate emotion on its own. The body is known to have this ability too. Whether activated by the brain or on its own, the body can secrete endogenous substances such as sexual and other hormones that, among their many functions, can induce or alter emotional experiences.

The ability of the brain to rapidly induce or alter emotional states through secretion of such endogenous substances can be an evolutionary advantage. Organisms are often overwhelmed when they are faced with situations that are beyond their capacity. The physiology of a person faced with overwhelming and inescapable trauma, such as torture, can become so dysregulated that it could lead to death, if it were not for endogenous biochemistry kicking in to regulate brain and body physiology to maintain some mental and physical capability to continue to cope with the threat. Such mechanisms are also often helpful in coping with ordinary life situations when strong emotional reactions might be counterproductive, as in a situation in which one is being evaluated unfairly by a supervisor. When emotional discomfort registers in the brain, the brain might be able to soothe that discomfort with the secretion of endogenous opioids. It makes sense that evolution would genetically hardwire such mechanisms into the developmental sequence of our physiology.

There are some who believe that the brain cannot recall an emotion generated through the body without involving the body again to some extent. But just as we can recall a stored visual image without involving the eyes, we should be able to recall a body experience without involving the entire body. The brain, with such a long history of evolution, has at least some innate capacity to make a quick prediction, based not only on the experience of this body in this life but on the experience of all the bodies of all the species that this body has evolved from as well. Body experiences become neural (brain) images with varying levels of aggregation and abstraction of body experience. These images exist in the physiology of the brain, its structure and its biochemistry. It is therefore not impossible to imagine evolution imprinting the brain with an innate ability to evoke certain experiences, such as universal basic emotions, in response to patterns perceived in the world through the five external senses as well as through the internal interoceptive sense.

There is precedent in the literature on emotions for such a possibility. The evolutionary perspective of Charles Darwin,[36] based on cross-cultural evidence for universal emotions, has been supported by studies from a long line of researchers, including Paul Ekman.[37] If evolution can program emotional displays in the body as innate tendencies, and emotional displays in the body can generate different emotional experiences with distinct neural patterns in the brain,[38] would it not be the next logical step in evolution to program in the brain a capacity to generate such emotional experiences independent of the body, to at least some extent? To enhance the brain's capacity to predict is to improve its chances of survival. The history of research on emotions offers more evidence for this ability on the part of the brain. The innate ability of the brain to generate emotions through its hardware, independent of body experience, is a fundamental feature in the theories of Walter Cannon,[39] Philip Bard,[40] James Papez,[41] Paul McLean,[42] Jaap Panksepp,[43] and Joseph E. LeDoux,[44] all important researchers who have studied the role of the brain in emotion.

To arrive at the best possible cognitive assessment of a situation, the brain uses both present and past experience. This is an efficient strategy. Evidence shows that the brain does the same with emotional assessment: it uses experience handed down by evolution as innate predispositions, along with past body experiences and current input from the entire physiology, including that of the brain. This is the comprehensive theory of the physiology of emotion that I subscribe to, a perspective I arrived at after a laborious study of the literature on the neurophysiology of emotions. In the process, I gained valuable insights that formed the scientific basis of the work of emotional embodiment.

Conclusion

The integrative view emerging from the more recent research on the physiology of emotion—that both the brain and the body play significant roles in the generation and experience of emotion—is supported and even extended by the findings in the field of psychoneuroimmunology, a relatively young field of inquiry dating back to the late 1970s. Psychoneuroimmunology research focuses on "information substances," chemical messenger molecules such as neurotransmitters or peptides, which circulate relatively freely among different systems of the body, including the brain, the autonomic nervous system, and the organs, through blood and fluids circulating between the cells.

When these molecules produced in one part of the body or brain reach another part of the body or brain, they bind themselves to special receptors on the surface of the target cells to alter the behavior of those cells. The information exchanges through this network account for 98 percent of all communication occurring in the body. In contrast, the information exchanges occurring in the nervous system account for a

mere 2 percent. The production cells and receptor cells for these messenger molecules are distributed throughout the brain and the body. In
the brain, they are concentrated in areas that traditional research on
the physiology of emotions has identified as having to do more with
emotion, leading researcher Candace Pert to describe these substances
as "molecules of emotion." Pert was the first scientist to discover opiate
receptors in the brain, as she toiled away night after night in a lab with
her baby strapped to her body. Pert was overlooked for the Nobel Prize
for her discovery due to gender politics in scientific circles.

Pert summarized her findings about emotions from her psychoneuroimmunology research in her 1997 book *The Molecules of Emotions: The
Science behind Mind-Body Medicine*. When asked whether an emotion is
a brain or body phenomenon, based on the findings on the dynamics of
various information substances in the brain and the body, she answered,
"Why, it's both! It's not either/or; in fact it is both *and* neither. It's simultaneous—a two-way street."[45] That is, the generation of emotion (for that
matter, the generation of cognition and behavior as well) involves both the
brain and the body. It does not make sense to talk of emotion, cognition,
or behavior as belonging dichotomously to either the brain or the body.

We can talk about the different roles of the body or brain in emotion
and its experience, but none of the body-specific or brain-specific roles
can account for the totality of the generation and experience of emotion.
The brain and the body can both be observed interacting and influenc-
ing each other all the time at the level of information substances. Physiological correlates or substrates of emotions in the form of information
substances, such as neurotransmitters and peptides, can be generated
first in the physiology of either the brain or the body. They can then set
off sequences or domino effects, either by themselves or by involving
other information substances that can quickly involve the entirety of the
brain and body physiology.

If the generation of emotion could be initiated in either the brain or the
body, it could also presumably be initiated in both places at the same time.
This possibility supports a dynamic network systems conceptualization of
the integrated nature of cells functioning across the brain and the body,

wherein an impulse can involve activating multiple nodes or places at the same time, or it can start in one node or place and spread to other nodes or places. The physiological impulse for an emotion can therefore be initiated in the brain and the body at the same time; or it can be initiated in the brain or the body and spread rapidly to the rest of the brain and body physiology.

We can see that the findings on the physiology of emotions we reviewed earlier, along with the hypotheses from the molecular research we just explored, support each other in a number of ways. When the brain is involved in generating emotion through its innate mechanisms or through recalling earlier experiences before it involves the entire body for a reality check, we can think of the emotional impulse as originating in the brain. When the brain is generating an emotion from the enactment of internal behaviors to maintain homeostasis and to manage energy and outer behaviors to cope with the situation, we can think of the emotional impulse as originating in the body. Because the generation of emotion likely involves prediction based on innate mechanisms, recall of past body experiences, and current input from the body, we can think of the emotional impulse arising in both the brain and the body at the same time.

In the next chapter, we will look at the evidence for how cognition, emotion, and behavior are intricately intertwined in the physiology of the brain as well as the body, and how emotion plays a central role in the triad of cognition, emotion, and behavior. In the subsequent chapter, we will examine all the known dynamics or mechanisms through which emotional experiences are generated and defended against, and the role they play in the formation of psychophysiological symptoms. The following chapter in part II will look at the factors that determine our affect tolerance (our capacity to tolerate emotions) and then present the scientific rationale for how using the larger container of the brain and body physiology, especially the body physiology, can build a greater capacity for emotions, especially unpleasant emotions. Using this larger container can in turn improve our cognitive, emotional, and behavioral functions as well as our health and well-being. The last chapter in part II will explore the different types of emotions and how we can access them to build a greater capacity for them.

6

Cognition, Emotion, and Behavior

Chapter summary: discusses the scientific evidence for how the body is involved in cognition, emotion, and behavior, how intricately interrelated the three are, and how embodying emotion can improve outcomes in all three spheres.

In the early chapters of this book, we saw examples of emotional embodiment being followed by changes in thought and behavior that helped individuals to deal better with situations that were causing them emotional difficulties. In this chapter, we will look more systematically at the science of how embodying emotions could help in improving all aspects of cognition and behavior in situations where difficult emotions occur.

The New Science of Embodied Cognition, Emotion, and Behavior

Cognition can be defined narrowly and identified solely with thinking; or it can be understood broadly to include mental processes of attention, focus, concentration, perception, thought, evaluation, memory, symbolization, language, etc. Behavior can be defined as what we do, do not do, or are unable to do; and how we express, do not express, or cannot express ourselves, vocally through language and sound, and nonverbally through facial and other body expressions such as posture and gesture.

There has been a virtual revolution in our understanding of the neuroscience of cognition, emotion, and behavior in the past twenty years. The research paradigm of embodied[1] and embedded[2] cognition studies the dependence of cognition on the body and the environment around it. The approach of enactive emotion explores emotion as a product of interaction of the brain, the body, and their environment.[3] These research approaches are discovering that our cognition, emotion, and behavior are functions of not only our brain but also our body, as well as the environment we find ourselves in; and that cognition, emotion, and behavior are ultimately inseparable in our experience as well as in the physiology of our body and brain. We will collectively refer to these new paradigms of research in cognitive and affective neuroscience and cognitive psychology, from which such important findings have emerged, as the science of embodied cognition, emotion, and behavior.

The Role of the Body and the Environment in Cognition

We saw in the last chapter how generation of emotional experience could involve the whole of our brain and body. It is relatively easy to establish that our behaviors (actions and expressions) are enacted through the body and are facilitated or constrained by the environment. What has not been obvious to us are the important roles the body and the environment play in cognition, over and above the roles they play in providing the brain with the energy to perform its various functions, including cognition. This is in part because scientific research has suffered from a basic but erroneous assumption that cognition has to do only with the brain. Before we look at the scientific evidence for the role of the body and the environment in cognition, let us intuitively and easily grasp how the brain, body, and environment could be involved in cognitive, emotional, and behavioral aspects of an ordinary but extremely important experience: bonding between a child and their birth mother.

The experience of mother–child bonding cannot be isolated to the brain alone. The experience of the relationship between mother and child involves their brains as well as their bodies as they interact in numerous and often intimate ways, including breastfeeding, from the very beginning of life. The quality of the experience of bonding in the body of the child, whether it is good or bad, depends very much on what is happening in the environment of the mother–child dyad: whether there is a supportive father, whether it is a time of war or peace, whether it is a time of plenty or poverty. Therefore, from the very beginning of life the cognitive, emotional, and behavioral aspects of a child's bonding experience involve not only the brain and the body, but also the bodies of others in the environment, as well as events in the larger body of the world in general.

Let us now see how the science of embodied and embedded cognition has teased out the role of the body and the environment in cognition.

How the Body Plays a Role in Learning

The brain learns about the body through the experience of the body. The brain also learns about the world through the experience of the body as it interacts with the world. This, in essence, is the philosophy of embodied and embedded cognition. A steady drumbeat of experimental evidence in cognitive psychology and neuroscience has established a scientific basis for these paradigms. Clinical research from body psychotherapy schools, especially Bodynamic Analysis, has contributed additional evidence from clinical settings. Let us examine a few examples of such research findings.

Learning the Alphabet and the Law of Inertia

The importance of the body in learning abstract symbols, such as the alphabet, was established through experiments demonstrating that young children who also practice writing the alphabet learn it faster than children who do not.[4] The importance of the body and the environment in learning a complex physics theory, the law of inertia, was established by an experiment we will discuss below. Before we examine the experiment, let us get acquainted with the law of inertia through an example.

If two objects, such as two balls, have identical weight and shape but differ in how their weight is distributed between their center and periphery, and if the two balls are rolled down an incline toward the ground at the same time, the law of inertia tells us that the ball with more weight toward its center will gather more velocity and reach the bottom faster than the ball with its weight distributed toward the surface. This is the law that figure skaters use to speed up their movements while spinning on the ice, when they draw their limbs in toward their core and curl their bodies inward. To slow down their movement, they simply do the opposite.

In the experiment,[5] two groups of undergraduate students who had signed up for a physics class were asked to predict which of two objects, a disc and a ring of equal weight and diameter, would reach the ground first if they were rolled down an incline at the same time. The disc's weight was concentrated more toward its center, and the ring's weight was concentrated more toward its edge. The experiment was conducted before the students had learned the law of inertia in the class. Both groups were given the same scenario and were asked the same question, but one group had to engage in an additional activity involving a plastic ruler and a binder clip. That group was asked to hold one end of the plastic ruler between their thumb and forefinger and move it up and down by flicking their wrists, first with the binder clip attached at the other end of the plastic ruler and then with the binder clip attached to the plastic ruler close to their fingers. Please note that when the binder clip is at the far end of the plastic ruler, it is analogous to the ring that had its weight distributed away from its center. The pencil with the binder clip close to the grip is equivalent to the disk with its weight concentrated toward its center. If you were to do this exercise yourself, you would find it more strenuous to flip your wrist up and down when the binder clip is at the end of the plastic ruler than when it is close to the grip. The law of inertia says the object with its weight distributed toward the periphery will encounter more physical resistance to its movement, which makes the movement slower.

The students were then asked to make their best guess as to which object, the disk or the ring, would reach the ground first. They expected the second group of students who played with the plastic ruler and the binder clip to learn the law of inertia implicitly through their body, by experiencing it as it interacted with the object. And that is what they found. The students in the group that had the opportunity to learn the law of inertia implicitly this way were twice as likely to answer the question correctly as the other group, even though they had not learned about the law of inertia before.

Learning through Psychomotor Movement

Psychomotor movement can be defined as bodily movement that assists in learning different psychological functions or capacities. In the somatic developmental psychology model of Bodynamic Analysis, the theory holds that children learn more psychological functions or develop more psychological capacities through the increasing number of psychomotor movements they are able to perform as their physiology matures. The empirical research done at the Bodynamic Institute in Copenhagen has resulted in a comprehensive theory of the psychological functions of the muscular system that correlates major muscle groups with their psychological functions through their psychomotor movements.[6]

For example, the biceps group of muscles on the front of the upper arm is involved in the action of bringing things we like closer to us. The triceps group of muscles on the back of the upper arm is involved in the act of pushing things we do not like away from us. When the environment is not attuned sufficiently to our needs—e.g., we are forced to take in things we do not want on a repeated basis, as in forced scheduled feeding of predetermined quantities of food in infancy regardless of what, when, and how much we need—it can lead to extreme rigidity or flaccidity in these muscle groups. The tendency toward abnormal rigidity or flaccidity in a muscle group interferes with its physical function and, in turn, its psychomotor function.

A child who undergoes such parenting in the first two years of life without subsequent corrective experiences could grow into an adult with a deep distrust of others or a despair of the world meeting their needs in an appropriate and satisfying manner. Because of this distrust or despair, such a person is prone to not reaching out to get their needs met and pushing away things that might be actually available to them. Cognitive, emotional, and behavioral experiences from childhood related to reaching out or pushing away often emerge in the process of working with these muscle groups. Working with such experiences is necessary to restore these psychological functions to an individual who has difficulties with them.

Let us now see how these findings from a body psychotherapy approach can help explain the results of an experiment in cognitive psychology in the embodied cognition research paradigm.

Let's Go Shopping in the Netherlands!

When we go to a grocery store, we usually have the choice of a hand basket or a shopping cart on wheels. Some of us spurn both these options and choose to use our God-given hands, at times out of a misplaced sense of pride because we imagine ourselves to be less consumerist than others. On our trips to a grocery store, we usually take a shopping list with us, either on paper or at least mentally. Some scientists in the Netherlands became interested in finding out if the choice of a hand basket or larger shopping cart influenced whether shoppers bought items they did not have the intention of buying when they went into the store.[7] These are often called impulse purchases, like the candy bar at the checkout counter—spur-of-the-moment acquisitions that shoppers often consider to be things that are not good for them and are ambivalent toward. The researchers were interested in finding out which group ended up buying more unplanned items on an impulse, those who used hand baskets or those who used shopping carts.

When I ask my students which group bought more unplanned items, I often get a very logical answer: those using shopping carts, of course, because they have more space to buy things they did not plan to get. The researchers actually found the opposite: those who use hand baskets are more likely to buy unplanned items! How does one explain that? Remember that choosing whether to buy something is an act of cognition, and we are discussing embodied cognition. The researchers obtained this counterintuitive result because different muscle groups are engaged in the use of the basket versus the cart, which affects shoppers' cognition in different ways. When we use the hand basket, the biceps muscle group—with the psychological function of bringing things we like toward ourselves—is more active. The heavier the basket gets, the more engaged the biceps become in order to keep it from dragging our arm and the rest of the body down to the ground. When we use the shopping cart, we use the triceps muscle group to push the basket ahead of us. The more the cart is loaded, the more engaged this muscle group is, with its psychological function of pushing things we do not like away from us.

Now, think of how many times in life we have used these two opposing muscle groups to bring things we like toward us and push things we do not like away from us. So, when faced with that chocolate bar at the checkout counter judiciously placed there to tempt us, we are more likely to give into the impulse of buying it if we are shopping with a hand basket rather than a shopping cart. Reading this piece of research made me think of all the times I have found myself walking down the aisles of a supermarket with my hands full of things I had not really planned to purchase, and wishing I had chosen to take a basket or a cart on my way in! The researchers did not study people like me, but if they had, they might have found an even stronger result. The more things I have in my hands, the more likely I am to use the biceps to clutch the things even closer to my chest, as I would hold a beloved!

The field of embodied cognition continues to reveal multiple ways in which the body is involved in different aspects of cognition. Research has consistently shown that exercise improves all brain functions, including all aspects of cognition such as attention and memory.[8] Basic cognitive functions of attention, focus, and perception depend on the physiology of the five senses in the body. Research has shown that posture affects cognition.[9] Research has also shown that body postures that are inconsistent with an emotion being experienced lead to decreased ability in the brain to cognitively process the emotions and their contexts, such as when subjects are asked to lean backward while processing attraction and to lean forward while processing aversion.[10]

The question is no longer whether the body is involved in cognition. The inquiry now focuses on the extent to which the body is necessary and involved in different types of cognition, such as abstract conceptual reasoning and its close cousin, language. To what extent can all language be reduced to body metaphors that can in turn be reduced to body experience? Does the brain need the body even in abstract conceptual reasoning of the highest order? To both questions, some respond with an affirmative "yes," while others dispute such a definitive conclusion. For a brief review of the field of embodied and embedded cognition, the reader is referred to the article by Winkielman et al. cited here.[11]

As with the research on emotion we discussed in the previous chapter, the roles played by the body and the brain in cognition continue to be debated, with evidence supporting the involvement of both. This suggests that an integrative view that they are both involved in different ways could provide the necessary reconciliation. In this integrative view, the body might be absolutely necessary to cognize things in early stages of childhood development and throughout our lives for certain functions such as perception and sense of connection in a relationship— probably for more things than we realize, coming from a brain-biased understanding of cognition as we do. But as we grow from child to adult and our capacity for abstract cognition of conceptualization, symbolization, reasoning, logic, inference, and language develop, perhaps there are some things about the world we can cognize through the brain alone. As Piaget states in his theory of cognitive development, the child becomes increasingly capable of abstract thinking.

It is possible that all of our knowledge of the world, regardless of the degree of abstract cognition involved in generating that knowledge, can be reduced to something we learned through the body at some point. Given that what we know about the world is insignificant in comparison to what we do not know about it, it may be true that the body is essential for additional learning about new things throughout our lives. It is also possible that we can learn new things about the world on the basis of what we have learned about the world through abstract modes of cognition, and the body might be necessary even in those instances for a reality check of the products of such abstract cognition.

Now that we have established the importance of the body in cognition, let us look at how the availability of the body for cognition—or, for that matter, emotion as well as behavior—might become compromised.

Hindered Body Implies Hindered Cognition

The body is involved in cognition on an ongoing basis in many ways and is necessary for a reality check of knowledge generated through abstract modes of cognition in the brain. But the body's availability for cognition could be compromised through the inhibition of emotion, behavior, or cognition itself. When a behavior can lead to severe adverse emotional consequences, such as pain, or unbearable cognitive consequences, such as severe dissonance, we might inhibit the body to inhibit the behavior and, in the process, compromise its availability for cognition. The body thus inhibited is also compromised for generating and coping with emotional experience, because emotion is potentially an entire body and brain phenomenon.

Similarly, when we inhibit the body to cope with unbearable emotional experiences (body defenses against emotions are the subject of the next chapter), we might end up making the body less available for cognition as well as behavior. For example, we might hold ourselves back from getting angry and pushing a person we love away when the person is abusive to us because of the emotional consequences of losing connection with the person, or because doing so is so contrary to our self-concept that it creates a very uncomfortable cognitive dissonance. Please note that even when the consequence of a behavior or emotion is cognitive, such as dissonance, it is ultimately the discomfort of the emotion generated by the dissonance that leads to inhibition of the body. Feeling bad is often a natural emotional reaction to cognitive dissonance, and inhibiting the body is one way to try not to feel the unpleasantness of it as well as to weaken the cognition of the dissonance itself, because cognition has been found to depend on the embodiment of the emotion associated with it. We will present the evidence for these assertions later in this chapter.

How might inhibition of cognition lead to the body being compromised for cognition, emotion, and behavior? Consider again the example of a victim of violent domestic abuse who suppresses the thought that the abuser does not care for them by inhibiting their fear, anger, and impulse to leave the situation. In this situation, inhibition of cognition compromises the body's ability to learn through emotion and behavior, and perhaps in other situations as well if the inhibitions in the body persist and the situation is ongoing. This is one reason why a traumatized person's mental functioning might show a decline across situations. Inhibition of cognition can take the form of constraints placed on the physiology of the brain itself, as in disabling the connection between the brain regions involved in the cognition, or inhibiting the neuronal patterns associated with the specific cognition.

For example, to sustain the cognition that the abuser is not all that abusive, the abused person's brain might suppress the connection between the reasoning part of the brain and the part that has memories of the repeated abuse that contradict the erroneous conclusion. The abused person's brain might also inhibit the pattern of neuronal firing associated with the correct conclusion that the abuser does not indeed care for them. Such physiological constraints in the brain can narrow not only cognitive possibilities but also emotional and behavioral possibilities (because they also depend on the brain). By extending to the body, these constraints can reduce the body's availability for optimal cognition, emotion, and behavior in the domestic situation, and perhaps in similar situations—and perhaps even in all situations, if the specific adverse situation is a constant presence in the person's life.

The dynamic systems perspective of the brain proposes that cognition, emotion, and behavior share brain physiology to a greater extent than in the functional specialization view, in which each function is allocated to a different brain area. From this perspective we can think of a cognition that is not allowed to occur as placing a constraint on the pattern of firing across the neurons, which is what embodies the cognition in the brain. The greater the number of disallowed cognitions, the more shut down and less available the brain is, not only for cognition but also for emotion and behavior, because they share the same physiology. In the same way, constraints placed on emotional or behavioral possibilities in the brain constrain the brain's cognitive possibilities too. And constraints on cognitive, emotional, and behavioral possibilities in the brain restrict corresponding possibilities in the body as well. Research shows that cognition, emotion, and behavior are highly interrelated in the brain and the body physiology, which is why constraints placed against one of the three—either in the brain or in the body—affect the other two. The embodied interrelationships among cognition, emotion, and behavior are further explored in the rest of this chapter.

How Lack of Emotional Capacity Can Compromise the Body's Cognition and Behavior

Whenever we inhibit cognition, emotion, or behavior in the brain or the body, we end up inhibiting the body in some way and compromising its ability to contribute to all three functions more fully. The main reason why we shut the body down or the body gets dysregulated is because we cannot tolerate the emotions, especially the unpleasant or unacceptable emotions, involved. The main reason why we inhibit certain cognitions or behaviors is because we cannot tolerate the emotional consequences of allowing them. For example, because I cannot tolerate the shame of being rejected, I cannot leave the person who is humiliating me or think of that person as being bad for me. Conversely, if I am able to tolerate the emotions (especially the unpleasant emotions) in a situation, it increases the likelihood that my body is more regulated, available, and connected to the environment so I can improve cognition and behavior in the situation, because I do not have to compromise my brain or body by shutting them down to cope with unbearable or unacceptable emotional experiences.

Therefore, the capacity to tolerate emotional experiences plays a central role in ensuring that the body and its connection to the environment are as optimally available as possible for cognition and behavior in the situation. Because emotional embodiment work increases the body's capacity for emotional experiences, it offers the possibility of improving a person's cognition as well as behavior in the situation by ensuring the body is more regulated, available, and connected to its environment for both functions.

Let us now examine the evidence from the science of embodied cognition, emotion, and behavior for improvement in cognition and behavior from optimizing and embodying emotion.

How Embodying Emotion Affects Cognition

Psychologist Paula Niedenthal became interested in finding out whether increasing the embodiment of emotion improved cognition.[12] Niedenthal and her colleagues set up an experiment in which subjects were exposed to emotionally charged stories. The subjects were divided into two groups: those whose facial muscles were prevented from participating in their emotional experiences while hearing the stories, and those whose facial muscles were allowed to function normally. (The facial muscles are well known for their role in emotion.) To make the facial muscles unavailable for one group, the researchers had those participants bite hard on a pen while hearing the stories, to make their facial muscles go into a fixed position. The researchers recorded patterns of neurons firing in the brain during the experiment, immediately after the experiment, and one or two weeks after the experiment, when the participants were asked to recall the emotional experiences along with the details of the stories they had been exposed to.

The researchers found that during the experiment, the brain regions involved in processing emotions and those involved in processing the details of the situation were less active in people whose facial muscles were constrained than in those whose facial muscles functioned normally. The same patterns were observed in recall tasks about the emotions and the situational details, immediately after the experiment and one or two weeks after the experiment. That is, people who could allow their facial muscles to be involved in their emotional experiences were observed to process the emotions and the situational details better in their brains during the experiment and during their noticeably better recall of the emotions and situational details during follow-up. These findings imply that the processing of emotions and their contexts, and the recall of both immediately afterward and one or two weeks later, are enhanced when emotion is more embodied than not.

Other studies have shown that preventing the embodiment of emotions of attraction and aversion by putting the body into postures that are contrary to the emotions they are associated with—leaning forward while processing emotions of aversion such as hate, and leaning backward while processing emotions of attraction such as love—interfered with the cognitive processing of the emotions and the situations involved.[13] These studies strongly suggest that the expansion of the emotional experience to as much of the body as possible can improve the function of cognition, especially in emotionally charged situations.

Emotional embodiment work involves this type of expansion. We will see in chapter 8 how it can increase the capacity to be with the emotion over a longer period of time. We saw the scientific evidence that embodying emotion can improve cognition about the emotion and its context. Increasing the time that a person can be with an emotion in the body because of an increased capacity to tolerate the emotion offers the brain more time to process the emotion and its context, and can only improve cognition.

Now let us look at how emotion and its embodiment can improve behavior in the situation associated with the emotion.

Emotion and Behavior

Emotion and behavior are inseparable as they emerge in our experience. Emotion provides the motivation to do or not do something. However, it is not possible to separate the emotion of "wanting to do something" or "having to do something" from the doing itself. It therefore makes sense that any attempt to suppress either emotion or behavior will suppress the other to some extent. Because emotion is an assessment of the impact of a situation based on cognition and behavior in relation to that situation, emotion depends on the behavior. This interdependence of emotion and behavior implies that dysregulation in one has the potential to dysregulate the other. Embodying emotion, because it regulates emotion, has the potential to regulate behavior. By the same logic, regulating behavior offers the promise of regulating emotion.

An example can help to ground these ideas. A person suffering from an eating disorder is often driven by unbearable emotions that consciously or unconsciously drive the disordered behavior. Giving in to the impulse of the addictive behavior reinforces the person's helplessness against the vulnerabilities that drive the addiction, driving them deeper into the unconscious. Making those vulnerabilities conscious, regulating them, and making them more bearable can help in regulating the compulsive impulse to binge or starve to avoid them. This can also give the brain more time to process the experience cognitively for more functional ways of coping with the situation.

In his book *Descartes' Error: Emotion, Reason, and the Human Brain* (1994/2005), Damasio offers evidence from research on people who have had accidents or surgeries that have injured parts of the brain associated with emotions to explore the effects of emotion on behavior.[14] The book challenges the conventional wisdom that emotions are opposed to reason. On the contrary, the evidence shows that lack of emotion is more likely than the presence of emotion to lead to irrational behavior. The book's fundamental evidence-based conclusion is that people make better behavioral decisions when they have more access to emotion. In addition, people generate more functional behavioral alternatives for action and expression to deal with a situation—and they are better at choosing the best behavioral alternative to act upon—when they have access to emotions. Conversely, the capacity to generate relevant alternative courses of action to deal with the situation and to choose better courses of action among the competing alternatives declines with the absence of emotion.

The amygdala in the lower brain is associated with generation of emotional experiences. Both Damasio and Joseph E. LeDoux[15] offer evidence that bilateral damage to the amygdala compromises the availability of emotion, which in turn negatively affects the person's behavior. The frontal lobes of the brain are involved in making emotional experiences conscious and in regulating them. Damasio presents evidence of compromised behavior in people with bilateral damage to the frontal lobes to show how affect regulation is important for improvement in behavior.

How can we reconcile these findings about access to emotion improving behavior with our common-sense notion that overwhelming and unbearable emotions cause people to commit crimes of passion or to act out against themselves or others through addictive or harmful behaviors? The answer lies in regulation. Behavior is better when emotion is available and worse when it is not; and when emotion is available, behavior is better when emotion is regulated than when it is not.

The evidence of how access to emotion and regulation of emotion affect behavior beneficially can be seen in longitudinal research studies that track people from childhood to adulthood and observe the relationship between a child's ability to feel and regulate emotion and their later success in their personal and professional lives.[16] Children with greater access to emotion and greater ability to regulate it turned out to be more successful in their personal and professional lives, countering the conventional wisdom that emotions do not belong in the workplace. In light of such findings, some school systems in the United States are bringing emotion experts into classrooms as early as kindergarten and first grade to teach children emotional intelligence—what emotions are, how to regulate them, how to communicate them, and so on. Because emotional embodiment work focuses on making emotion more available and regulated, it offers the possibility of regulating behavior to make it more functional and optimal in situations in which difficult emotions arise.

The Simultaneity and Sequentiality of Cognition, Emotion, and Behavior

One topic of inquiry in the science of embodied cognition, emotion, and behavior is whether these three elements arise simultaneously or sequentially in the physiology of the brain and the body; and if they are sequential, in what order do they arise? There are several seemingly irreconcilable points of view on this topic, each supported by evidence. Let us examine this controversy before we attempt our own reconciliation. Even though it is hard to argue that some form of evaluation, conscious or unconscious, has to precede emotion, findings reveal that cognition—including initial attention to the environment even before perception occurs—is strongly influenced by emotion.[17,18] This evidence supports the view that emotion is the starting point, followed by cognition and behavior. Then, there is the equally evidence-based point of view that behavior precedes emotion as well as cognition.[19] The conventional wisdom, of course, holds to the classical sequence of cognition first, emotion second, and behavior third.

Evidence has also been presented to show the simultaneity rather than the sequentiality of cognition, emotion, and behavior[20] and the inseparability of the three at the physiological level in the brain and the body.[21,22] To underscore the inseparability of cognition and emotion, some have gone so far as to view emotion as a form of cognition.[23] When we examine our experience closely, we can see that the three are inseparable even in the simple experience of wanting something. The emotion of attraction, a favorable evaluation of the object involved, and the impulse to move toward or otherwise act in relation to the desired object, however slight, are all implicit and inseparable in the experience. Yet, at other times, we can observe the three arise in the classical sequence of cognition-emotion-behavior. So we have seeming contradictions even within our awareness of these elements of our experience. We can also observe in our experiences that cognition, emotion, and behavior bounce off each other, sometimes simultaneously, sometimes in one sequence and sometimes in another, like balls on a billiard table.

A comprehensive discussion of these issues is beyond the scope of this book. However, the seeming contradictions appear to have to do with the level at which the researchers are studying cognition, emotion, and behavior. If they are studying these phenomena as the physiological or energetic processes in the brain and body physiology that precede the experiences of cognition, emotion, and behavior, it is more likely that they find them arising simultaneously. If they are examining them at the level of more symbolic representations of these experiences in the brain or the body, they are more likely to find different sequences among them. If the researcher's preferred starting point is influenced by their prior theoretical disposition that orders cognition, emotion, and behavior in a certain sequence, they are bound to find evidence supporting that theoretical disposition at one level of representation or the other.

To restate, the deeper the level of the physiology that is explored, whether at the neuronal, molecular, or quantum energetic level, the more support there appears to be for the inseparability and simultaneity of the origin of cognition, emotion, and behavior. The more these phenomena are studied in the brain than in the body, and the more they are studied at the representational level than at the physiological level in the brain or the body, the more likely it is that different sequences will be discovered among them. This is how it is possible for there to be inseparability and simultaneity on the one hand and different sequences in their occurrence on the other.

Summary

Figure 6.1 encapsulates the discussion of cognition, emotion, and behavior in this chapter.

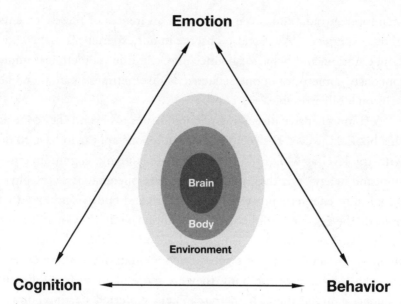

FIGURE 6.1 Embodied Cognition, Emotion, and Behavior. Cognition, emotion, and behavior depend equally on the brain, the body, and the environment. They influence each other, often simultaneously; but emotion appears to be primary, as it is a strong mediator of both cognition and behavior.

Cognition, emotion, and behavior arise together in the brain and body physiology and can be observed to affect each other in different sequences as they become more recognized as seemingly separate phenomena in the brain. Emotion has a stronger influence on cognition and behavior for two reasons:

- Cognition and behavior are influenced in every moment by the emotional state of the organism.

- It is the unbearability of emotional consequences of cognition and behavior that leads to the brain and the body shutting down, which in turn compromises all three.

Therefore, emotional embodiment work offers the potential for improved regulation and function of cognition, emotion, and behavior, increasing the odds of the person successfully coping with the situation.

7

Physiological Dynamics Involved in Generating and Defending against Emotional Experiences

Chapter summary: presents all the ways in which physiological defenses can form in the brain and body physiology to cope with and defend against difficult emotional experiences.

In this chapter, we will explore a variety of physiological dynamics, such as constriction and arousal, that might be involved in generating and defending against emotional experiences. As we shall see, all the physiological dynamics identified in this chapter can be involved in generating an emotional experience or in defending against it. Each of these dynamics can also be involved in generating one emotional experience while defending against another emotional experience at the same time.

An understanding of these complex physiological dynamics, and of whether they are contributing to generating or defending against an emotional experience in a specific situation, can be particularly helpful for therapists who use tools such as touch and awareness of body sensations to work directly with the brain and body physiology to change physiological states, in order to change emotional and other psychological experiences. Such understanding can help improve the work of all therapists to identify and target specific physiological dynamics for manipulation to change psychological experiences such as cognition, emotion, and behavior; and to ensure that physiological dynamics, such as constriction, are not always mistaken as defenses against emotional experiences and targeted for removal, with the risk of loss of significant emotional and other psychological experiences.

Please note that an understanding of all these complex physiological dynamics is not necessary to do good emotional embodiment work. Therefore, this is perhaps the most optional chapter in the book for the technically challenged.

The Concept of Physiological Defenses against Emotions and Other Psychological Experiences

The notion that physiological dynamics or states such as constriction can form in the brain and body physiology as a defense against emotions and other psychological experiences has been present in body psychotherapy approaches going back to the therapy of Wilhelm Reich.[1] The use of such tools as breath, movement, and exercises to remove physiological defenses and access the psychological experiences being defended against has been an integral part of body psychotherapy treatments ever since.[2,3] Constriction of the musculature is a physiological state that is often seen as a physiological defense. For example, one might constrict the muscles of the arm to inhibit the boundary-setting behavior of pushing a loved one away, for fear of losing the relationship. Over time and with enough repetition, someone who does this might not only lose the impulse to set boundaries through the arms but also inhibit the cognitive possibility of boundary setting from ever reaching consciousness, as it could lead to inner conflict between one's cognition and one's behavior. One can also imagine emotions associated with experiences of boundary violations, such as hurt, betrayal, and anger, being inhibited along with the cognitive and behavioral experiences around boundary formation.

Constriction of the arm muscles is not the only way through which one could inhibit cognitive, emotional, and behavioral experiences around boundary setting. Flaccid states in the arm muscles involved in setting boundaries or lowering of arousal or energy in the arms are other ways in which these experiences can be defended against.[4]

When emotional experiences are unacceptable or unbearable, physiological defenses can form against them. Even pleasant emotions such as love and sexuality can become unacceptable because they might be associated with unbearable consequences of unpleasant emotions such as fear and shame. Inhibition of muscles in the pelvis such as the iliacus, which is associated with psychomotor actions involved in sexuality, can keep one's sexuality at bay.[5] Inhibition of sexual glands from secreting the sex hormones of testosterone and estrogen can also produce the same effect. When emotional experiences become unbearable, physiological defenses can form against them.

Emotions can become unbearable in one of two ways. First, emotions can become unbearable when they push the brain and body physiology toward extremes threatening the organism's very survival. For example, in the phenomenon called "fright death," one has a fatal heart attack from excess fear. I once read an account about a boy who went camping with his family at Big Bear Lake, California. One morning the boy came out of his tent and ran straight into a black bear—and his heart just stopped, never to beat again. High levels of fear are associated with a very high level of stimulation of the heart's natural pacemaker and the cardiac musculature by the sympathetic nervous system. At very high levels of sympathetic stimulation, far beyond normal range, there is a risk of electrical malfunction either in the pacemaker that regulates the heartbeat or the musculature that regulates the strength with which the heart pumps blood.

In such instances, the parasympathetic nervous system could kick in and inhibit the heartbeat and the pumping of the heart from reaching levels dangerous to one's survival. Unfortunately, the parasympathetic nervous system could also overcorrect the problem and stop the heart for good in the middle of an experience of terror.[6] So we can manipulate physiological dynamics such as constriction and arousal to defend against emotional states that threaten our survival by generating out-of-the ordinary and dangerous physiological conditions.

The second way in which physiological defenses against emotional experiences could occur has to do with clinical evidence showing that people might resort to physiological defenses against emotional experiences even when there is no threat whatsoever to the survival of the brain and body physiology. Because unpleasant emotional experiences are by definition states of stress and dysregulation of the brain and body physiology, they are inherently painful, and they lower a person's sense of their well-being. For this reason, we are programmed to avoid unpleasant emotional experiences and seek pleasant emotional experiences instead. This, as discussed earlier, is Freud's pleasure principle. The ability to tolerate unpleasant emotional experiences varies considerably in the population, as does the engagement of physiological defenses against emotional experiences. We saw clinical examples of this variation in affect tolerance levels, and cases involving severe psychophysiological symptoms like asthma even at low levels of emotional suffering, in the cases presented in chapters 1 and 2.

From the discussion so far, it might appear that physiological dynamics or states such as constriction that are involved in physiological defenses against emotions serve only one function: minimizing or eliminating life-threatening or unbearable emotional experiences. However, upon closer examination, we can see that such physiological dynamics might be involved in generating other emotional experiences at the same time. This is because when we try to get rid of an emotional experience, we are trying to create another emotional state. For example, a successful defense against anxiety produces calm or a sense of neutrality, both of which qualify as emotions in the broadest definition, along with changes in one's sense of well-being. So, to be accurate, we have to say that the physiological dynamics engaged in reducing anxiety are defending against anxiety or generating calmness, or both. Therefore, we have to specify the emotion and the situation (to make sure that it makes sense to experience the particular emotion in the situation) to determine whether a physiological state such as constriction or arousal is involved in defending against an emotion or in generating one.

Defense Mechanisms as a Coping Strategy

In this chapter, we are interested in creating a useful framework for under-standing and working with physiological states within the brain and body physiology that contribute to generating and defending against emotional experiences. Our emotional experiences in a situation are derived from the sensations of all the physiological states generated in the brain and body physiology by all the ways in which we are coping with the situation, and from the sensations of the direct physical impact of the situation on our brain and body physiology. Because physiological dynamics or states that give rise to emotions arise in the execution of all of the coping strategies and from the direct impact of the situation on the physiology of the brain and body, let us quickly review all the coping strategies we might employ in a situation including the one we just saw—what body psychotherapists call physiological defenses against emotional experiences.

We saw in chapter 5 that our emotions are assessments of the impact situations have on our well-being. When we are faced with a situation, we respond to it in ways that maximize our well-being and minimize threats. Such adaptive responses, which we call our coping strategies or mechanisms, are generated through a large number of physiological changes in the brain and body physiology. We will refer to the physio-logical changes generated by the execution of the different coping strat-egies or mechanisms as physiological dynamics or states associated with our coping mechanisms. The various coping strategies we might employ to deal with a situation are:

a) predictions of emotions from recall of previous experiences in similar situations in the brain;

b) predictions of emotions in the form of instinctual emotional responses hardwired into our brains by evolution;

c) physiological changes initiated in the brain and the body to mobilize energy, such as through faster breathing and circulation, to provide fuel for behaviors such as expression and action to cope with unfavorable situations or to take advantage of favorable situations;

d) physiological changes initiated in the brain and the body by the enactment of behaviors, such as expression and action, to cope with unfavorable situations or to take advantage of favorable situations; and

e) physiological changes initiated in the brain and the body to ensure their survival or to cope with the stress of psychologically and physiologically intolerable experiences that arise in the course of implementation of the other coping strategies.

Let us look at each of these coping strategies in a simple example. If I am in an automobile accident, my brain predicts emotional consequences in terms of how the accident could affect my well-being by recalling emotional experiences from similar experiences in the past—e.g., coping strategy (a)—and by activating instinctual survival circuits hardwired in the brain through evolution (b). The predictions based on past experience and instinctual brain circuitry also include optimal energy mobilization and behavioral response strategies given the situation. Based on these predictions and on evaluation of current information from the environment, my body mobilizes energy (c), and it uses that energy in behaviors such as turning the wheel to the right to guide the car off the road and avoid further collisions (d). I realize that I cannot avoid hitting a tree on the side of the road, even though I might have avoided hitting other vehicles on the road. The impact of the crash against the tree affects my entire brain and body physiology in a shocking manner (direct physical impact of the situation on the brain and body physiology).

As I lie dazed after the impact, my heart is racing too fast for its own good, so that physiological defenses are engaged to slow it down so I do not have a heart attack and die (e). The fear I have of dying is too much to bear; thus, physiological defenses against the fear are engaged to numb the brain and the body physiology so I can be calmer until help arrives (e). Emotions that the brain generates in this situation involve sensations arising from the physiological changes in the brain and body physiology resulting from the execution of all these coping strategies and the direct physical impact of the situation on the brain and body physiology.

With regard to defending against emotions, coping strategy (e), we saw earlier that a physiological dynamic involved in implementing this strategy, such as constriction or arousal, might also be contributing to the generation of another emotion. In each of the seven categories of physiological changes or dynamics we will discuss at length below, we will also see that the same reality applies. That is, none of the physiological dynamics grouped under the categories to follow might be exclusively generating or defending against emotions. For example, the coping strategy of external behaviors directed at the world (d), such as action and expression to deal with a dangerous situation, could be contributing to generating the emotion of anger while defending against the emotions of fear and helplessness. As another example, high arousal contributing to the emotion of confidence in a situation could very well be a defense against the feeling of helplessness.

If we were to encounter the physiological dynamic of constriction in the brain and body physiology in a situation, it would be difficult to attribute it exclusively to one of the coping strategies (a) through (e) or the direct impact of the situation on the brain and body physiology, because more than one coping mechanism at the same time could be using constriction. For example, if we are involved in fighting in a dangerous situation, we are likely to be constricting our musculature to move in order to fight (d). It is also possible that we might be using constriction of our musculature to brace our body to reduce or manage suffering from the blows that are landing on it (e), the sensations of which are also an input for the construction of emotion in the brain.

If things are so complicated—if it really is very difficult to say with certainty whether a physiological dynamic such as constriction is in the service of generating or defending against emotion—how can body psychotherapy approaches claim that physiological dynamics such as constriction in the breathing muscles, the diaphragm, the intercostals, and the abdominal muscles always defend against emotions? The claim is valid because the abovementioned breathing muscles have the general psychological function of managing emotions.[7] Therefore, it is possible to make such a general statement as long as one overlooks the fact that constriction of the breathing muscles to block certain emotions, such as agitation, might make the person feel other emotions, such as calmness.

Also, body psychotherapies usually specify the situation, the emotion, and at times even the behavior, and only then describe a constriction as blocking the emotional experience to make their statement valid. For example, when a child is traumatized for coming into power in the terrible twos, a typical way in which the child might hold power back is by hyperconstricting or hypoconstricting its diaphragm to stay out of trouble. A child experiencing a threat to their existence in the pre- and perinatal period of development might constrict their eyes to hold back the emotions of terror and rage.[8] In both of these examples, these defenses are specific to the emotions and the situations they arise in, making them useful in diagnosing and treating clients with power and existential issues.

In the next section of this chapter, we'll elucidate seven categories of psychological dynamics that could be involved in generating or defending against emotional experiences. These categories offer body psychotherapists a comprehensive framework for developing theories of physiological defenses against psychological experiences, including emotions, in specific life situations. They can also help psychotherapists guard against mistakes some might make in always treating physiological states such as constriction as defenses that need to be gotten rid of.

For the majority of psychotherapists who are beginning to work with the brain and body physiology and who might find this framework too complex, there is no need to be concerned. They can follow a simple rule: when working with an emotion in a situation, they can assume that the emotion is defended against in the places wherever the emotion is not a conscious experience in the brain and body physiology. This is because an emotion, especially an overwhelming one, has the potential to be present throughout the entirety of the brain and body physiology. One does not have to know what specific physiological dynamic, constriction or arousal, is involved in blocking the emotional experience in a part of the brain and body physiology. They can simply work with the usual tools such awareness, intention, breath, self-touch, or therapist's touch where possible, to undo the defenses in that area to expand the emotional experience to that area.

Now, let us turn to detailed discussion of each of the seven categories of physiological dynamics that might be involved in generating or defending against emotional experiences: constriction/deconstriction dynamics, arousal/charge dynamics, movement dynamics, function dynamics, biochemical and bioelectrical dynamics, dynamics of stress, regulation, and dysregulation, and electromagnetic and quantum mechanical energy dynamics.

Physiological Dynamics Involved in Generating or Defending against Emotional Experiences

When I set about developing a framework for classifying all possible physiological dynamics or changes that could contribute to generating or defending against emotional experiences, I intended for the framework to be of as much practical use to clinicians as possible. I used the physiological dynamics that have been already identified in the literature on the physiology of emotions, body psychotherapy, and energy psychology as a place to start and build from. To the extent possible, I wanted a chosen physiological dynamic to be as observable as possible in the awareness of therapists and clients so that they are manipulable in clinical work.

To be clear, the term "physiological dynamics" refers to general categories of physiological changes in the brain and body physiology that result from implementing any of the five coping strategies—mechanisms (a) through (e) discussed earlier—in a situation, and the direct physical impact of the situation on the body and brain physiology. We will see that the categories are not mutually exclusive but rather are overlapping and interdependent. For example, movement, a separate category of observable physiological changes, cannot occur without constriction/desconstriction dynamics in the musculature, another category of observable physiological changes in our framework.

1. Constriction/Deconstriction Dynamics

All things in our brain and body physiology, from the muscle at the macro level to the cell at the micro level, constantly constrict and deconstrict to facilitate a variety of functions: movement, breathing, moving food through the digestive tract, and so on. From the body psychotherapy point of view, constriction and deconstriction are often, if not always, involved in implementing one or more of the five strategies (a) through (e) involved in coping with a situation or in the direct physical impact of the situation on the brain and body psychology.

I have found that the easiest way to demonstrate the role of the body in generating and defending against emotional experience when I am teaching is to have people in the class collapse their upper body to the front, which deconstricts some muscles on the back and constricts some muscles in the front in the upper half of the body. I then ask them to say aloud, "I am feeling confident now," to notice their bodies feeling exactly the opposite because of the collapse of the upper body to the front. I follow this up with having them put their upper body in the opposite position, upright and even leaning backward slightly, and have them say "I am not feeling confident now," to have them experience their body countering their statement and generating exactly the opposite emotional state. The collapsed state supports the generation of the emotion of diffidence and defends against confidence; the upright state does the opposite, supporting confidence and countering diffidence. This shows clearly that, in order to answer the question of whether a constriction/deconstriction dynamic is contributing to generating an emotion or defending against it, we need to specify the emotion first. This is also true for every one of the six other physiological dynamics we will discuss below.

Almost all body psychotherapy approaches have focused on the role of the voluntary muscular system in generating and defending against emotional experiences. Earlier systems, such as Reichian Therapy[9] and Bioenergetic Analysis,[10] focused on its defensive role; later systems, such as Bodynamic Analysis, emphasized its defensive as well as its generative functions in relation to all psychological experiences, including emotions. In the empirically derived psychology of muscles in Bodynamic Analysis, the major muscles are assigned their psychomotor functions as well as their psychological functions.

The ability to constrict and deconstrict a muscle over its range is theorized as optimal for the muscle's availability for its psychomotor and psychological functions. Habitual constriction or desconstriction toward the extremes, leading to hyperconstriction or hypoconstriction of the muscle, are considered to be defensive in nature in relation to psychomotor functions and the generation of psychological experiences. Hypercontraction is associated with holding back the impulse, and hypoconstriction is associated with the loss of impulse toward the psychomotor functions and psychological experiences of cognition, emotion, and behavior associated with the muscle. For example, hypoconstriction or flaccidity in the triceps muscle group can inhibit the psychomotor action of setting boundaries by pushing people or things away. Hypoconstriction in the triceps can also inhibit cognitive, emotional, and behavioral experiences and memories in relation to boundary setting. For this reason, when we have clients push us away with their arms, cognitive, emotional, and behavioral experiences around boundary setting often emerge. The work done by Ekman and colleagues at the University of California, Berkeley, in the tradition of academic research that started with a multicultural study of the role of facial muscles in emotion by Charles Darwin, has established how different patterns of constriction/deconstriction of facial muscles can contribute to generating and defending against different emotional states.[11]

Earlier body psychotherapies, such as Reichian Therapy and Bioenergetic Analysis, focused on breaking down rigid or highly constricted muscles that were deemed as physiological defenses against access to emotions and other psychological experiences the clients needed to work with. Later body psychotherapy approaches, such as Bodynamic Analysis,[12] focus on restoring a wider range of movement possibilities in hyperconstricted or hypoconstricted muscles that are deemed as defenses against psychomotor and psychological functions of cognition and emotion, and of behavior associated with the specific muscles.

It makes sense that many body psychotherapy approaches focus on the muscular system. The voluntary nature of the skeletal muscular system and its availability near the surface of the body make it more accessible for manipulation through touch or voluntary movement. The sensations of the muscular system are also more available to introspective awareness than those of the viscera or the nervous system. The viscera (organs, glands, and blood vessels) depend on the voluntary muscular system to carry out vital biological functions, such as breathing, circulation, and digestion, on which the survival of the central nervous system areas of the brain and spinal cord depend. Therefore, working with the voluntary muscular system can facilitate physiological and therefore psychological changes in the viscera and the central nervous system.

Of the five dynamics (a) through (e) involved in coping with a situation, the first two—recalling emotional experiences in similar situations, and generating instinctual emotional reactions—can be thought of as having more to do with the brain than the body, even though it is likely that they affect the body to some extent. The three other coping mechanisms that have more bearing on the body are behavioral changes initiated internally to generate energy, external behavioral changes enacted to deal with the world, and physiological defenses initiated throughout the brain and body physiology to manage overwhelming emotional experiences to ensure survival and reduce unbearable suffering. The constriction/flaccidity dynamic, and indeed any of the other physiological dynamics that will be discussed in this chapter, can occur in the execution of any of these three coping mechanisms; they can also result from the direct physical impact of the situation on the brain and body physiology.

Most, if not all, of the coping strategies, as well as the direct physical impact of the situation on the brain and body physiology, are likely to be present in every situation. Because of this complexity, it is difficult if not impossible to determine which coping strategy or strategies an observed physiological dynamic such as constriction might be contributing to, and whether it is contributing to the generation of or defense against an emotional experience.

2. Arousal/Charge Dynamics

The physiological dynamic of arousal/charge, which can also be made conscious as an experience, is an important component in generating and defending against emotional experiences. When something, such as arousal, contributes to an emotional experience that can be made conscious within or observed from the outside, it becomes possible through awareness or other means, such as medication, to alter the emotional experience. According to the dimensional theory of emotions,[13] arousal and valence are the two basic dimensions of all emotional experiences. Arousal refers to whether the property of arousal is high or low, and valence refers to whether an experience feels good or bad. For example, anxiety and thrill are both high-arousal emotions, but they differ in that anxiety feels bad and thrill feels good. Depression that feels bad and calmness that feels good are both low-arousal emotions.

Variations in arousal or charge, the sensations of which become an input into the construction of emotion in the brain, arise internally in the brain and body physiology as the brain goes about generating arousal in some places and then distributing it to other places where it is needed as fuel for the execution of external coping behaviors such as expression and action. Arousal and its variation can be experienced throughout the physiology in the brain, spinal cord, nerves, organs, glands, blood vessels, muscles, fascia, and skin. For example, in order to supply the energy for a vigorous manual effort, the aroused brain guides the autonomic nervous system to generate energy through organs, glands, and blood vessels and distribute it to the muscular system so it can carry out the effort. The increase in arousal can be felt as a conscious experience in each of the places involved, and it can be interpreted as motivation when one is favorable toward the act and as pressure when one is unfavorable to it.

Arousal is a slightly ambiguous term that can also refer to the increase in the tone in the nervous system, without a clear understanding of whether such arousal implies an increase or decrease in energy. The tone is defined as the rate at which a nerve is firing. An increase in tone in the sympathetic nervous system, often referred to as an increase in arousal in the sympathetic nervous system, often implies an increase in charge or energy. An increase in the tone or arousal in the parasympathetic nervous system, on the other hand, often implies the opposite—the lowering of charge or energy. "Charge" is therefore a clearer term, with low and high charge corresponding to lower and higher energy states.

As we saw earlier, increase or decrease in charge can be consciously experienced in every part of the physiology. And, as with constriction dynamics, charge dynamics in the physiology can contribute to the generation of an emotional experience or to the defense against it. If an emotional experience could be challenging survival or is simply too much to bear, the brain might manipulate the energy dynamics to increase or decrease charge in order to defend against the emotional experience. For example, it might increase charge to create mania to ward off the pain of depression, or it might decrease charge to generate depression to defend against an unbearable experience of anxiety characterized by high charge.

Please note that, as with the constriction/deconstriction dynamic, one cannot determine how an arousal/charge pattern in the physiology is contributing to the generation of emotion, or to the defense against it, unless we specify the emotion, as well as the situation the emotion is a response to. We might need to know the situation in order to know whether the emotion is a defense or might be reasonably expected in the situation. For example, if we repeatedly encounter anger in relation to a loss with no vulnerabilities on the horizon, and we find a high charge in the physiology associated with it, then it would be reasonable to conclude that the arousal contributing to the habitual anger is serving the purpose of defending against the painful and unbearable vulnerabilities that usually go with a loss.

Charging the physiology through breathing or movement has long been used to break through defenses against emotional experiences in some therapy approaches. Breathing, especially rapid breathing, increases charge. Movement, especially when vigorous, compels increase in energy mobilization and charge in the physiology. Both breathing and movement that increase charge challenge the inhibitions against emotional experiences in organs involved in cardiovascular and respiratory functions, such as the lungs and the heart; muscles involved in breathing and in movement in the rest of the body; and inhibitions in the nervous system against breathing and movement.

3. Movement Dynamics

Movement is essential for our survival. One kind of movement or another is involved in our actions and expressions that help us cope with situations in the world; in our vital biological functions, such as breathing, cardiovascular function, and digestion; and the exercises we do to maintain our health. Therefore, it makes sense that movement dynamics plays an important role in generating our emotional experiences and in defending against them.

This is a good place to pause and point out that the seven physiological dynamics we are exploring in this chapter are not independent of each other. For example, movements of skeletal muscle and smooth muscle are brought about by constriction and deconstriction dynamics in the muscles involved. Arousal or charge dynamics involve movement or constriction dynamics. For example, for blood to be diverted from digestive organs to skeletal muscles to charge the muscles for action, blood vessels have to be dilated or deconstricted in the muscles and constricted in the organs.

When we move our muscles, we allow them to participate in generating, enhancing, and processing our emotional experiences. As we saw in the experiments conducted by Paula Niedenthal at the University of Wisconsin–Madison, preventing facial muscles from movement during emotional experiences compromises the processing of emotional experiences in the brain.[14] Inhibition of movement can contribute to emotional experiences as well. Emotions such as helplessness and despair are often associated with the inability to move, caused by inhibition of movement. Movement during sexual acts usually enhances the pleasure derived from it. However, inhibition of movement is not always associated with decrease in emotional intensity because other physiological dynamics, such as charge, in combination with inhibition in movement can bring about greater intensity in emotional experience. For instance, we can hold ourselves back by holding back movement in the muscles even as we continue to charge them with energy, creating an explosive charge of the emotion of desire.

As with constriction and arousal dynamics, we can only determine whether movement or inhibition of movement is contributing to an emotion or is a defense against it after we specify the emotion and the situation associated with it. For example, if we move our facial muscles into a smiling position, we cannot know whether we are doing so to counter and defend against the rage we have brewing within us or to genuinely express our liking for a person, without knowing what the relationship situation is at the moment and what emotion we are referring to with respect to the movement of the facial muscles toward a smiling position.

Movement therapy and dance therapy are therapeutic modalities that use movement itself to undo defenses in the brain and body physiology against movement, to increase the range of possibilities in movement and thus to increase the range of possibilities in our cognition, emotion, and behavior. Psychomotor therapy uses movement informed by knowledge of specific psychomotor movements of different muscle groups to undo defenses against those very movements to enhance specific cognitive, emotional, and behavioral possibilities. Because the functions of the viscera and the central nervous system are quite dependent on the voluntary muscular system, movement of these muscles has also been found to be effective in increasing the health and range of function in those systems.[15]

4. Function Dynamics

Functions performed by the brain and body physiology can be classified into purely biological functions measurable through physiological metrics, such as heartbeat and breath rate, as well as psychophysiological functions such as posture, gesture, and facial expressions that, in addition to their role in biological functioning, have psychological purposes. The three layers of the brain and body physiology—the central nervous system, the viscera, and the muscular system—are involved in a large number of biological functions. In fact, each of the seven physiological dynamics presented in this chapter, such as constriction, arousal, and movement, are biological functions that can also be used for psychological purposes. The purpose of having an additional category of function dynamics is to capture some of the other major biological and psychophysiological processes that are worked with in psychotherapy to facilitate psychological processes.

BIOLOGICAL FUNCTIONS

Breathing: Breathing is perhaps the biological function that is most often manipulated in therapy to regulate emotional experiences in both body-oriented and less body-oriented psychotherapy approaches. The evidence-based cognitive behavioral therapy of systematic desensitization often uses a relaxation protocol involving the breath to treat symptoms of PTSD. Relaxation protocols that involve conscious breathing patterns are commonplace in the treatment of anxiety. Meditation and yoga often use conscious awareness and manipulation of breath for various purposes, including regulation of psychological experiences of cognition, emotion, and behavior.

Patterns of breathing, such as rapid chest breathing, are used to break through physiological defenses against psychological experiences, including emotions, in therapeutic approaches such as Reichian Therapy, Bioenergetics, Rebirthing Therapy, and Holotropic Breathwork.[16] A person might use breathing consciously or unconsciously to generate an emotional experience, regulate it, or defend against it. Slowing down one's breathing and making it more measured can help in combating the emotion of anxiety or serve as the basis of the emotional experience of calmness. Again, one cannot really say whether a breathing pattern is contributing to an emotion in a situation or is in the service of regulating or defending against an emotional experience unless we know the emotion and its context.

Heart rate: The heart rate, the number of times the heart beats per minute, plays an important role in all of our emotional experiences. The heart rate is an important, if not the most important, contributor to arousal or charge, which characterizes all pleasant and unpleasant emotional experiences along a continuum from low to high. We cannot manipulate the heart rate as directly as we can regulate the breath rate, the number of times per minute we breathe in and out. But we can indirectly manipulate the heart rate to some extent through the breath. Research has shown that those who are more capable of being consciously aware of their heart rate and can report the number of times their heart beats per minute are more aware of a larger range of emotional experiences than those who cannot report their heart rate.[17]

Heart rate variability (HRV), a computation based on the difference in the rate at which the heart beats during inhalation (more) versus exhalation (less), has emerged as a measure of heart health and as an indicator of balance between the sympathetic and parasympathetic branches of the autonomic nervous system. HRV is now being used clinically to measure outcomes in the treatment of PTSD. Because HRV can be tracked relatively easily with applications on smartphones, it is used in biofeedback to manage stress and unpleasant emotions. Higher HRV scores are associated with pleasant emotions, such as love, and lower HRV scores are associated with unpleasant emotional experiences. This may be caused by the fact that unpleasant emotional experiences, by definition, involve more stress and dysregulation in the brain and body physiology. As with the breath rate and heart rate, variations in HRV can be involved in generating as well as defending against emotional experiences. Again, HRV's exact role in a situation can only be known when we know the details of the situation and the specific emotion involved.

PSYCHOPHYSIOLOGICAL FUNCTIONS

Posture: Posture, the particular way in which we hold our bodies, can tell the world a lot about who we are. We consciously or unconsciously communicate our mental states to the world all the time. Whether we sit with our chest open and our arms at our sides or with our chest closed and our arms crossed in the front of us can communicate to the world how open or closed we are to the person and the communication we are engaged in. Such a posture also affects our ability to be open and communicate with the other person nonverbally, electromagnetically, or quantum mechanically through interpersonal resonance. Postural analysis is a formal tool in body psychotherapy approaches going back to their beginnings, in the psychology of Wilhelm Reich.[18] It is used to determine a person's character—their habitual ways of thought, feeling, and behavior—from their usual body postures in different life situations. Postural analysis is something we do all the time unconsciously or consciously to some extent. For those who wish to delve more deeply into this subject, the book *Embodying Experience: Forming a Personal Life* by Stanley Keleman is a good beginning.[19]

Posture not only communicates our thoughts, feelings, and behavioral intentions to others; it can also generate, constrain, and defend against them. The use of posture, gesture, facial expressions, and other body expressions to generate and embody suitable cognitive, emotional, and behavioral tendencies is common in acting classes. Forward-leaning postures are associated with emotions of attraction, and backward-leaning postures are associated with emotions of aversion. Putting people into forward-leaning postures and having them process situations that involve emotions of aversion and into backward-leaning postures to process emotions of attraction significantly alters the brain's ability to process the emotions as well as the situations in which they arise.[20] Again, as with all other dynamics, whether posture is being used to generate an emotion or defend against it depends on our knowledge of what the emotion is and the situation we find it in.

Gesture: Gesture, like posture, can communicate our cognitive, emotional, and behavioral dispositions to others as well as generating them or defending against them. Often, I bring this point home to participants in my classes by having them reach out with both their arms and say "I hate you" or "I do not want you." This gesture usually communicates longing for another person and is used in the psychomotor act of

reaching out to the other person to fulfill that longing. The class participants laugh when they realize that what their body is doing generates a
strong emotional state that overrides the emotional state they are trying
to generate in their brain by saying "I do not want you." It is also good
exercise to convince people of the role of the body in emotional experience. Please note that gesture, posture, facial expressions, and other
body expressions can also be used to conceal our inner states or deceive
others. For example, we might be able to convince others of our confidence with an upright posture, which usually communicates confidence,
while hiding the diffidence we might feel deeper in our body. The extent
to which we actually end up believing our manufactured confidence
depends on the degree to which we can shut down the cries of diffidence
from deeper within us.

Dennis Slattery, a professor specializing in imaginal psychotherapy at
Pacifica Graduate Institute in Carpinteria, California, where I earned my
PhD in clinical psychology, is the author of the book *The Wounded Body:
Remembering the Marking of Flesh*. One morning Slattery woke up with an
inspiration that important gestures in dreams could be the portals through
which one could access the core emotions in the dreams.[21] He then went
about having his clients identify gestures they thought were important in
their dreams, enact the gestures, and hold them in place while they processed their dreams. Lo and behold, his inspiration proved to be right, and
another method of working with dreams was born.

Facial expression: The role of facial expression in emotion has been
extensively researched. Charles Darwin was the first to scientifically
establish that facial displays communicate our inner emotional states
to others.[22] The understanding that facial expression also plays a role in
generating and defending against emotional experiences came later.[23]
We can infer the emotional states of others not only by observing their
facial expression but also by mirroring their facial expressions with our
own faces and generating corresponding emotional states in ourselves.
More than other parts of the body, the face is programmed to mimic the
faces of others from immediately after birth. Inhibition of involvement
of facial musculature in emotion has been shown to disrupt the brain's

processing and recall of not only the emotion but also its context, i.e., the details of the situation that gives rise to the emotion.[24] Making sense of an emotional experience in the body by connecting it with the face is considered to be an important milestone in our development from childhood to adulthood.[25,26] Because the facial muscles generate a wider range of expressions than the rest of the body, facial expression helps to bring greater clarity to the physical or emotional experience in the body and to differentiate it further; for example, physical pain can become emotional anguish.

The polyvagal theory of the autonomic nervous system shows us that the facial muscles can be more quickly energized and moved than other muscles in the body through the ventral vagal nerve's action on the heart's natural pacemaker.[27] This makes it possible for the facial muscles to act more rapidly in generating or defending against emotional experience. Research with people who have had Botox treatments that immobilize parts of the facial musculature for cosmetic reasons shows that such treatments can reduce depression by reducing the ability of facial muscles to generate negative emotions.[28] So, given the face's special place in the physiology of emotions for all of the above reasons, it makes much sense to work with the face in therapy.

Vocalization: In addition to body expressions such as twisting, turning, pushing things away, or pulling others toward oneself, children express their emotions early on primarily through facial expression and vocalization of sounds before they learn to express their emotions through words. Vocalization, in addition to its function of communication, provides the child relief and regulation by discharging some of the arousal fueling the emotion. Vocalization serves all the purposes that are attributed to facial expression. Mothers can distinguish different emotions in the cries of a child from very early on. Through mirroring their cries, mothers can generate the corresponding emotional states in themselves. Vocalization, like facial expression, helps to integrate the head and neck area and the rest of the body in emotional experience. It can also help in clarifying and differentiating emotional experiences in oneself and others.

We can tell that vocalizations generate and enhance emotions by observing the obvious pleasure children derive from vocalizing. Inhibition of expression of one's experience through words or vocalization inhibits the physiology in the throat and can be a powerful physiological defense, not just against the expression of emotional experiences but also against generating them. We can see this in our everyday experience of being able to come into our emotions as soon as we start to share our experiences with others. The throat musculature is similar to the facial musculature in its ability to generate and defend against emotions. According to the polyvagal theory of the autonomic nervous system, the actions of the face and throat musculature (forming what Porges refers to as the "social engagement system") are highly coordinated with the functioning of the heart and the lungs through the ventral vagal nerve in emotional and other experiences.[29]

Research on psychophysiological symptoms has shown that they are driven by a combination of adverse experiences in childhood and a low capacity for sensing and expressing one's emotions.[30,31] In human development, nonverbal vocalization and facial expression of emotion precede verbal expression of emotion through words. Therefore, I decided to experiment with the following intervention in the treatment of psychophysiological symptoms: imagining someone else or oneself expressing the discomfort in the psychophysiological symptom in the body through vocalization or facial expression, and then actually doing the vocalization or facial expression if necessary, with the therapist mirroring and supporting both modes of expression. It worked! I found that this intervention can offer many benefits. It can give the person relief, help them understand the more differentiated emotions involved, integrate the head and neck area and the rest of the body in emotional experience, and help to expand the emotional experience throughout the body to increase the person's ability to tolerate the emotional experiences to resolve the symptoms.

Vocalization of emotion is a rudimentary verbal as well as nonverbal expression of the emotional experience. Because 95 percent of any expression is said to be nonverbal, vocalization offers the possibility of initiation of nonverbal expression and expansion of emotion throughout the body.

5. BIOCHEMICAL AND BIOELECTRICAL DYNAMICS

Biochemical and bioelectrical dynamics are the very basic dynamics that drive all other physiological dynamics identified in this chapter, with the exception of some electromagnetic and quantum mechanical energy dynamics that we will discuss at the end of this chapter. The brain, the spinal cord, and the somatic and autonomic nerves that regulate the body communicate through bioelectrical impulses that are both preceded and succeeded by biochemical changes. There are a large number of biochemical agents produced in the brain and the body. Neurotransmitters such as dopamine, hormones such as insulin, steroids such as testosterone, and a large number of peptides are examples of biochemical agents or "information substances" that are constantly coursing throughout the brain and body physiology to initiate all kinds of physiological changes.

Biochemical and bioelectrical dynamics happen largely outside of our conscious awareness. What we are aware of as physiological changes are the effects of these biochemical and bioelectrical dynamics. It is seldom the case that we can change biochemical and bioelectric dynamics by bringing them into our conscious awareness. We can, however, influence them by becoming aware of the physiological changes they cause. For example, we can affect biochemical and bioelectrical dynamics in our brain and body physiology by regulating our breathing patterns. Even though we can seldom influence these dynamics by direct observation, there are a couple of reasons why we are including them in the discussion of physiological dynamics. First, I want to provide a comprehensive list of physiological dynamics that contribute to generating and defending against emotions. Also, there are therapeutic interventions that do try to influence biochemical and bioelectrical dynamics, such as psychoactive medication in psychiatry, psychoactive agents such as DMT in psychedelic therapy, and nutrition in naturopathy.

The role of biochemicals (neurotransmitters such as dopamine and serotonin, and hormones such as testosterone and estrogen) in emotional experiences is well documented, as is their role of activation or inhibition of bioelectrical activity in the brain and the rest of the nervous system in generating, altering, and defending against emotional experiences. For example, the research done by Helen Fisher and her colleagues at Rutgers University has shown that emotions of lust, love, and attachment involved in experiences of romantic love appear to be driven by different sets of biochemicals.[32] Lust is driven by increases in the sex hormones of testosterone and estrogen, love is driven by increases in dopamine and norepinephrine and decreases in serotonin, and attachment is driven by increases in oxytocin and vasopressin.

Bilateral dysfunction of the amygdala (which is part of the emotional brain), as measured by reduction in electrical activity in the area, is associated with the lack of conscious experience of fear. Transcranial magnetic stimulation therapy (in which magnets are positioned on opposite sides of the skull to change the electrical activity in the areas of the brain in between them) and craniosacral therapy (where the therapist's hands are placed on opposite sides of the skull or one side of the skull to change the dynamics in specific brain areas through the electromagnetic and quantum energy fields created by the therapist's hands) seek to increase, decrease, or otherwise influence the bioelectrical functioning of the targeted areas for the better.

As with all physiological dynamics discussed earlier, the role of biochemistry and bioelectricity in an emotional experience, whether it is facilitating or inhibiting, requires knowledge of what the emotion is and the context in which it has risen.

6. DYNAMICS OF STRESS, REGULATION, AND DYSREGULATION

The physiological dynamics of stress and the physiological dynamics of regulation and dysregulation are aggregates of a large number of individual physiological processes that break all the way down to biochemical and bioelectrical dynamics at the cellular level. One reason why they are included in this framework of physiological dynamics involved in generating or defending against emotional experiences is because all pleasant and unpleasant emotions can be characterized by levels of stress, regulation, and dysregulation. That is, unpleasant emotions are characterized by higher levels of stress and dysregulation, and pleasant emotions are characterized by lower levels of stress and higher levels of regulation.

Another reason to include these aggregate dynamics is because they are amenable to introspection as conscious experiences in our physiology that we can then manipulate through awareness and other tools such as self-touch. We can track higher levels of stress and dysregulation in our awareness as something that feels bad, not okay, and overwhelming—and lower levels of stress and higher levels of regulation as something that feels good, okay, and manageable—as meaningful sensorimotor emotions in relation to situations. Tracking body experiences at such aggregate levels can often be more efficient, not only in capturing any possible meaning but also in regulating or transforming the experiences, than when we track the individual physiological dynamics that contribute to them. This is analogous to the difference between trying to lift a table by grabbing opposite sides of its top or by one of its four legs.

Tracking body sensations associated with individual physiological dynamics, such as heartbeat, can be very helpful in regulating physiological and psychological experiences. However, the meaning of such microlevel experiences and whether they are contributing to or detracting from emotional experience in a situation are not always clear, unless we know what the emotion is in that situation. Because tracking of microsensations tends to downregulate the physiology from dysregulation to regulation, we run the risk of regulating away unpleasant emotional experiences that are, by their nature, states of stress and dysregulation. Tracking the stress, regulation, and dysregulation dynamics at the aggregate or macro level, as opposed to tracking the more meaningful states they might be contributing to, also poses this risk but to a much lesser degree than tracking them at the micro level of their constituent parts or components.

As we saw earlier, when we track the level of stress, regulation, and dysregulation at the aggregate level, we track the qualities of feeling good or bad, okay or not okay, and agreeable or disagreeable. These can be meaningful experiences in relation to the situation we find ourselves in, and they therefore qualify as emotions in themselves—sensorimotor emotions at a very basic level. They could be contributing to more complex emotions such as companionship or loneliness. When they are unpleasant states of stress and dysregulation, they could just be psychophysiological symptoms arising from the person's inability to cope with and tolerate emotional experiences. They could also be defenses against more appropriate emotions in the situations wherein they arise. For example, it is possible for a person to become thoroughly disorganized or even go crazy to avoid facing the reality of a painful situation.

For all these reasons, when tracking aggregate experiences of states of stress, regulation, and dysregulation, one has to be careful not to always treat them as psychophysiological symptoms to be regulated downward and away through medication or by other means such as detailed tracking of body sensations. One has to use discrimination, in relation to the situation wherein the experiences arise, to determine whether they are emotions in themselves, whether they are contributing to more complex emotional states, whether they are defenses against appropriate emotions, or whether they are psychophysiological symptoms. We will return to this topic in chapter 9 when we look at different types of emotions.

Please note that states of apparently decreasing stress and increasing regulation can also be defensive in intent. For example, it is not uncommon for what appears to be a state of low stress and even great regulation to arise in the physiology in the face of an overwhelming experience through the secretion of biochemicals such as opioids and endorphins as a defense.

7. Electromagnetic and Quantum Mechanical Energy Dynamics

Energies of the electromagnetic spectrum that are produced in one place in the physiology, such as the heart, have been observed to affect another place, such as the liver, by traveling directly between the two locations outside the nervous system.[33] Biomagnetic and bioelectric energies from the heart and the brain are also known to affect each other directly, communicating outside the nervous system through the connective tissue matrix. Such energies have also been observed to travel between two bodies to influence each other. These energies from outside of the body are certainly capable of playing a role in our emotional experiences as part of the impact a situation is having on us, because they have been known to affect even gene expression at the cellular level.[34]

The therapeutic method of transcranial magnetic stimulation involves placing two magnets on opposite sides of the skull to stimulate bioelectromagnetic energy patterns being generated in the brain, to improve physiological and psychological functioning. Methods and devices for working with other parts of the body, such as organs and muscles, through manipulation of their electromagnetic fields have also been developed.[35] Bodywork and energy work modalities also work with these energies to facilitate or change physiological and psychological experiences. The experiences of the brain and body physiology resulting from the stimulation of these energies by other parts of the brain and body physiology or coming from outside it can contribute to generating or defending against our emotional experiences.

Our brain and body physiology also exists at the quantum level of subatomic particles, and physiological dynamics at the quantum level can contribute to the generation of and defense against our emotional experiences. Energy and energy psychology models, especially from the East, have numerous theories about how changes in quantum energy patterns affect our brain and body physiology. They offer a number of methods for working with such quantum energy patterns to facilitate various psychological experiences, including emotion.[36] For example, in one theory, quantum energies concentrate toward the center of the body along the spine to regulate and defend against unbearable emotions and other experiences in the brain and body physiology.[37] Expanding and balancing the quantum energies throughout the brain and body physiology can undo defenses in them against emotions and other psychological experiences, thus making our physiological and psychological experiences more regulated and bearable.

In the next chapter, we turn to a discussion of factors that play a role in affect tolerance—our ability to tolerate and stay with difficult emotional experiences—and we examine why expanding the brain and body physiology to expand emotional experiences within it can help to increase our capacity to tolerate and stay with even higher levels of difficult emotional experiences for longer periods of time, without forming psychophysiological symptoms.

8

Emotional Embodiment and Affect Tolerance

Chapter summary: discusses factors that determine affect tolerance, and discusses how expanding the brain and body physiology to expand emotional experiences in it can quickly contribute to improving a person's capacity for tolerating them.

The most important assumption in emotional embodiment work is that emotional embodiment—expansion of the emotional experience to as much of the brain and body physiology as possible—brings about greater affect tolerance: the enhanced capacity to bear and stay with a difficult emotional experience over a longer period of time, which is often required for successful resolution of past traumas. In this chapter, we explore how that might be possible, especially for unpleasant emotional experiences that our brains are innately programmed to resist. Throughout this chapter, the combined physiology of the brain and body will be referred to simply as the physiology. The terms "body physiology" and "brain physiology" will be used when there is a need to distinguish between them.

The Basic Physiology of Pleasant and Unpleasant Emotional Experiences

As we saw in chapter 5, emotions are assessments of the impact of a situation on a person's well-being. Pleasant emotional experiences are movements in the direction of improvement in one's well-being. In essence, pleasant emotions result from increases in states of regulation, or decreases in states of dysregulation, in the physiology. On the other hand, unpleasant emotions are movements in the direction of worsening in one's well-being. They are, in essence, increases in states of dysregulation and decreases in states of regulation in the physiology. We breathe with greater ease, are less stressed, and feel an increase in our well-being when we are experiencing love in a secure relationship. We breathe with difficulty, are more stressed, and feel a decrease in our well-being when we feel the hurt from the breakup of the same relationship.

Experiences of states of regulation in the physiology are inherently more pleasurable. Experiences of states of dysregulation, on the other hand, are inherently more painful. For this reason, evolution has programmed us to avoid unpleasant emotional states and seek pleasant emotional states to maximize our chances of survival.[1] Unpleasant emotional experiences, as states of dysregulation, threaten our survival by compromising our physiology. Conversely, pleasant emotional experiences, as states of regulation, improve our physiology and enhance our survival. One reason—perhaps the most important reason—why we have much difficulty in tolerating and being with unpleasant emotional experiences has to do with the fact that they are inherently painful. It is much easier to be with the pleasure of a wedding engagement than with the pain of a divorce!

A Simple Model of the Physiology of Regulation and Dysregulation

The physiology of regulation and dysregulation, which as we saw in chapter 5 is also the physiology of emotion, is extremely complex. It is the subject of inquiry in a large number of disciplines, including medicine. For our purpose, to understand how expanding the physiology to expand the emotional experience can make the emotional experience more bearable, we need a model of the physiology of regulation and dysregulation. So, let us build a simple one.

The regulation and dysregulation of the physiology can be understood in terms of certain flows that are vital for the physiology's health and functioning. First is the flow of blood. Blood carries basic nutrients such as oxygen and glucose, regulatory biochemicals such as hormones, immune agents such as white blood cells, information such as blood sugar level, and waste products such as carbon dioxide, from one part of the physiology to another. Second is the flow of information back and forth between the brain and the body through the sensory and motor nerves of the somatic and autonomic nervous systems. This flow is essential for the brain to gather information about the body and to regulate the body based on that information.

The third flow is the interstitial or extracellular flow: the flow of fluid between the cells, through which nutrients such as minerals and messenger molecules such as peptides are carried from one part of the physiology to another.[2] The fourth flow is the lymphatic flow, which plays a role in managing fluid levels in tissues, absorbing fat from the intestines, protecting the body from invaders by producing and distributing immune cells such as white blood cells, and removing waste products.[3] The fifth flow is the flow of measurable electromagnetic energies from one part of the physiology to another, which are now known to play a role in regulating the physiology.[4] The sixth flow is the flow of quantum energies at the subatomic level between one part of the physiology and another that are involved in generating and regulating experiences in the physiology.[5,6]

Whether the physiology is regulated or dysregulated, overall or in part, depends very much on the state of these six vital flows from one part of the physiology to another. When these flows are relatively unobstructed, we can imagine that the level of regulation and the person's well-being would be on the high side, with lower levels of stress. On the other hand, if there are significant disruptions in one or more of these vital flows, one can expect dysregulation, disease, and reduction in one's well-being, with higher levels of stress. Because the physiology is an integral unit wherein every part depends on every other part for its functioning, the level of overall regulation, health, and well-being throughout the physiology could be diminished when these vital flows are hamstrung even in one or a few areas of the physiology. Disruption in the vital flows can also be expected if there is significant damage to one or more parts of the highly interdependent physiology.

Through the lens of this simple model of regulation and dysregulation, unpleasant emotional experiences, because they are states of dysregulation and high stress, can be expected to involve disruptions in one or more of the six vital flows in one or more parts of the physiology. Pleasant emotional experiences, because they are states of greater regulation with lower levels of stress, can be expected to involve less disruption in these vital flows among different areas of the physiology.

One might wonder if unpleasant emotional experiences always involve disruption in one or more of the six vital flows that have been identified as having to do with regulation and dysregulation in the physiology. After all, we saw in chapter 5 that emotional experiences can be generated in the brain alone through neurotransmitter action or through recall of prior emotional experiences. Even in such instances, disruptions of the vital flows can occur. Unpleasant emotional experiences generated in the brain might elicit physiological defenses against them in the brain physiology itself, which can lead to disruption in the essential flows within the brain physiology and between the brain and the body physiology. The emotional experiences generated in the brain physiology can also elicit defenses against emotions in the body physiology, such as reduction in one's breathing to decrease oxygen to the brain, to ease the emotional intensity there.

As brain-generated unpleasant emotional experiences extend to the body (which they often do), it is hard to imagine situations in which physiological defenses against emotions activated in the body would not lead to disruption of the vital flows in the body physiology. One might also think of the possibility that unpleasant emotional experiences could be created without involving any disruption in the vital flows in another way. For example, painful experiences could theoretically be generated through the stimulation of pain receptors that are distributed all over the body, without any disruption. However, physiological defenses such as constriction and numbing almost always occur in response to pain and do disrupt the vital flows of information and substances from one part of the physiology to the other.

The Effects of Physiological Defenses against Emotions on the Physiology of Regulation

As we saw in chapter 7, when we are coping with a situation with everything we have, our emotional experiences could become too much for us to handle, and they could start to compromise our ability to continue coping with the situation. This might happen because the dysregulation in our physiology could become so extreme as to threaten our very survival, as when our heart rate might go so high as to risk a heart attack; or our brain might be unable to bear the emotional experience because its threshold or limit for tolerating suffering is exceeded, as when the pain in the heart from a breakup is simply too much. The disruption caused by the threat to one's survival in the first instance, and the distraction from the unbearable suffering in the second, could interfere with and compromise our cognitive and behavioral processes involved in coping with the current situation.

We saw in chapter 7 that in order to prevent overwhelming emotional experiences from compromising our ability to cope with a situation, nature has provided us with a number of physiological defenses to manage them. For example, endogenous opioids, secreted as a defense against overwhelming emotions such as debilitating terror and helplessness in an extremely dangerous situation, can make a person feel paradoxically calm and collected so they can plot their escape cognitively and behaviorally. Such physiological defenses against extreme emotional experiences in the course of coping with difficult situations throughout our lives are indeed adaptive. They can be seen as additional coping mechanisms to make sure our emotional experience (our assessment of the impact of a situation on our well-being) does not in itself become disruptive of our ability to continue to cope with the situation through cognition and behavior.

However, physiological defenses against emotions come with a price. They tend to disrupt the vital flows and therefore dysregulate the physiology. For example, constriction dynamics can inhibit blood, lymph, and interstitial flows. Inhibition of respiratory and cardiovascular functions can also disrupt these three flows. Biochemical dynamics such as numbing can disrupt the flow of information through the nerves—information that needs to go between the brain and the body for the brain to sense and regulate what is happening in the body. However, these dynamics save the day in that they help prevent unbearable emotional experiences from overwhelming our cognition and behavior. Given the alternative— threats to our physiological and psychological survival—it is a small price to pay in the short run. However, physiological defenses against emotions can cause physiological and psychological dysfunction if they persist over the long term.

Not all physiological defenses against emotions might disrupt the vital regulatory flows. For example, arousal or charge as a defense against depression cannot be thought of as inhibitory of any of the vital flows, even though prolonged use of it can stress the physiology, create unpleasantness, trigger inhibitory defenses such as constriction and numbing, and in turn disrupt the vital flows. Most physiological defenses against emotions, such as constriction of tissue and movement, and inhibition of various biological functions, tend to be inhibitory and are therefore disruptive of vital regulatory flows.

We use the physiological and psychological defenses at our disposal to cope with unbearable experiences. Inhibitory physiological defenses against emotional experiences, such as constriction and numbing, are often biologically expensive because, as we have seen, they tend to disrupt the vital flows that regulate our physiology. Psychological defenses against emotional experiences that use our cognition and behavior to protect us might be less expensive. We can at times cognitively convince ourselves that our abusive partner is not really all that bad, so as to help ourselves feel less bad. Or we might just use work as a behavioral defense to feel good and avoid feeling how lousy our relationship is making us feel. However, we cannot continue to cope with an ongoing difficult situation such as a bad marriage in the long run only cognitively and behaviorally without physiological consequences.

We are less capable of using cognitive and behavioral defenses when we are children than when we are adults. For this reason, when children encounter traumatic situations, they are more likely than adults are to freeze and dissociate, as opposed to fighting, fleeing, or reasoning their way out of it. Children who have not had the necessary support and opportunity to work through their childhood traumas emotionally are also more likely to become adults who are prone to psychophysiological symptoms.

Our focus here is on how physiological defenses affect the physiology of regulation in terms of the vital flows that govern it. Our physiological defenses against overwhelming experiences in the middle of a crisis can unfortunately persist beyond the event, increasing the level of dysregulation in the physiology. They can kick in automatically if similar situations trigger unresolved emotions stemming from the original event. For example, a child can develop asthma from shutting down the respiratory physiology to manage the overwhelming experience of separation from their mother.[7] Just to be clear, please note that a child can develop asthma for many reasons, including allergies. And not all children separated from their mothers develop asthma as a psychophysiological symptom. Still, the child who develops asthma from the stress of separation from their mother might continue to have asthma attacks as an adult whenever there is a threat of a loss in relationship, if the adult has not worked through the trauma of the original separation.

The patterns of defense engaged during the loss can also become generalized and form automatic defensive reaction patterns to any event that causes significant stress, in relationships or other contexts. The constriction pattern on the right side of my cranium—resulting from my birth, in which I nearly died, along with my mother—continues to kick in and cause discomfort and dysfunction when I am stressed beyond a certain point, no matter the source of stress. In the field of pre- and perinatal psychology, the twisting constriction of the structures of the spine in the womb into a dysfunctional scoliosis pattern is believed to be a defense mechanism instinctually employed to manage overwhelming unpleasant emotional experiences, such as existential terror and fragmentation. In all these ways, physiological defenses against emotions can persist—like the emergency brake engaged in a dangerous road condition staying on after the danger has passed—and can thus contribute to psychological and psychophysiological symptoms, until there is no longer a reason for them to be triggered to defend against unbearable experiences.

How does one ensure that physiological or psychological defenses against overwhelming emotions used in difficult situations do not cause pathologies? A standard answer in psychology is that we have to resolve the emotions involved by working with the situations they arise in. To complete an emotional experience such as a heartbreak, so that we are not constantly defending against it by shutting our heart down as soon as it rears its ugly head from the unconscious, we need to get ahold of that experience and process it to the point that we have a sense that we can bear it. At that point we can get to a sense that we can live through it or we have lived through it, it is behind us, and we could live through it again if it were to happen again. Also, when we can tolerate the experience, it becomes possible to stay with the experience without shutting the brain and body physiology down. That way we can process the experience more optimally, not only emotionally but also cognitively and behaviorally. As we saw in chapter 6 on cognition, emotion, and behavior, the more unencumbered the physiology of the brain and body, the more functional all three can be.

How Undoing of Physiological Defenses against Emotions and Expanding the Emotional Experience in the Physiology Make It Easier to Process Unresolved Emotional Experiences

The primary reason we use psychological and physiological defenses against emotions is because they are painful. Even when we are defending against pleasant emotions such as love and power, as well as unacceptable cognitions and behaviors, we do so because of emotional consequences that we expect to be unpleasant. Emotional experiences are painful because of the levels of physiological dysregulation and stress that define them. To work with unresolved emotions contributing to our symptoms in therapy, we often need to make them conscious to begin with. That usually involves looking at the details of the situations in which they arise, working to undo the psychological and physiological defenses in their way, and providing the necessary external understanding, validation, and support to experience them for as long as might be necessary.

What we are asking of ourselves and those we are trying to help is to meet the necessary suffering of their unresolved emotions in the short run in order to reduce the unnecessary suffering from their symptoms in the long run. In the short run, that means we are increasing the level of dysregulation, stress, and distress in the physiology that define the unpleasant emotional experience.

No one likes to suffer if they can help it. I can personally vouch for that. So when we work with unresolved emotions that contribute to our symptoms, we are trying to push a boulder uphill. We are trying to increase the level of inherently painful physiological dysregulation, increasing distress in the physiology. We are, in short, asking for trouble. Psychological and physiological defenses can be expected to kick in and push the boulder downhill, countering our efforts to deepen the emotional experience toward its resolution. The physiological defenses that are engaged, to the extent that they inhibit the vital regulatory flows, will also subject the physiology to additional dysregulation, stress, and distress, even if it might appear on the level of conscious experience that there is some relief from the distress resulting from the attempt to reduce the unpleasant emotional experience through the defenses.

When we work to reduce physiological defenses against emotions that are adding to dysregulation in the physiology, and we are at the same time engaged in generating unpleasant emotional experiences in the same physiology, we are in effect reducing one source of dysregulation, discomfort, and distress in a person's experience. The more places in the physiology we remove the physiological defenses that are disrupting the vital regulatory flows, the less they contribute to the dysregulation, discomfort, and distress in accessing the unpleasant emotional experience, and the greater the person's ability to tolerate the expansion of the emotional experience in the physiology, even when it is painful.

This is one way in which emotional embodiment work increases affect tolerance (the ability to tolerate an emotional experience over a longer period). It can be likened to the experience of a person whose arms are being pulled in opposite directions. If one side stops pulling, the suffering would immediately be a lot less. We can verify this for ourselves next time we are having a painful physical or emotional experience. If we turn inward, we can find the pain as well as a felt sense of resistance to the pain. By simply saying to ourselves that we accept the pain for what it is, we can surprise ourselves with a drop in the level of suffering compared to just a moment ago. In moments of suffering, I try to remember and practice to the best of my ability (often unsuccessfully!) the wisdom I lavish upon others by reminding myself of the following statement: the resistance is half the suffering.

Another reason why emotional embodiment work increases affect tolerance has to do with the expansion of the emotional experience to as much of the body as possible. Emotion is an assessment of the impact of a situation on the entirety of the brain and body physiology, especially for overwhelming emotional experiences that motivated a person to resort to psychological and physiological defenses against the experiences at some point. Expanding the impact of a situation, even if it originally affected one part of the physiology more than another, distributes the impact's burden and makes it more bearable.

As an example, a car hit me on the right side of my body barely a week after I started my first doctoral study at Northwestern University. After the accident, while I was walking I would start to feel fear and unease on the right side of my body when it was exposed to the street. That emotional response would get stuck as a result of the left side of my body bracing along with the right side, as it did during the accident, leaving me anxious and uncomfortable for a long time. For the resolution to happen, the defensive reaction of bracing, which involves

constriction of tissue and movement, had to ease so that the vital regulatory flows could carry the information of the impact from the right
side to the left side. I resolved the issue by managing to get my fear and
unease to spread to my left side. To personally verify this dynamic, next
time you are in your dentist's office getting a shot, try to imagine relax-
ing your body to let the pain disperse, as opposed to constricting your
neck and gripping the chair with your hands, and discover for yourself
that it is an easier experience.

There is yet another way in which emotional embodiment work
might increase affect tolerance: by increasing the ability of different parts
of the physiology to help one another by facilitating the vital regulatory
flows among them. It is not uncommon for a physiological defense, such
as constriction or numbing in one part of the physiology, to interfere
with the exchange of regulatory information between that part and the
rest of the physiology, disrupting the regulatory processes between the
part and the whole and increasing the level of dysregulation, stress, and
distress locally as well as globally. From this perspective, undoing physiological defenses against emotions to integrate and coordinate the functioning of different parts of the physiology by improving the regulatory
flows among them could improve one's ability to tolerate the emotional
experience. Such integration could be expected to reduce the level of
regulation, stress, and distress throughout the physiology, even as one is
trying to process an unpleasant emotional experience.

Energy Psychology's Take on Why Expanding Emotional Experiences in the Physiology Makes It Easier to Tolerate Them

In energy psychology approaches such as Polarity Therapy, difficulties in
accessing and managing psychological experiences such as emotions are
theorized to arise from an uneven distribution of quantum or subatomic
energies in the brain and body physiology.[8] Whether these quantum
energies belong to the depths of the physiology or issue from an independent body interacting with it (an assumption in some approaches),

all of our experiences, physiological as well as psychological, are believed to arise from these quantum energies stimulating the physiology. When defenses in the quantum energy fields are worked through and the energies are more evenly distributed, there is less dysregulation, stress, and distress throughout the physiology, even when stimulating unpleasant emotional experiences in the physiology. The more even stimulation of the physiology by a more balanced quantum energy pattern distributes the emotional experience more evenly in the physiology, making it more bearable.

Why Unresolved Childhood Experiences Are Harder to Tolerate

A client once sought my help to alleviate her suffering from a constant fear she had had ever since childhood. This fear made her constantly look for a reason for it in her current life and engage in one activity or another to fix it. We used one of the objects of her fear that she identified—that she could die from an illness—to evoke the fear, and then we worked to get her to distribute the fear to more of her physiology until she could tolerate and stay with it. Then she could clearly see that the fear was nothing less than the fear of dying itself. What amazed her was that she could experience it throughout her brain and body physiology and observe that her mind was not spinning to come up with a reason for it or an action to fix it. Given the relative ease with which she could now handle a fear she had suffered from all of her life, she wondered why she had found it hard to fully grasp, let alone to stay with, until then.

After joking that this was because I would not have gotten the credit then, I set about exploring answers to the interesting question: why, every time I succeed in processing an overwhelming childhood emotion, do I find it to be somewhat of an anticlimax?

There is more than one reason for this paradoxical experience of finding that a long-avoided childhood experience is surprisingly not as hard to resolve as one had expected, given a long history of difficulty in resolving it. First, at the time of the experience, the child is less capable of tolerating it because of the child's immature physiology and psyche, with fewer cognitive and behavioral resources to cope with the experience. The child's affect tolerance threshold (the intensity of experience they can bear) is rather low, and the defenses that are readily employed are more physiological than psychological. The experience is buried in the unconscious, along with its physiological defenses in tow, to which more psychological defenses get added in later years, and marked as extremely dangerous and intolerable to go anywhere near. So when something now triggers it to the surface of consciousness, the physiological defenses as well as the later psychological defenses tend to engage rather quickly, even before the actual emotional experience is fully out the door. In a way, it is like putting a child in front of a closet door and asking them to open the door, and the child freaks out because they think there is a monster inside the closet. One has to use the adult ego to gently persuade the child ego to open the door and find that the actual experience is not as bad as the child might have imagined it to be.

The second reason why resolution may feel anticlimactic is that what is recalled is not exactly what one might have experienced back then in its original form. For example, no matter how hard I try, I cannot fully recall and reenact in my physiology the awful experiences of nearly dying in my birth and coming close to having cerebral palsy, with my skull crushed and stuck in a birth canal too small for my head, with the umbilical cord wrapped around my head, and with my mother—to whom I was still physiologically connected—on the verge of death herself. It is as though the child ego is expecting and guarding against that original experience, all that terror, fragmentation, and death anxiety, and not the pale symbolic emotional summary of it. So when recalled in the adult physiology in the here and now, it cannot be anywhere as intense, dreadful, or consequential as the child's original horrible experience, in flesh and blood, on the verge of death. Hence the relief when it is actually finally experienced as a weak version of the original.

The third reason why this type of resolution ends up being not as bad as expected is the predominant use of physiological defenses to guard against primal experiences from childhood, and their activation when we try to access the experience to work with it. They can kick in quickly and cause much disruption to the vital regulatory flows, stirring up a lot of dysregulation, stress, and distress when we actively try to go back to that experience. To use an earlier metaphor, there are more people trying to push the boulder downhill when we are trying to push it uphill. Getting rid of those folks who are well-intentioned but outdated—i.e., getting rid of the physiological defenses—makes it so much easier to move the boulder up the hill. Without the dysregulation, stress, and distress they cause, the emotional experience and its impact can disperse more through the present-day adult and more capable body. This can make the experiences of the watered-down version of the original experience that is behind the defenses more tolerable to be with. It can also get us to a place where we can resolve it successfully, with mastery, while being amazed at how and why it took us so long to get there.

Other Factors That Contribute to Affect Tolerance

We have seen how emotional embodiment can contribute to affect tolerance by decreasing dysregulation, stress, and distress in the processing of unpleasant emotional experiences that are, by definition, states of dysregulation, stress, and distress. Apart from emotional embodiment, there are other factors that contribute to a person's ability to tolerate emotions. The two most important factors that contribute to affect tolerance are a) the support we have for our emotions from others, and b) our own attitudes toward emotions. Let us look at each briefly.

Emotional support from others: The support one has for one's emotions from others is perhaps the most important factor determining a person's ability to experience and tolerate emotions. Research shows that the ability of a child to experience, identify, express, and tolerate a large range of emotional experiences is very highly correlated with corresponding abilities in the child's primary caregivers.[9,10] This can take the form of support from others in the present, or it can take the form of support from others in the past that the individual has internalized.

One's attitudes toward emotion: A person's attitude toward an emotion is an important factor in determining the person's capacity to experience and tolerate the emotion. There can be any number of such attitudes. For example, some people resist unpleasant emotions because they believe it is unhealthy to dwell on them. Some believe men should not show any vulnerability and women should not experience anger. Some people do not understand that unpleasant emotions are inherently difficult to experience because they are states of stress and dysregulation in the brain and the body, and that one has to override the innate resistance to unpleasant emotions to experience and process them for healing to take place. The more educated a person is about the role of emotion in physical and mental health, the more functional the person's attitude toward emotional experience is likely to be. Please note that the two factors discussed are related to each other. The more support one has for an emotion growing up, the more functional one's attitudes toward an emotion are likely to be.

Affect Tolerance, Symptom Threshold, Level of Body Expansion, and Formation of Psychophysiological Symptoms

Given the level of support we have for our emotions from others and the functionality of our own attitudes toward emotions, affect tolerance can be imagined as a function of the level of emotion (subjective assessment of whether it is high or low), the level of intensity (subjective difficulty in tolerating emotion), and emotional embodiment, as in the following diagram (figure 8.1). We can also see how symptom threshold, or the level of suffering at which a psychophysiological symptom forms in a person, might be increased and psychophysiological symptoms might be resolved through emotional embodiment.

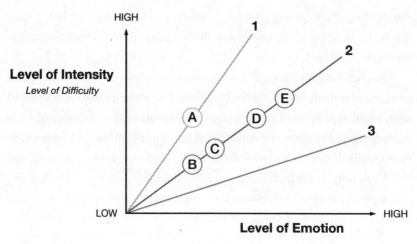

FIGURE 8.1 Relationship between Affect Tolerance and Emotional Embodiment

Figure 8.1 presents the relationship between the level of emotion (horizontal axis) and the level of intensity (vertical axis) as a function of the level of expansion of emotion in the physiology (lines 1, 2, and 3). Please note that the level of emotion and the level of intensity are not independent of each other. A person is likely to find higher levels of emotion to be more intense.

Lines 1, 2, and 3 represent increasing levels of emotional embodiment or expansion of emotion in the body and brain physiology. In general, the more embodied an emotion, the lower the level of intensity for every level of emotion. Line 1 corresponds to a scenario where emotion is least expanded in the body. Here, every level of emotion is experienced with higher levels of intensity than on lines 2 and 3, which correspond to higher levels of emotional embodiment. Point A refers to the limit or threshold beyond which psychophysiological symptoms form in a part of the body. When the body is expanded by undoing the physiological defenses against emotion to expand the experience of emotion in the physiology, this allows the person's affect tolerance profile to shift to a flatter line, 2, where every level of emotion is experienced with less intensity than on line 1.

What combinations of level of emotion and intensity of emotion might a person report after emotional embodiment work, on line 2, without forming the psychophysiological symptom? Here are some reports we typically hear from people who go through emotional embodiment work. In one scenario, the person might report the same level of emotion with less intensity overall and in every part of the physiology involved in the expansion of the emotional experience (point B). As we have mentioned before, when you lift the same load with two arms instead of one, both the overall strain and the strain on either arm are less than if one arm were to carry all the weight.

In another scenario, the person might report a higher level of emotional experience with less intensity in all the parts involved (point C). The load is heavier, but there are now two arms instead of one, and both the overall difficulty and the local difficulty in either arm are still lower than before.

Or the person might report a much higher level of emotion than at B and C, but the overall intensity, as well as the local intensity in every part involved in the expansion, might still not exceed the symptom threshold at D. Interestingly, at E the person might report a higher level of emotion and even a higher level of intensity than at D without forming the symptom. How might that be possible? Let us look for the answer in terms of the symptom threshold.

The threshold on line 1 is at A. In the immediate aftermath of emotional embodiment work that moves a person from line 1 to line 2, where is the new symptom threshold likely to be? It would seem that it has to be between B and D, at least in the short run, because the intensity or psychophysiological difficulty in some part of the body and brain physiology cannot be higher than at A, the symptom threshold on line 1.

There is yet another possibility that we run into as an outcome from emotional embodiment work. A person could well end up with a symptom threshold that is even higher on line 2 than point D, point E for instance, if not in the short run then in the long run. What this means is that in the more expanded and regulated brain and body physiology represented by line 2, even combinations of higher levels of emotion and higher levels of intensity, at A or D, might not trigger the psycho-physiological symptom. This can happen in the session itself, which can immediately become the basis for a new threshold, such as E on line 2, especially if the client is held at that level for a long time in the session for habituation or imprinting (depending on your theoretical point of view) for the new level of symptom threshold to be established.

Alternatively, the new threshold E on line 2 can be established over time. Just as a person who does weight training is able to lift increasingly more weight over time without injuring any muscles or increasing his or her body weight, the psychophysiology of a person who is doing emotional embodiment work with higher and higher levels of emotion and intensity without forming symptoms can develop the ability to experience higher levels of emotion and higher intensity overall, or in all parts of the physiology involved in the emotional experience, without forming a symptom.

Because the level of intensity or psychophysiological difficulty rises steeply with the level of emotion on lines such as 1, which represent lower levels of expansion and regulation in the body, we can expect people with potentially lower levels of body expansion due to stronger psychological and physiological defenses to have lower symptom thresholds. We can expect people with flatter lines—such as 3, representing abilities to experience higher levels of emotions with relatively lower levels of intensity—to have relatively higher thresholds in terms of combinations of levels of emotion and levels of emotional intensity.

In conclusion, please note that a number of factors, including a person's environment, might determine how much of the body can be expanded, how much emotion can be generated, and how much a person can tolerate emotional experiences without forming symptoms. We often find that we have shorter fuses when we are with our parents than with our friends, when we are hungry, or when we are sick. A person might have greater capacity for one emotion, such as anger, than for another emotion, such as sadness. So it is important not to think of an individual's capacity for emotion or affect tolerance as fixed, as though it were independent of the environment or particular emotions.

In the next chapter, we will discuss different types of emotions, some familiar and some unfamiliar, to enlarge our understanding of the range of emotional experiences we are capable of.

9

Different Types
of Emotions

Chapter summary: presents and discusses different kinds of emotions, including the always present but often overlooked sensorimotor emotions, with the aim of helping people to find emotions as quickly as possible to embody them.

Finding Emotion

Emotional embodiment work requires that emotions are available as conscious experiences. From teaching in over twenty countries spread across five continents, I have found that the general impression among a majority of mental health professionals around the world is that it takes time and a great deal of effort to get clients to experience their emotions, and that a relationship of trust has to be built over time between therapist and client for clients to feel comfortable enough to share their intimate emotional experiences. Emotions are indeed very intimate and shy things. Therefore, it makes sense that they could take a long time to emerge in relationships, therapeutic or otherwise. However, there is something about this perceived wisdom and widespread adherence to it among mental health professionals that has not always sat well with me.

You could say I am a therapy junkie. Even though I have had one Jungian analyst, Richard Auger in Los Angeles, as a constant companion for personal growth for more than twenty-five years, I have seen many other therapists as a client in the different therapeutic modalities in which I am trained. While I could not go anywhere near an emotion with some of them, even after spending a fair amount of time with them, there were others who were able to get me there rather quickly, sometimes even during the first session.

Looking back on what distinguishes these categories of therapists from each other, two things stand out. The therapists with whom I could access my emotions relatively quickly were those who were interested in my emotions from the very beginning, seemed to know many emotions, and had many ways to support me to come into them. They were likely to be body oriented in their practice and knew how to work to undo physiological defenses about emotions, defenses I did not know I had. These were also the therapists with whom I was able to establish a trusting relationship faster than with those who took longer to address my emotions, perhaps to establish a good enough relationship before broaching the topic. These reflections made me think of a psychological chicken-or-egg problem: which comes first in a relationship—emotion or trust?

Over time, I have evolved into the kind of therapist who believes that emotion can come first; that it is possible to engage clients emotionally from the very first session; and that how quickly a client can get to their emotions really depends on the therapist. It is true that there are clients who need a long-term relationship with their therapists to start to trust them with their emotional experiences; but an assumption that it is necessary for all clients is something I can easily and confidently quarrel with. In the course of developing emotional embodiment work, I have been looking for all kinds of things to teach therapists to help their clients to access their emotions faster. I have found that teaching therapists that there exist more types of emotions and a larger number of emotional experiences than we are taught in graduate school, teaching them about the language of emotions, and teaching them about how we experience them in our bodies is extremely important in building their ability to help their clients find emotions faster.

This chapter is about the different kinds of emotions and the larger number of emotional experiences we are capable of, what they feel like in our brain and body physiology, and the language we can use to elicit them, so we can more readily identify emotions in ourselves and those we work with, not only to heal but also to live a richer emotional life with a larger range of pleasant emotional experiences. Research has shown that those with greater emotional granularity—those who report a larger number of emotional experiences, with more nuance and differentiation— are more psychologically resilient.[1,2] Throughout this chapter, we will refer to the entirety of the brain and body physiology simply as the physiology, using the terms "brain physiology" and "body physiology" to make a distinction between the two when necessary.

A Broader Definition of Emotions

To generate a longer list of emotional experiences and build a wider net to catch them as quickly as possible, we first broaden our understanding of emotions to include emotions, feelings, affects, motivations, drives (such as sexuality), attitudes (such as positive, negative, or ambivalent), and temperaments (such as optimism and pessimism). Even hunger in the presence of a loved one and the lack of appetite in their absence can qualify as an emotion, as it reflects the impact of the environment on our well-being.

Researchers have drawn different distinctions among these terms for different purposes. Damasio defines all emotions as unconscious and a feeling as a conscious experience of an always unconscious emotion.[3] In the literature on emotions, emotions and feelings are understood as short-lived, more intense experiences in relation to specific situations. Moods are understood as less intense emotional experiences that have longer lives, often without a relationship to any specific situation. Temperaments, such as melancholic, are considered to be even longer-lasting than moods. Drives, such as hunger and sexuality, are thought of as instinct-driven calls for action. Of late, even attachment behaviors are considered to be drives that ensure our survival. "Affect" is a broader term that is understood to include emotions, feelings, and moods. We will refer to all of these experiences—short term and long term, less intense and more intense, more specific and more general—as emotions, as Candace Pert does in her book *The Molecules of Emotions*, so as to have a wider net to catch them.[4]

The Basic Emotions Approach

If we were to ask someone for a list of the most important emotions, the following emotions are most likely to be on their lists: happiness, sadness, fear, anger, shame, and guilt. This is because, from the very beginning of Western scientific research on emotions—which, we could argue, started with Charles Darwin—there has been an interest in and focus on identifying a set of emotions called basic or primary emotions that human beings share in common regardless of our culture, the expression of which can be easily detected on our faces, if not in our voices. There are many lists of basic emotions, and the emotions listed above appear in almost all of those lists.

Paul Ekman built on Darwin's research and initially listed happiness, sadness, fear, anger, surprise, and disgust as the six basic emotions.[5] He subsequently added amusement, contempt, contentment, embarrassment, excitement, guilt, pride in achievement, relief, satisfaction, sensory pleasure, and shame, to take the total number of basic emotions up to seventeen.[6] In one paper, Ekman even went as far as describing all emotions as basic.[7,8] The list compiled by Richard and Bernice Lazarus has sixteen emotions: aesthetic experience, anger, anxiety, compassion, depression, envy, fright, gratitude, guilt, happiness, hope, jealousy, love, pride, relief, and shame.[9] Alan Cowen and Dacher Keltner offer twenty-seven basic emotions: admiration, adoration, aesthetic appreciation, amusement, anger, anxiety, awe, awkwardness, boredom, calmness, confusion, craving, disgust, empathic pain, entrancement, excitement, fear, horror, interest, joy, nostalgia, relief, romance, sadness, satisfaction, sexual desire, and surprise.[10]

I do not mean to make your reading tiresome (which is another potential emotion!) by hitting you with one list after another. In fact, I have chosen to exclude some of the lists in the literature. The purpose of this exploration is twofold: first, to get you started constructing a broader vocabulary of emotions. How many of the emotions listed so far can you recognize in yourself or others? And how do you experience them in your physiology? Second, I want you to recognize that these lists might not account for all of your emotional experiences. For instance, you may not be able to find an emotional experience, such as loneliness, that you might be particularly aware of.

There are indeed a large number of emotional experiences. The Emotion Annotation and Representation Language proposed by the Human-Machine Interaction Network on Emotion (HUMAINE) classifies forty-eight emotions into ten categories, such as negative, forceful, positive, and lively.[11] In her book *The Book of Human Emotions: An Encyclopedia of Feeling from Anger to Wanderlust,* Tiffany Watt Smith offers a list of 154 emotions around the world in alphabetical order, with some emotions that have no parallels in the English language.[12] (Please see appendix A for the lists of emotions from the HUMAINE project and Smith's book.) A good webpage with additional lists of emotions and their associated meanings can be found at www.emotionalcompetency.com.[13]

Why learn so many emotions and their associated meanings? Why not just stick to a limited number of basic emotions? If these questions arise in you, please remember that the more you can differentiate emotional experiences in your physiology through language, the more granular (i.e., differentiated) they become, and the more you can regulate them. These lists might be a good place to start. As you go from one emotion to a related emotion, such as from sadness to grief, notice how the experiences of these emotions differ in your body.

You might notice that many more emotions are listed in the two lists in appendix A than in the lists of basic emotions we have seen. At the start, basic emotions were understood as universal emotions, experiences shared by all cultures and expressed especially through our faces and voices. They were not intended to capture all of our emotional experiences. To answer the question of how a limited number of basic emotions are related to all of our other emotional experiences, some followers of the basic emotions approach came up with the answer that a limited number of basic emotions are the ingredients of all our emotional experiences, as a few primary colors are the basic ingredients of all the colors we find in the world.

The wheel of emotions developed by psychologist Robert Plutchik, as illustrated in figure 9.1, is perhaps the most sophisticated of the models developed in this tradition.[14]

In this diagram, Plutchik's eight basic emotions are in the middle concentric circle: joy, trust, fear, surprise, sadness, disgust, anger, and anticipation. The eight basic emotions are combined in dyads and triads to arrive at secondary and tertiary emotions that can in turn be combined further to arrive at all of our emotional experiences, according to this theory. The words on the outer edges of the wheel, between two

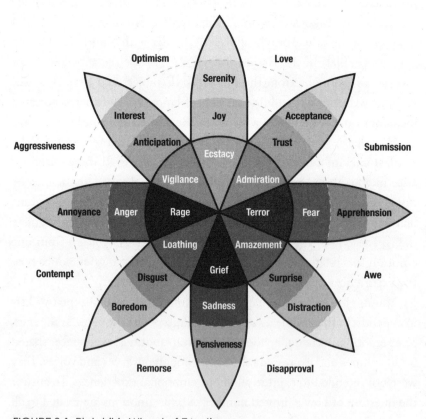

FIGURE 9.1 Plutchik's Wheel of Emotions

leaves, are secondary emotions arrived at by combining the two primary emotions represented by the leaves. For example, contempt is arrived at by combining anger and disgust. That appears to make sense. However, disapproval as a combination of sadness and surprise does not make as much sense. Would not anger be one of the components of disapproval? The idea that all of our emotional experiences can be arrived at by a combination of a limited number of basic or primary emotions quickly runs into such difficulties.

Plutchik's wheel of emotions model can be considered to be a combination of the basic emotions approach we have seen so far and the dimensional approach to emotions that came later, which we will discuss next. In each leaf of Plutchik's model, arousal increases as you move from the outside to the inside, generating emotional experiences of greater intensity. For example, fear with lower arousal is apprehension; fear with higher arousal yields terror. All emotional experiences vary along the dimension of arousal. This is a characteristic of the dimensional approach to emotions that distinguishes all emotional experiences in terms of two or three basic qualities, such as arousal.

The Dimensional Approach to Emotions

The dimensional approach to emotions is focused on capturing fundamental dimensions that characterize and differentiate all emotional experiences. For example, the circumplex model by James Russell arranges emotional experiences in a circle around two dimensions, arousal and valence (the degree to which an emotion is experienced as pleasant or unpleasant), as in figure 9.2. Calmness is a pleasant emotion characterized by low arousal or activation. Positive excitement is also a pleasant emotion but with a high arousal. Fatigue and tension are both unpleasant emotions at the opposite ends of the arousal or activation continuum. Russell, like other dimensional theorists, describes the valence dimension as the "core affect," which is "the neurophysiological state consciously accessible as simply feeling good or bad, energized or enervated."[15]

189

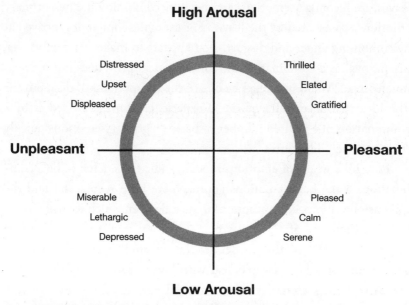

FIGURE 9.2 The Circumplex Model of Emotions

The Constructionist Approach to Emotions

As opposed to the basic emotions approach, which holds that evolution has built distinct physiological patterns for different emotional experiences into the architecture of the brain and the body, the constructionist approach to emotions posits that emotions are constructed in the present. Different constructionists emphasize different factors that contribute to the construction of emotions in the present. Social constructionists ignore biology and emphasize the importance of social roles, such as mother and father, and beliefs such as atheism, in the construction of emotions. According to psychological constructionists, emotions are not hardwired in the brain or the body but are constructed in the present from more basic ingredients such as thoughts and body experiences. Neuroconstructionists focus on how experience, in shaping the wiring of the brain, contributes to the construction of emotions in the present. The theory of constructed emotion by Lisa Feldman Barrett, combining social, psychological, and neuroconstructionist approaches, is the one used below in the discussion of differences between the basic emotions and constructionist approaches to emotions.[16]

Contrast between the Basic Emotions Approach and Constructionist Models of Emotion

In the basic emotions approach, every emotion is believed to have a distinct physiological pattern in the brain as well as the body. The number of basic emotions is limited, and all emotional experiences can be arrived at by a combination of two or more basic emotions. Therefore, the total number of emotional experiences is also limited in the basic emotions approach. In the constructionist approach, every situation first leads to predictions of likely emotion (impact of the situation on a person's well-being) in the brain, based on recall of past experiences stored in the brain. This prediction is then updated with current experiences of one's physiology in the situation. The brain then perceives very general physiological patterns (dimensions) in the updated information and links them to concepts in language, such as "it feels like a dagger in the heart," to arrive at emotions.

The constructionist approach disputes the theory that there are universal emotional experiences across cultures. The constructionist approach also does not believe that there is a distinct physiological pattern in the brain or body physiology for every emotion across all cultures. It is not that the constructionists do not allow for any body patterns in the construction of emotions by the brain. Rather, the constructionists hold that the physiological patterns used by the brain to construct emotions are very general in nature, such as arousal and valence, as we saw in the circumplex model of emotions.

Constructionists posit that the lack of uniformity across cultures and even subcultures in emotional experience is due to variations in physiological experiences in different contexts, and in language concepts used to describe them. An important difference between the basic emotions model and constructionism is that there is no limit on the number of emotions possible in the constructionist theory of emotions. Because we are interested in the possibility of embodying emotions in as much of the physiology as possible, it is important to note that the concept that generating emotion involves the entire brain and body physiology is the constructionist approach. This is also true in the basic emotions approach, at least among those who allow a role for the body in emotional experience.

A More Expansive View of Basic Emotions

Basic emotions such as happiness, sadness, fear, anger, disgust, and surprise are extremely important. As we have seen, most basic emotion theorists believe that there are universal emotional experiences across cultures that are easier to express through facial and vocal expressions. The more they looked for emotions in facial and vocal expressions, the more they found. Babies are known to have the innate ability to express basic emotions through facial and vocal expression shortly after birth, and discerning mothers are known to be able to recognize these emotions from early on, meaning that these expressions make it easier for others to know what we are going through emotionally.[17,18,19] Also, when we ask people what they are feeling, they usually respond in terms of such basic emotions. So it makes sense that we start exploring where we are emotionally or what others are going through emotionally with questions about the more easily available basic emotions that might be reasonably anticipated in a situation.

In the constructionist paradigm, the more complex, differentiated, and nuanced emotional experiences are called "specific instances of emotion." In the differentiation of all emotional experiences (specific instances of emotion) along the basic physiological dimension from good to bad (valence), we can see that a "good feeling" or a "bad feeling" is a basic or core quality in all emotional experiences, something our brain can construct or abstract and report faster than the more complex emotional experiences themselves. In fact, as we will argue in the section on sensorimotor emotions later in this chapter, a good feeling or a bad feeling is even more basic than the basic emotions such as happiness and sadness, and it qualifies as a basic emotion because whether a person is feeling good or bad can also be easily discerned in a person's facial or vocal expression, unless of course they are concealing it for some reason.

Why are basic emotions, such as sadness, easier to access than more granulated (complex, differentiated, and nuanced) emotional experiences, such as despair or the feeling of a knife twisting in the heart from a betrayal? Why is there so much research and evidence for specific brain locations and circuits for basic emotions, such as fear and anger? Why do they have more distinct physiological patterns in the face or the voice? The standard answer from the basic emotions approach to these questions is that evolution has chosen them and hardwired them into our brain and body physiology as quick, instinctual emotional reactions to different situations, to give us a survival advantage.

Yet how does one reconcile that answer with the evidence we have seen in chapter 5 that the brain is also capable of making emotions in other ways—by recalling past emotional experiences in similar situations to predict emotional responses to current situations, or by marrying specific or general patterns in the information on a situation's impact on the physiology with language concepts? I struggled with this question for some time. And the answer I came to was relatively simple: basic emotions—whether they are generated through instinctual emotional circuits laid down by evolution in the brain or the body, or through recall of past emotional experiences, or from matching broad patterns of current information from the physiology with language concepts—are quick takes on the impact of a situation on our well-being, requiring less information processing from the brain than more complex emotions, which require more time and neurological resources to generate, if not make conscious.

It is well known that our brain is capable of arriving quickly at overall impressions of situations as good or bad, favorable or unfavorable, before it processes the situation thoroughly, and that it takes more time and neurological resources to arrive at a confirmation, a revision, or a more complex understanding of the initial impression. The amygdala, part of the so-called limbic brain, has been identified as an important structure involved in such rapid information processing.[20] When the brain receives from the physiology complex information on the impact of a situation, it can use this ability for rapid information processing to get a quick take on how the situation is impacting us as well as how to respond to the situation. For example, we might quickly process a situation as unfavorable and respond to it with fear or anger, only to revise it later as requiring neither, upon further processing. As long as the initial emotional assessment or response such as happiness is not totally contradicted by subsequent analysis, all the subsequent detailed assessments of the impact—that is, all the subsequent emotions—will have happiness as a basic quality or dimension.

We can think of a basic emotion such as happiness and sadness as an underlying common quality or theme across a large number of similar instances of emotion (to use the language of the constructionists). A basic emotion can be arrived at before the construction of more complex emotions, as a quick take on the impact of the situation through instinctual emotional reactions in the brain or the body, from recall of past emotional experiences in the brain, or through quick processing of current information from the physiology. It could also be abstracted from the more complex emotions after their construction, as the brain is known to have the ability to abstract common qualities among similar experiences.

Let us illustrate these ideas with an excellent framework of emotions put forth by Gerrod Parrott at Georgetown University.[21] Parrott's list of basic emotions consists of love, joy, surprise, anger, sadness, and fear. He groups the other emotions into secondary and tertiary emotions, arriving at a grand total of 146 emotions. (This list is also useful for building our vocabulary of emotional experiences, organized into categories that make it easier to learn them.) You might have noticed that a secondary emotion such as affection is also listed as a tertiary emotion here. This is because Parrott's model is in the form of a tree. Here, a secondary emotion is not a combination of primary emotions, and a tertiary emotion is not a combination of secondary emotions, as in the theory of basic emotions. Love is akin to a major branch of the tree of emotion; secondary emotions such as affection and lust are the smaller branches off the love branch; and tertiary emotions such as attraction and affection are still smaller branches off the affection branch. Affection appears as a secondary emotion as well as a tertiary emotion probably because affection is an emotion that can be experienced in so many different ways.

When we examine the secondary and tertiary emotional experiences associated with a basic emotion, we can see that the basic emotion is a basic or core quality in all of them. For example, sadness can be seen as a common quality that can be abstracted from depression, despair, hopelessness, gloom, glumness, unhappiness, grief, sorrow, woe, misery, and melancholy; or it can be arrived at prior to them as a quick take on the impact of a situation through instinct or history, and accorded the status of a basic emotion. In the same way, anger can be seen as a common quality in instances that generate rage, outrage, fury, wrath, hostility, ferocity, bitterness, hate, loathing, scorn, spite, vengefulness, dislike, and resentment, or it can be arrived at prior to them through instinct or history, and labeled as a basic emotion. When the basic emotions are arrived at prior to the generation of more differentiated versions of them, they might also prime the brain and make the analysis of current information from the physiology more efficient. For example, if happiness were triggered as a quick take by instinct or from historical data, the brain might first look for patterns that have happiness as their core quality in the current physiological information and in the search for language concepts to describe them.

TABLE 9.1 Parrott's Framework of Emotions

PRIMARY EMOTION	SECONDARY EMOTION	TERTIARY EMOTION
Love	Affection	Adoration, affection, love, fondness, liking, attraction, caring, tenderness, compassion, sentimentality
	Lust	Arousal, desire, lust, passion, infatuation
	Longing	Longing

(continues)

TABLE 9.1 Parrott's Framework of Emotions *(continued)*

PRIMARY EMOTION	SECONDARY EMOTION	TERTIARY EMOTION
Joy	Cheerfulness	Amusement, bliss, cheerfulness, gaiety, glee, jolliness, joviality, joy, delight, enjoyment, gladness, happiness, jubilation, elation, satisfaction, ecstasy, euphoria
	Zest	Enthusiasm, zeal, zest, excitement, thrill, exhilaration
	Contentment	Contentment, pleasure
	Pride	Pride, triumph
	Optimism	Eagerness, hope, optimism
	Enthrallment	Enthrallment, rapture
	Relief	Relief
Surprise	Surprise	Amazement, surprise, astonishment
Anger	Irritation	Aggravation, irritation, agitation, annoyance, grouchiness, grumpiness
	Exasperation	Exasperation, frustration
	Rage	Anger, rage, outrage, fury, wrath, hostility, ferocity, bitterness, hate, loathing, scorn, spite, vengefulness, dislike, resentment
	Disgust	Disgust, revulsion, contempt
	Envy	Envy, jealousy
	Torment	Torment
	Suffering	Agony, suffering, hurt, anguish

PRIMARY EMOTION	SECONDARY EMOTION	TERTIARY EMOTION
Sadness	Sadness	Depression, despair, hopelessness, gloom, glumness, sadness, unhappiness, grief, sorrow, woe, misery, melancholy
	Disappointment	Dismay, disappointment, displeasure
	Shame	Guilt, shame, regret, remorse
	Neglect	Alienation, isolation, neglect, loneliness, rejection, homesickness, defeat, dejection, insecurity, embarrassment, humiliation, insult
	Sympathy	Pity, sympathy
Fear	Horror	Alarm, shock, fear, fright, horror, terror, panic, hysteria, mortification
	Nervousness	Anxiety, nervousness, tenseness, uneasiness, apprehension, worry, distress, dread

The Missing Emotions: Simple and Complex Sensorimotor Emotions

We saw earlier how it is expedient to initiate our inquiry with basic emotions such as happiness and sadness for a number of reasons. Unfortunately, basic emotions such as fear and anger are subject to social inhibition, especially because they are easy to express through our face and voice, unless of course we were fortunate enough to have plenty of support from others to express them while growing up. However, if we look closely at the statements people make when they seek our help, most of the time they are saying they need our help not to feel as bad as they have been feeling. "Feeling bad" is an emotion because it is an assessment that some situation in their life is having an adverse effect on their well-being, which is our definition of emotion. We can start the process of embodying that emotion by expanding it to as much of the body as possible. In James Russell's dimensional theory of emotions that we saw earlier, feeling good and feeling bad are the polarities along the dimension of valence, but they are not identified as emotions in themselves or presented as such in the various lists of emotions. This probably explains why we might overlook them when our clients tell us they are feeling quite bad in the situations in which they find themselves.

We just saw above how basic emotions such as happiness and sadness can be thought of as abstract qualities of categories of emotions whose generation can precede or succeed more detailed emotions. We also saw how basic emotions might be quick first responses to situations from memory or activation of instinctual emotional circuits, and how they lend themselves to facial and vocal expressions recognized around the world. What about feeling good or bad? Whether one is going to feel good or bad in a situation is easy to access. These feelings are easy to express on one's face and in one's voice. It is easy to detect them in facial and vocal expressions of others, at times with greater ease than basic emotions such as sadness and happiness. They are easier to recall from memory. They are likely to have been built into instinctual emotional brain circuits, as we are often able to quickly come up with statements such as "I have a good/bad feeling about this" before we can differentiate them into more specific emotions.

So, feeling bad is the most basic of all unpleasant emotions, including basic emotions such as sadness and fear; or it is their core quality, generated before or after a variety of unpleasant emotions. Clients tell us they are feeling bad in the very act of seeking our help to alleviate their suffering. When other emotions are difficult to access because of social inhibition, we can go to this very basic emotion of feeling bad to start the process of emotional embodiment. We can tell them we understand that they are seeking help because they feel bad enough about something, and then we can ask them where in their body they feel bad, to start the process of embodying it.

If we can address what is in the core of any unpleasant emotion that makes it hard to tolerate the emotion, locate it in the body, and expand it to develop a capacity to tolerate it, we can build a capacity for all unpleasant emotions that have this universally undesirable quality in their core, and we can make it easier to allow them into our awareness and be with them. This is exactly what I often find when I am working with people who come in and have no access to the basic emotions such as sadness or fear. Linking their awareness of feeling bad in the body or brain physiology to facial expressions and vocalizations often helps them reach the next level of basic emotions such as sadness and fear. There are other emotions that are equivalent to feeling bad; feeling unpleasant, uncomfortable, painful, awful, terrible, overwhelming, and stressed are examples of other basic emotions that can be used instead of the simple emotion of feeling bad, and one of them might resonate with some people more than the simple emotion of feeling bad.

When we look at the lists of emotions, not only do we rarely find simple physical states such as good and bad; we also find other simple and more complex physiological states that can easily qualify as emotions. Feeling empty when a loved one is not around and feeling full when they are; feeling fragmented or together in one's sense of self; feeling satisfaction or dissatisfaction, stressed or relaxed, pleasure or pain, weak or strong, and numb or alive are examples of relatively simple physiological states that qualify. More complex examples of this kind of emotion can be found in descriptions such as:

I feel as though I have been run over by a truck.

It felt as though she stabbed me in the heart and turned the knife a few times.

My body feels like a black hole.

The body felt like a rotting corpse infested with live maggots.

To counteract the distaste of these rather unpleasant examples (and to make sure you do not drop this book), how about these:

My body felt so sweet, as though it were my favorite chocolate.

My body felt as though it were being streamed with wave after wave of grace.

I felt as solid as a mountain.

We find such expressions abundantly in fiction and poetry, but rarely in our clinical settings, probably because the psychological literature on emotions generally excludes them, and because the body and its experience are by and large excluded in most psychological approaches.

What shall we call this type of emotion, which is more common and frequent in our experience than those we find on the lists—a name that will draw attention to itself and stick in one's mind so it is not forgotten? We can call them "body emotions"; but then, are not all emotions of the body? I think I read somewhere that such psychologically meaningful physiological states could be called "sensorimotor emotions," but I have not been able to backtrack and locate the source. Did I make it up? I am not sure. But when I use the term in my classes, it gets people's attention. They start to differentiate it from other types of emotions and give it the importance it deserves. So, I have stuck to the term "sensorimotor emotions" to describe these emotions.

Sensorimotor emotions can be building blocks of other emotions. For example, loneliness is often experienced as an unbearable physiological experience of emptiness. Sensorimotor emotions can also be the sources of abstraction for better-known emotions. For example, happiness can be abstracted from states of pleasure or satisfaction. Sensorimotor emotions can also combine with basic emotions to offer better explanations of how some emotions might be constructed. For example, if emotions can be arrived at by combining other emotions, the experiences of despair or helplessness are better captured through the combination of sadness and loss of energy than from any combination of basic emotions.

If a person is not able to identify emotions in an adverse situation, we can guide that person to look for basic sensorimotor emotions such as feeling bad, awful, painful, stressful, upset, or unpleasant, in the brain or body physiology. At times, even when no other emotions emerge, embodying these basic sensorimotor emotions might be adequate to resolve the presenting symptoms. If they do not resolve, how do we go from these simple sensorimotor emotions to other emotions? Let us explore, first by discussing a bit of interesting information on the physiology of emotions as a background for our exploration.

Facial Affect System

In the physiology of emotions, the face and throat physiologies are somewhat special, as they have evolved to play multiple roles with respect to emotions. They are specialized to express emotions through facial expressions and vocalizations. They can express the many basic emotions, such as happiness and sadness, as well as simple sensorimotor emotions, such as pain and pleasure, soon after birth. Emotions are expressed through the face and throat physiology more than through other parts of the body physiology. Through facial and vocal expressions, we communicate our emotions to others and get the necessary help to regulate them. There is also some relief, or even pleasure, experienced from the very act of expressing emotions.

The face and throat physiologies are powerful generators of emotional experiences as well as defenders against them. If you doubt this, assume an unhappy face or voice and make the following statement: "I am happy now." Experience for yourself the powerful contradiction between your happy statement and the unhappiness you have just generated in the face and the throat. Because our faces and voices can mimic the faces and the voices of others, they can help us physiologically simulate and generate the emotional experiences of others within us. Other parts of the physiology can do this as well, but not nearly to the same degree. Further, facial and vocal expressions of emotions are almost always accompanied by nonverbal expression and expansion of emotion in more of the brain and body physiology. Inhibiting the participation of facial muscles in emotional experiences is known to inhibit emotion processing and recall in the brain.[22]

In the physiology of emotions literature, there is a distinction between the facial affect system and the visceral affect system.[23] According to this theory, the facial affect system is designed to express the emotional experience in the visceral affect system. The integration of these two affect systems is considered to be a developmental achievement in the growth of a human being, a development that is aided by caregivers. The lack of integration of the two systems is a fertile ground for psychophysiological symptom formation. When I read this theory, I wondered whether the facial affect system, which I expanded to include the throat, could be used to increase the range of emotional experiences—to increase emotional granularity, so to speak—in those whose emotional range is limited to simple sensorimotor emotions such as pain and pleasure (or to basic emotions such as happiness and sadness, for that matter). I also wondered whether the facial affect system could be used to resolve psychophysiological symptoms in those who are known to have had early adverse childhood experiences and limited capacity for emotional experiences.

To find out, I developed the following interventions and tried them on myself and my clients. When all a client could sense was a simple sensorimotor emotion of a bad feeling, discomfort, or pain in response to a situation, I first helped them expand the emotional experience in the body physiology to see if developing a capacity for it helped the client to get to more differentiated emotional experiences, more complex sensorimotor emotions, basic emotions, or other complex emotions that are the close cousins of the sensorimotor emotion.

If that intervention did not lead to more complex emotions, or if I could not get the client to expand emotion in the body physiology, I invited them to imagine someone else or themselves expressing the generic feeling in their body through facial expression or vocalization. Sometimes I would even have them actually express it on their face or in a vocalization, while I would mirror their facial expression or vocalization with my own, to support them and to get a sense of what they might be feeling. For those who are extremely inhibited, imagining someone else express the feeling facially and vocally, or just imagining themselves expressing the feeling that way, is often less threatening than doing it outwardly right away. This is how I found out that these simple manipulations of the emotional physiology of the face and throat areas could quickly lead to the emergence of more differentiated emotional experiences and to surprisingly quick resolution of long-term psychophysiological symptoms.

Bringing It All Together

We have expanded the range of possible emotional experiences by adding simple and complex sensorimotor emotions to the traditional simple and complex emotions on various lists. We have differentiated the physiology of emotions into the brain, the body, and the face and throat, the primary physiology of emotional expression. Let us now look at some ways in which we can bring them all together to find emotional experiences and embody them as quickly as possible.

Emotions can be generated in either the brain or the body first, or in both places at the same time, and they have the potential to spread throughout the brain and body physiology, if unimpeded.[24] As we saw in chapter 7, their flow can be impeded by any number of psychological and physiological defenses that can remain in place or get reactivated whenever those emotional experiences get stimulated again, leading to cognitive, emotional, behavioral, and psychophysiological symptoms. The primary physiology used in emotional expression, the face and throat, can be used as an efficient bridge to bring together as well as to differentiate emotional experiences that arise in the brain or the body.

When the emotional experience is limited to the brain, we can expand it into the face and the neck through facial expression and vocalization. There is evidence that doing this improves the brain's ability to process the emotion and its context, to differentiate them as well as to remember them.[25] That is, the face and throat physiology can help us in understanding, decoding, and differentiating the emotional experiences that originate in the brain. It can also potentially increase the expansion of the emotion into the rest of the body because nonverbal expression and expansion of emotion in the body usually accompany the verbal (this time vocal) expression of it.

Expansion of the emotional experience into the rest of the body is very important. If emotional experiences are confined to the brain alone, they could be just reflective of our instinctual and historical emotional reactions. If they are not reality-tested against current information from the physiology, they are bound to be less than optimal, leading to inappropriate cognitive, emotional, and behavioral responses. So facial expression and vocalization, by connecting the brain and the rest of the body beyond the face and throat areas, can help in integrating the brain and body physiologies in emotional experience.

In the other direction, when the body physiology is contributing to emotional experience, the activation of the face and throat physiology through facial expression and vocalization can help the brain process the information from the body physiology for its emotional significance. The face and throat physiology can be a major bridge in expanding emotional experiences in both directions, from the brain to the body and vice versa.

We now turn to the methodology section, in which the concrete steps of emotional embodiment are presented in greater detail.

PART III

PRACTICE:
The Four Steps of
Emotional Embodiment

In this part of the book, we will take a more systematic look at the nuts and bolts of how to go about the process of embodying emotions. We can use this information to work with emotions in our clients and, to a certain extent, ourselves.

If you are not a therapist, please note that you need to seek the help of a mental health professional if you find yourself in a difficult place in your practice of embodying your emotions. This advice also applies if you are a therapist, for two reasons. First, working with your emotions by yourself can go only so far. All of us need emotional support from time to time, from at least one other person, to resolve our emotions. Nature has just set it up that way. It is easier and quicker to process emotions with the support of others than on one's own. Second, only the most basic information for the practice of embodying emotions is provided here. More detailed technical information in relation to emotional embodiment work is presented in the Integral Somatic Psychology (ISP) professional trainings, which are limited to those working in the helping professions. Regardless, I hope that as many of you as possible, in various therapy modalities as well as other walks of life, find the material in these chapters to be of immediate use for navigating the choppy waters of emotional experiences in yourselves and those you serve.

The process of emotional embodiment has been conceptualized as involving four steps: 1) the situation; 2) the emotion; 3) the expansion; and 4) the integration. Please note that the four steps need not always be implemented in the sequence they are presented. As is often the case, it is possible that a situation might warrant going back and forth between the steps or starting with a later step in the sequence. It is better to look at these four steps as ingredients for an emotional embodiment session that need to be added to the mix as and when needed to keep the process on track, rather than as a rigid sequential protocol. We will examine each of the steps in the four chapters that follow.

When I conceptualized the practice of embodying emotion in four steps, I did not think I would have to write much on the first two steps. I assumed that the tasks of zeroing in on a situation, eliciting a relevant emotion, and keeping it alive by providing adequate support would be second nature to most psychotherapists and that I would have to write more on the more technical steps of expansion and integration. To my surprise, for whatever reason, what I found in country after country is a common difficulty in helping clients find a relevant situation to focus on and then guiding and supporting them to access and stay with an emotion in relation to the situation. Expansion and integration of brain and body physiology without emotion would only regulate unpleasant emotion away if a therapist did not continue to refer to the situation and support the emotion, as often as necessary. Even though the four steps have not been clearly defined for you yet, please keep in mind the importance of the first two steps throughout the process of embodying emotion.

As a medium for communicating how to go about the practice of embodying emotion, a book containing words and pictures is limited at best. To overcome this limitation, we have set up free secure online access to videos of complete demonstration sessions of emotional embodiment work, as well as shorter illustrative videos of the steps involved in the practice of embodying emotion. To gain access to this free online resource, please visit www.integralsomaticpsychology.com, then click "Books," then "Embodying Emotion," and then "Resources" in successive dropdown menus, and register.

10

The Situation

Chapter summary: shows how important details of a situation or context can be used to evoke and maintain an emotional response, for the purpose of embodying it.

When we are working with an emotional difficulty to resolve it, the work is almost always in relation to a particular situation. Therefore, in working with emotions, it is important to stick to one situation as much as possible, unless of course it is helpful to refer to other situations. It is possible that triggering many situations from memory when we are working with an emotion in one situation can make the emotional experience simply too much to handle. It could also dissipate the emotion as the brain gets busy with the distraction of processing the many cognitive and behavioral aspects of the other situations. In some people, the brain's attempt to distract from the focus on an unbearable emotion or its frantic search among other situations for a solution to end the suffering in the first situation can even become a defense against staying with an emotion. We will see in the next chapter that when we are working with an emotion in one situation, other emotions can pop up in rapid succession, either as a sign that the current emotion is too much to bear or as a pattern of avoiding the suffering involved in staying with one emotion. Therefore, in emotional embodiment work, as a general rule we stay with one emotion in one situation at a time, unless of course there are reasons not to.

An emotion can be thought of broadly as an assessment of the impact of a specific situation, or a series of situations, on a person's well-being. One's reaction to a situation depends on the person's understanding of the situation. It is contingent upon what the person thinks is feasible in terms of what can be done to cope with the situation. For example, if I have my computer bag stolen at a train station, my emotional reaction would vary depending on whether I think my passport is also in the bag and whether I remember that I just made a complete backup of my computer that very morning. It would also depend on whether I have enough resources through insurance or other means to replace the computer. So it can be said that one's emotional reaction to a situation is determined by one's cognition of the situation and one's behavior (perceived as feasible) in the situation. According to Barrett, the brain rapidly simulates a number of emotional reactions to a situation based on a variety of cognitive and behavioral predictions, and it chooses one as the most feasible reaction on the basis of past experiences in similar situations and constant updating of information about the current situation.[1] Please note that none of these processes need to be conscious. Some of it can be, but they are unconscious more often than conscious.

When clients come to us, it is usually to seek relief from a situation that stresses them emotionally. In order to help them, we need to first support them to clarify their understanding of the situation and of the feasible coping behaviors available to them. It is possible that their emotional difficulty might resolve just from cognitive or behavioral change. This might be true not only for emotional experiences that have to do with the present but also for those that have to do with the past. Guilt that one feels in relation to another person can at times be resolved through a heartfelt apology, whether the incident in question is recent or far in the past. Understanding that another person had a good reason for separating from you that had nothing to do with you, for example, can contribute to your healing, whether it happened last week or forty years ago.

In general, emotional difficulties that have to do with the present are more resolvable through cognitive and behavioral change than those having to do with the past. For example, in a current situation involving domestic violence, cognitive and behavioral change can be seen as immediate and feasible remedies for emotional suffering. A cognitive change from "he beats me because he is jealous" and "he is jealous because he loves me" to "not everyone who loves is either as jealous or as physically abusive" is a step in the right direction. Changing from "I cannot imagine leaving the relationship" to "I have made concrete plans to leave the relationship in a day or two and there is no going back" is a positive behavioral development in the dire situation. Both can shift the way one feels in the current situation.

However, even in ongoing situations, some might have to work through the unpleasant emotional consequences standing in the way of necessary cognitive and behavioral changes. For example, one might have to work to manage the fear that might surge when one contemplates leaving the abusive situation. Given the increasingly lower levels of capacity for affect tolerance in the general population, emotional embodiment work might even be necessary in a large percentage of cases where the situation causing the difficulty is still active.

Please note that a situation of domestic violence is often complex. For example, there are many other reasons, such as finances, that might prevent a person from leaving an abusive relationship; and love is not always present in situations of battery. I add this caution so that no reader, especially one who has experienced domestic violence, is confused by the very limited example I have presented above.

The need to increase capacity for the emotional experience is all the greater when the situation causing the emotional distress is in the past. The inability to get over a past relationship, despite having replaced it with another one, is an example of a situation where there is no way around having to do the hard emotional work. Otherwise, healing changes in one's cognition (believing that the current partner is in no way inferior to the one that got away) and in one's behavior (spending more time with the current partner as opposed to avoiding her) might not be possible. This would especially be the case when the person shut down the brain and body physiology to cope with an intolerable emotional experience in the past and has not been able to resolve it ever since, because of a lack of capacity to tolerate the emotional experience of processing it. Because cognition and behavior also depend on the body (we saw how in chapter 6), the body that is shut down from intolerable emotion would make it difficult to change cognition and behavior to resolve the emotional difficulty.

More often than not, when people go to therapists for help, the symptoms they seek relief from (physical, energetic, cognitive, emotional, behavioral, or relational) have emotional difficulty as their cause. The evidence-based therapeutic modality of emotion-focused therapy approaches all mental health issues as emotional problems.[2] Often, what looks like a person's reaction to a situation in the present is actually the person's reaction to a situation in the past that the current situation has triggered deep within the person's unconscious. That is what transference reactions are all about—the stuff that is usually worked through in therapy or as a result of reflections from close friends.

When people are emotionally distressed, they can usually pinpoint one or more situations as the cause, but sometimes they do not know what is causing their distress. It is possible that their unconscious is trying to manage their distress by hiding the connection between their emotional suffering and a situation in their present or past that might be more clear to others around them. Or they may just report a psychophysiological symptom and say they have no idea what might have caused it. For example, a person might report that they have been depressed and do not know why. Or, one might present asthma as a possible psychophysiological symptom after medical examinations had failed to produce an organic cause, such as allergy. A person might also present cognitive symptoms, such as noticeable difficulties in their ability to remember or plan, or behavioral symptoms, such as no longer having the motivation to get up early in the morning to continue writing their book—a symptom I can attest to—with no knowledge of the symptom's source. They might present a physical symptom such as chronic pain and even insist that there is nothing psychological about it, even after they have pursued many medical options in their quest for a cure and have come up empty.

Usually, with a little bit of inquiry, we can find a situation in the present or the past as a place to start in searching for the cause of a symptom. There are some questions that are particularly helpful in unearthing situations that might have some link to a client's suffering. We can ask questions such as the following:

- How long have you been suffering from this emotion or symptom?

- When did you start to notice that you have this problem or symptom?

- Did anything out of the ordinary happen to you or a loved one around this time?

- What significant life changes did you experience in your life around this time?

- In your work life or in your personal life, did you experience a setback or a loss of a person, relationship, or job?

- In which situations do you find the symptom increasing, and what situations appear to help in decreasing your suffering?

In a real-life case of a person who suffered from depression, it turned out the cause was a recent breakup. He did not think the relationship had anything to do with the depression because he was really not all that involved in the relationship, and he had been the one to end it. In the real-life case of a woman who reported asthma with no medical diagnosis or psychological condition as its cause, it turned out again that it had to do with the ending of a relationship a year prior. She had broken up with a man whom she said she had loved more than anyone else, because he had disappointed her in some way. Again, she did not think her asthma had anything to do with it, because it was she who had ended it. The example of her treatment through emotional embodiment and the surprisingly quick outcome can be found in chapter 2.

Sometimes, merely connecting an emotional reaction in a current situation with a past situation, which would be a cognitive insight or change, is adequate to resolve the symptom. Here is a real story that provides a dramatic example. A young woman who was having a psychotic episode called her mother during the episode and said, "Mother, I am standing next to an open window on the sixteenth floor of a high-rise building. I am going crazy. Unless you tell me what I need to know, I am going to jump."

Here is what her mother said in reply: "Please do not jump. Please sit down and hear what I have to say, as this could come as a shock to you. Your father had another family in a neighboring town—a family with children—the whole time you were growing up."

We have known since the time of Sigmund Freud that family secrets can cause tremendous upheaval in the psyche and can result in severe mental illness. Thus, when the young woman heard what her mother had to say, she became clear, got down from the window, and was cured of her psychotic episode.

Here is a less dramatic example from couples therapy. A man became convinced that his wife was cheating on him, and he started thinking about hiring a private detective to follow her. The couple's therapist knew the man well because he had seen him separately in individual therapy for a while, and the therapist discerned that the intensity of the husband's jealousy might have been triggered by a current stressor in the husband's life: the possibility of job loss. The therapist reminded the husband that he had witnessed such episodes of jealousy between his parents too many times, and he suggested that the fear of losing his job might be somehow triggering it now. That led to the man snapping out of his emotional trance and reacting to the current situation with his wife differently.

Given the intensity of the emotion involved, I would have thought this situation needed deep work with the emotion to change the cognition. So when I heard this story from a colleague, I was reminded of the power of cognition in bringing about change.

At times, linking a present situation to the past resolves the issue in the present. Pointing out to a client that their reaction to their wife appears to be a known reaction to their mother might be enough to change the reaction to the wife. Sometimes this helps to get the person to a place where they can start to process the emotions involved, now that their intense reaction to a person in the present is somewhat lessened. With the insight that the reaction to the wife might have to do with past experience with the mother, the client might calm down enough and become agreeable to working with the emotion that is now less intense.

Often, to get to a past situation that is triggered in the present but is buried deep in the client's unconscious, or to get a real felt sense of connection between the present and the past that is needed for a therapeutic change, it is necessary to embody the emotions in relation to the present situation. An example of the first instance is a woman who, after embodying her suffering from jealousy caused by her suspicion that her husband is cheating on her, can shift her attitude toward her husband upon recognizing that this jealousy is a feeling she often used to feel in almost all her close relationships. An example of the second instance is a man who, after acquiring a capacity to tolerate the fear of dying triggered by his girlfriend leaving him, states that he had always known that his inability to let go of his girlfriend had to do with his traumatic separation from his own mother as an infant immediately after birth, but he had not been able to "feel" the connection to such an extent before.

When a client is very upset about a situation, if the upset cannot be resolved by working with cognition, emotion, or behavior in relation to the current situation, therapists often look for a past situation that might be triggering the present activation. In emotional embodiment work, the question often arises as to which situation to work with—present or past—when both possibilities are available. Here, the general rule is to work with the situation that is more emotionally evocative. It makes sense to work with the situation that is more emotionally charged to begin with, to develop a greater capacity for emotions in that situation, so that the person is in a better position to work with the other situation emotionally, because that might be the situation that really holds the key to the resolution of the problem. If both situations are emotionally evocative, one has to apply further discrimination. At times, people who have had a lot of therapy have a tendency to regress to familiar situations from the past, with familiar emotional experiences. This could even be a defense against experiencing the pain resulting from what is happening in the current situation. In such instances, it makes sense to choose to work in relation to the present situation. I usually try to work with the present, not the past, unless of course the involvement of the past and the need to work with it becomes clear in working with the present.

If one is unable to discover a situation that might have a relationship to the symptom, one can look for any situation in the person's life that is stressful emotionally or otherwise to begin the process of embodying emotions. People with a tendency to form physiological symptoms, such as chronic pain, in relation to psychological problems might find it difficult to come up with emotionally meaningful situations to work with, partly because such people also tend to have poor access to emotions, limited psychological insight into their situations, and insufficient understanding of the connection between their psychological and physiological conditions. In these and other cases where it is difficult to locate a situation to work with, we can take the person's detailed history—their history of adverse experiences in childhood as well as adulthood, and the support they did or did not have as children for their emotional experiences—and use this information as the basis for guiding the client toward emotionally difficult situations.

One can also work with the client's dreams, as dreams tend to efficiently capture what is going on in a person's life. Dreams with an emotional charge can serve as situations in the search for emotions to embody. They show the ability of the unconscious to handle emotional experiences that are hard to process consciously. I once worked with a woman who could not make the commitment to marry her long-term boyfriend because of her enmeshment with her mother. The woman was shaken by a dream in which she repeatedly stabbed her mother to death. Processing the sheer horror and other intense emotions she accessed through the dream, with the support of the class in which I worked with her, helped her finally make the commitment to marry a few months later.

Speaking of dreams and embodiment, when you wake up from a disturbing dream that you cannot remember, try the following: grab the disturbed feeling with your awareness and expand it in your body so as to create a greater capacity for it. When I do that, I almost always retrieve fragments of the dream, if not the whole thing, back into my awareness.

If all efforts to identify a relevant situation, past or present, come up short, we can use the distress that drove the person to seek our help as the initial emotion to embody, moving forward from there. We saw in chapter 9, which discussed different kinds of emotions, how we can start at the very basic level of sensorimotor emotions of feeling bad or feeling stressed in the brain or the body physiology. We can then use the specialized emotional physiology of the face and the throat to express the emotion vocally and through facial expression, to differentiate such simple primitive emotional experiences into more complex ones. We can also use vocalization and facial expression in this way in cases where we have a situation to work with, but emotions are hard to come by because of lack of affect development or social inhibition. In either instance, the embodiment of emotion can lead to situations emerging from the unconscious that have a bearing on the person's suffering.

Here is an example that illustrates both instances. I once worked with a person who was suffering from a great deal of stress. We knew this stress probably had to do with a recent breakup, so we had a clear situation. But working with the situation and trying to tie it to the stress went nowhere, with strong psychological and physiological defenses in place against the emergence of other emotions involved. In this context, sensing the discomfort and pain of the stress and moving it toward vocal and facial expression not only helped the person access more differentiated emotions, such as sadness and loneliness; it also led to the person making a clearer connection between the distress and the breakup, as well as a connection between current emotions and childhood situations that made the present experience of separation all the more unbearable. This helped the person process both the distant and the recent situations in the here and now.

Sometimes people report emotions without a situation attached to them. In the process of embodying emotions that emerge first, situations arise sooner or later, which can then be used to keep the emotions alive or to evoke other emotions. Once a situation is identified, we can gather concrete details about the situation to zero in on another specific emotional reaction to a specific aspect of the situation, which we can then work with. The situations and their details then help to keep the emotion alive as we work to embody them further, if necessary. When working this way, we need to mention the situation's details as often as necessary to keep the emotional response on track and prevent it from dissipating. Repeating statements about situational details, such as "You saw your child lying in a pool of blood after the accident," helps keep whatever emotion you are working with alive. Details of a situation can also help in managing the level and intensity of an emotional experience. When we need to reduce the level of emotion and its intensity, we can refer less often to the emotionally charged details, and we can refer to them more if we need to increase the level and intensity of the emotional experience.

The situational details can also be helpful in evoking emotions in other ways. They can give us information on how we might be using cognitive, emotional, and behavioral defenses against emotions. If we felt angry then and continue to feel angry now, we might be stuck in anger as a defense against vulnerable emotions. If we did not act to protect ourselves physically then and are unable to do so now, challenging ourselves to act physically in ways to protect ourselves now can enable us to access the anger and embody it so we can get to a place of empowerment. If we try to ignore a person's abusive behavior toward us by limiting our cognition, with thoughts such as "I deserved to be treated badly," we can challenge such cognition to grasp the abuse so we can move from self-blame and shame and toward anger on the way to resolving the situation.

Emotional reactions are specific. They are specific to a specific understanding of a specific aspect of a situation and what we perceive as feasible in terms of behavior to cope with that aspect of the situation. Therefore, the more concrete the clients are in terms of cognitive and behavioral details of the situation, the more likely we can help them to arrive at the specific emotional reaction to work with. For example, if a client is upset about not having good experiences in relationships and wants help to change this difficulty, we have to clarify whether we are talking about personal or professional relationships. If we are dealing with personal relationships, we have to ask about which specific personal relationship or relationships they are having difficulty with. We have to ask about details of the specific personal relationship: what is the other person's name, how long they have been in relationship, what aspects of the relationship are troublesome, etc. We have to ask about the details of a specific interaction or instance that was troublesome that serves as an example of the difficulty they have in that aspect of the relationship, in order to get to a concrete emotional reaction to work with.

The client's reply to this level of specific, detailed inquiry might be as follows: "I have difficulty in personal relationships. At the moment I am most troubled in my relationship with my wife. The sexual aspect of the relationship is what is most troubling to me. Specifically, my wife does not respond to the extent I wish she would, and that upsets me. Let me give you a recent example. Last Thursday, after the kids were asleep, I started to have a sexual impulse toward my wife. When I reached out with sexual desire, she batted my hand away. It upset me. I thought that this is a hopeless situation. I just gave up, turned away from her, and tried to calm myself to sleep." We now have a specific upset, an emotional reaction to work with.

The more we can get clients to describe the situation that bothers them, and the more concrete the details of the situation are, the more likely they will have an emotional reaction we can work with. There are of course exceptions to every rule. Sometimes clients come in highly upset or anxious without much insight into what is triggering these reactions from the unconscious. It is possible that trying to get clients to understand where such reactions are coming from might be helpful in managing the extreme reactions. In other instances, as we have seen, such attempts to help the client understand the situation might fail, or they might only alleviate suffering for the time being. In such cases, as we have already mentioned, deeper work with the embodiment of the emotion available might be necessary to bring about change in the client's understanding of the situation and their suffering.

During an emotional embodiment session, once the situation is defined and its details are known, one does not have to go through all the details again each time. Doing so could be distracting as the brain busies itself with cognitive and behavioral aspects of the situation. It is sufficient to use certain key phrases that connect crucial, emotionally evocative aspects of the situation with the emotion itself. You can use statements such as "the pain you felt in your heart as you saw him with his new wife," "the fragmentation you felt when your boss told you that you were no longer wanted," "the terror you felt when you realized that all exits were blocked," or "the shame you felt when your father slapped you."

11

The Emotion

Chapter summary: shows different ways to support others in accessing their emotions and staying with them so they can embody their emotions.

In the first step in the process of embodying emotions, we saw how important the details of a situation are for the formation of an emotional response. However, the details of the situation alone are not enough to evoke the emotional response. We know this from our everyday experience of people who have an adequate grasp of the details of the situations they find themselves in, but who, at the same time, report no emotional responses. There can be many possible reasons for this condition. For example, some people might have unhelpful attitudes toward emotions; others might not know how to label or express their emotional experiences. Let us look at the different ways we can support others so they can overcome these and other blocks in the way of their emotions, to help them access their emotions and stay with them so the emotions can be embodied.

Providing Support for Emotions

In general, people who have had support for their emotional experiences while growing up are more likely to experience and report emotional experiences to others. Research has shown that the most important determinant of the capacity for emotions observed in children is the capacity for a range of emotions in their parents.[1] Children internalize (introject) their important caregivers' attitudes toward emotions as their own. As a result, they can have supportive or non-supportive attitudes toward attending to and reporting their emotional experiences. In addition, no matter how supportive their internal attitudes toward emotions are, people in general have difficulty attending to and reporting their emotional experiences if there is inadequate support for their emotions in the people immediately around them. Therefore, for people to allow themselves to experience and express emotions, supportive attitudes toward emotions from those around them are just as important as having their own supportive attitudes toward emotions.

In order to work with emotional responses in clients, therapists have to explore the situation so as to guide them to the details that are most likely to evoke the emotional responses, providing whatever external support clients need for experiencing and expressing their emotions. Emotional support can take so many different forms, but the most important ingredient in supporting other people emotionally is the caring we are able to bring to the impact a situation is having on them. That is, we have to communicate to the other person that we care about the impact the situation is having on that person. We communicate that we care by bringing sympathy and empathy to the suffering of others.

Sympathy and Empathy

With sympathy, we communicate that we care that someone is suffering by making statements such as "It must be really hard emotionally to go through what you are going through," "I cannot imagine how much you have suffered in this situation," "I feel bad when I see you suffer," "I wish you did not have to suffer so much," and so on. Sympathy is showing compassion for the suffering of another and caring for the other.

With empathy, we show that we care even more by finding a way to experience the suffering of others in ourselves. Peter Fonagy, a significant contributor to attachment theory, calls the ability to experience the emotions of others in our bodies "embodied attunement."[2] According to Fonagy, mothers who can experience the emotions of their children in their bodies are better at regulating their children emotionally. When we share another person's emotional experiences in our own bodies when we are with them, we provide them the best possible support for their emotional experiences. Through empathy, we can also help others articulate what their emotional experiences are by experiencing and articulating their emotional experiences in ourselves first. This can help people feel really understood. We will see in chapter 14 on interpersonal resonance all the ways we can experience the emotions of others in ourselves.

Other Ways of Supporting Emotions

Here is a list of practical ways we can support emotions, including examples of statements we can make that provide each type of support:

- We can educate people about the important role emotions play in our lives.

    "Emotions give us important information on how situations affect our well-being."

- We can address common negative misconceptions people have about emotions, to help them achieve a more nuanced and accepting understanding of emotions.

    "People often avoid emotions because they have heard that emotions are irrational. Emotions can indeed lead to irrational cognition, like 'no one loves me,' or irrational behavior, like the impulse to hurt the person who abandoned me, when I cannot tolerate the vulnerable emotions from being abandoned. However, if I can develop the capacity to tolerate emotions by embodying them, my cognitive and behavioral responses to being abandoned are more likely to be rational."

"Adults often tell children it is not okay for boys to cry or for girls to be angry. That is not correct. That is probably what they heard from adults when they were children too. Sadness and anger are both valid emotional responses for boys, girls, men, and women."

- We can validate others' emotional states as real and appropriate to the situation.

    "Of course anyone in your situation would feel what you are feeling. I would too."

- We can support emotions in others by deeply listening to them and reflecting what we hear back to them.

    "I hear that you are very sad."

    "I hear that the situation with your children is very difficult for you now."

- We can provide information on the different kinds of emotions listed in chapter 9 so that they can look for a larger range of emotional experiences.

    "When people think of emotions, they often only look for basic universal emotions such as happiness and sadness. There are so many emotions that we miss because they are not generally recognized as emotions. Did you know that just feeling bad about a situation is a legitimate emotional response to that situation?"

- We can bring to them a rich and expanded vocabulary of simple and complex emotion-related words and phrases to help them describe and differentiate their emotional experiences.

    "Does your shame feel like your inside has become rotten?"

    "Does your hurt from the breakup feel like your heart has splinters of glass in it?"

    "Does the betrayal feel like the person stabbed you in the heart?"

- We can offer a checklist of all possible emotional reactions to a situation, from personal experience as well as the experiences of others, drawing from life, therapy, art, and literature.

  "When I work with people who have gone through early losses, I often run into shock, hurt, sadness, grief, despair, resignation, and anger. I also know these emotions from processing my own losses."

- We can mirror the verbal, vocal, facial, and other body expressions of others as a way to understand, share, support, and regulate their emotional states.

  "As I listen to you describe what you went through, as I assume the expression on your face and your body posture, I am overcome with profound grief."

- We can be vulnerable with others with our own emotions, to make it safer for them to come forth with theirs.

  "I also experience shame. At times, I feel like I am the least worthy person in the whole world."

  "When I see you suffer, my heart feels like crying."

- We can teach them how to manage overwhelming emotional experiences to make it safer for them to go into them next time, making use of all the techniques described in chapter 13 in the section on managing extreme emotional states, such as:

  "Please open your eyes and orient to the present."

- We can model for others the different ways in which emotions can be expressed and communicated through verbal, vocal, facial, postural, gestural, and other body expressions. We learn from others how to express our emotions throughout our lives.

- We can teach them how important it is to get support for our emotional experiences from others throughout our lives, and how to go about getting such support.

- We can support others by understanding and regulating their emotional experience through interpersonal resonance, in all the ways described in chapter 14.

- We can demonstrate how they can manage their emotional experiences through cognition and behavior.

    "Do you notice whether your emotional experience changes when you understand the situation differently?"

    "Do you observe any change in your emotional reaction when you think of this different way to handle the situation?"

- We can educate them about the benefits of embodying emotions.

    "Expanding the emotional experience to as much of the body as possible can help us not only in regulating our emotions by making them more tolerable but also in improving our cognition and behavior in the situation."

- We can show them how to work with their physiological and energetic defenses against emotions to expand and regulate their emotional experiences, in all the ways described in chapter 12.

Working with Innate Defenses against Unpleasant Emotions

Human beings are averse to pain and attracted to pleasure, as Freud noted in describing his pleasure principle. Unpleasant emotional experiences are painful by their very nature because they are generated from stress and dysregulation in the physiology. Unpleasant emotional experiences are opposed to an organism's health, well-being, and survival. Therefore, we all have an innate psychophysiological tendency to avoid them. We can call this a psychophysiological tendency because it is in part physiological and in part psychological. Knowing this is the case will not eliminate this innate tendency, which is part of our makeup throughout our lives. We just need to accept it and work around it when we need to process painful emotional experiences.

This innate tendency to avoid suffering is hardwired in all of us and is a constant presence in every moment of our lives, like our very shadows. When I wake up from a bad dream, the dream itself has often disappeared from my awareness, leaving behind only the unpleasant emotional experience associated with it. I get up, check my phone for email, read the latest news, all in order to suppress the lingering unpleasant emotional turmoil in my system and drive the dream content back deeper into the unconscious. At times, I remember that the development of capacity for an unpleasant emotional experience can lead to cognitive and behavioral clarity. And then I reluctantly turn my attention to the unpleasant experience to embrace it and embody it, to have fragments of the forgotten come back into my awareness.

Emotions are more often predictions of what situations mean for our well-being than they are assessments of the actual outcomes. Either way, they are important sources of information for our well-being and survival. Predictions and actual experiences of unpleasant emotions are all the more important information for us to learn from, to improve our chances of well-being and survival for the present as well as the future. We have seen that when emotions are more embodied, they can help us be more regulated as well as improve our cognitions and behaviors in the situation. This enhances our ability to cope with the situation in the present as well as in the future when we run into the same emotions in different situations. Therefore, emotions in general and unpleasant emotions in particular have important adaptive value for our well-being and survival.

Clients usually come to us because they are suffering and want an end to their suffering. Most of them think going deeper into the suffering by embodying it makes no sense and runs counter to their innate resistance to suffering. Unless clients are informed about the tremendous benefits of embodying their unpleasant emotions, they are not going to understand why they need to overcome what feels like a natural resistance to suffering of any kind.

Sometimes we are able to reduce their suffering through cognitive and behavioral changes that do not entail much suffering. We know this is possible because we learned in chapter 6 that cognition, emotion, and behavior are inseparable if not intertwined aspects of a singular life experience. Therefore, we can potentially operate on one of the elements to change the other two elements. At times, we are able to help clients reduce their suffering through regulating their brain or body physiology, taking medication, or engaging in somatic practices.

When physiological, cognitive, and behavioral strategies do not reduce their suffering or are taking too long to make a difference, that is a good time to introduce them to the idea of emotional embodiment and to educate them about its various short-term and long-term benefits. This is also a good time to educate them about the innate resistance we all have to unpleasant experiences, and the need to override that resistance so we are more open to embodying difficult emotions, not only to resolve current symptoms efficiently but also to be more resilient to them on future occasions. The more often they can do that, the easier it would be for them to override their innate resistance to suffering to embody unpleasant emotions in the future.

Educating clients as well as therapists about the innate resistance to suffering in all of us and the need to face and work with unpleasant emotions is an important, if not the most important, aspect of helping clients to embody unpleasant emotions. It is also important for getting therapists past their own innate resistance to work with unpleasant emotions in their clients.

Psychological Defenses against Emotions

Emotions, especially unpleasant ones, can be painful. In general, we do not want to experience the suffering of unpleasant emotions; nor do we want those we care about to experience them. In relationships, we might try to minimize our awareness of the negative impact we have on each other, in order to not feel guilt or shame or to maintain the perception that relationships are better than they actually are. People can also have difficulty embracing pleasant emotions. There can be familial or social prohibitions on the experience and expression of emotions such as pride, joy, love, and sexuality.

Since its beginnings, psychology has been studying and cataloging the different methods or defenses we use to push away unbearable or unacceptable experiences, not only of emotion but also of cognition and behavior. It is important to remember that all psychological defenses are coping mechanisms that are employed to keep unbearable or unacceptable experiences at bay, and that we might continue to use them out of habit even when we no longer need them. To help others access emotions and embody them, it is important that we know how to recognize a psychological defense, interpret it for the client or educate them about it, and work with some of the more common defenses.

Following is a list of common psychological defenses against emotions, including explanations of how each one works:

Repression: When we repress our emotions, we prevent them from even entering our conscious awareness in the first place. They are pushed out of awareness unconsciously. Not being able to recall that one has ever been angry with one's mother is a clear example of repression.

Suppression: When we suppress our emotions, we consciously try to push them away from our awareness. As soon as one remembers an instance of being angry with one's mother, consciously pushing the memory away by trying not to think about it or to forget it in another way, such as thinking about something else, is an example of suppression.

Denial: Imagine that someone is talking about their mother with an angry tone of voice or facial or body expression. If you were to ask that person whether they were angry and they denied it, that would be an example of the coping mechanism of denial. Please note that just because another person can see signs of anger in me, that does not mean I am aware of it myself. I can deny it because I am not aware of it, or I can deny it even though I am aware of it because I do not want to focus on it or express it, because it feels unsafe for me to admit to it.

Displacement: When we're angry at our boss but we direct that anger toward our spouse at home, this is an example of the defense of displacement.

Projection: When someone describing a scary event perceives the fear only on the faces of those listening, this is an example of projection.

Reaction formation: When you are angry with someone and force yourself to be nice to that person instead, this is an example of reaction formation. When one has lost a love object, being angry all the time without feeling the love or feeling the love all the time without being angry are common examples of reaction formation.

Sublimation: When one chooses exercise to get rid of one's anger at a superior at work on a regular basis, it is an example of sublimation. One burying oneself in one's work in order not to feel the emptiness of a personal life without meaningful relationships is another example of sublimation. In sublimation, one does something that is neither damaging to oneself nor to others, as a way of not feeling unpleasant emotions.

Rationalization: When someone you are attracted to turns you down, and to avoid the pain of rejection you use the logic that you were not really all that attracted them, this is an example of rationalization.

Intellectualization: When people focus on thinking about a situation rather than on how they feel about it, as when people focus on psychologically analyzing those who have rejected them to avoid feeling their feelings about the rejection, this is an example of intellectualization. This example shows how multiple defenses can be used in the same situation to push away unpleasant emotions. When people convince themselves there is something wrong with the person who rejected them so they can arrive at the logic that there is nothing wrong with them, thus preventing them from feeling the shame or inadequacy that people often experience when they are rejected, this is an example of rationalization. In that they are focusing so much on the intellectual pursuit of analyzing the other person rather than feeling what they feel about being rejected, they are also using the strategy of intellectualization. Another way in which they could use intellectualization in order not to feel their emotions around rejection is by using spiritual statements, such as "God loves everybody all the time. Therefore, nobody is ever rejected at any time. God is love. I am one with God. Therefore, I am love."

Compartmentalization: When people feel compassion for one group of people in a situation and not for other groups of people in the same situation, they are using the strategy of compartmentalization.

Here they could be using logic, such as the notion that other groups do not believe in the same God, to rationalize why other groups of people do not deserve compassion. Slave owners rationalized that enslaved people were not really humans in order not to feel compassion toward them. Another example of compartmentalization is when people block having feelings about what happens to them at work but allow themselves to feel what happens to them at home. Compartmentalization is also happening when people allow themselves to feel feelings about one person in a situation but not about another in the same situation, as when a child is angry at the father who physically abused the child but not at the mother who was present but did not help the child, with the rationalization that the mother was too afraid to intervene.

Conversion: This is when uncomfortable feelings are turned into physical symptoms such as pain. Physical conversion symptoms can mimic serious medical symptoms, such as paralysis. Psychophysiological symptoms are physical symptoms that form when a person is not able to handle psychological experiences, such as emotions. When psychophysiological symptoms form, it is not always the case that they are formed in order to avoid experiencing difficult emotions in the situation. It could just be that the person's physiology is not able to handle the overall stress from the situation, and that alone can lead to the formation of psychophysiological symptoms. In addition, it is possible for psychophysiological symptoms to form from the physiological and energetic defenses people use to cope with unpleasant or unacceptable emotions in a situation, as we saw in chapter 7 on physiological defenses against emotions. For example, when a child constricts their breathing muscles on a regular basis to avoid feeling anger at their abusive father, this can lead to the development of a serious breathing difficulty for which medical help proves ineffective. An example from my own childhood!

The concept of conversion defense can also be applied to situations where one emotion is used defensively to cope with another emotion that is more intolerable or unacceptable. The energy of the more unbearable or unacceptable emotion is also channeled into the defensive emotion. The use of anger to guard against vulnerable emotions such as hurt and shame is a good example. The use of sadness instead of anger, especially in women, is another example of emotional conversion as a defense. Because one emotion is substituted for another, this defense strategy could also be called substitution defense. The difference between conversion or substitution and displacement is that in displacement, the emotion meant to be directed at one person is directed at another person, whereas in emotional conversion or substitution an emotion is changed into another emotion within the same person. The conversion can also be from feeling an emotion to expressing it, as when a person cries for relief when sad or angry. When the energy behind one emotion is converted into its opposite emotion, as when hate is turned into love, this is also an instance of reaction formation.

Regression: Imagine an adult who experienced severe abandonment as a child that they have not really worked through and come to terms with. Whenever that adult experiences a loss, the experience of emotions associated with the current loss is simply too much. The triggering of the unresolved emotions of loss from childhood drops the person down into a child ego state, where it is even more difficult to tolerate the emotions from the current loss in adulthood. In this state, one might find relief by crying or curling up, as when a child used to sucking its thumb for comfort goes back to sucking its thumb after a traumatic experience. This way of coping with unbearable or unacceptable emotions is called the regression defense.

Deflection: A less-known defense from gestalt therapy, deflection is when people distance themselves from their emotions through humor, generalizing, theorizing, debating, asking questions, and other distractions.

Confluence: Also from gestalt therapy, confluence is when children identify with their parents' emotional states and are unable to differentiate their emotions from those of their parents in order to avoid conflict and unpleasantness. They might as adults be unable to come into their emotions and differentiate them from those of their partners, as in couples therapy, for fear of conflict and unpleasantness.

Dissociation: Dissociation is another defense that is used to cope with overwhelming emotional experiences. Three types of dissociation have been identified in psychiatry.[3] In *primary dissociation,* cognitive elements such as visuals of the trauma are screened out of awareness in order to manage the emotional overwhelm they can trigger, as when visual memories of childhood sexual abuse are repressed. *Secondary dissociation* disconnects a person's awareness from the unbearable emotions of the trauma, as when a person feels numb or has out-of-body experiences during sexual abuse. Often mediated by internal chemicals such as analgesics and opioids secreted during times of stress to help manage difficult experiences, secondary dissociation can include altered states such as feeling paradoxically euphoric while being injured. In *tertiary dissociation,* traumatic experience is compartmentalized as in dissociative identity disorder (formerly known as multiple personality disorder), where one or more compartmentalized parts of the personality carry the cognitive, emotional, and behavioral memories of the trauma and other parts remain apparently unaware of them or are aware but unaffected by them.

The various psychological coping mechanisms or defenses against unpleasant or unacceptable emotions are not separate watertight categories. One or more defenses might be used in the service of another. For example, repression of an emotional experience might be supported through sublimation, deflection, rationalization, or intellectualization. Rationalization, the use of logic to defend against emotion, can be thought of as a special instance of intellectualization, the use of one's intellectual capacity to keep an emotion at a distance. Compartmentalization of experience is involved in tertiary dissociation within dissociative identity disorder. Also, a person might use multiple defenses in the same situation to cope with the enormity of the unbearable suffering. For example, a person might use intellectualization as well as projection to cope with a difficult experience, as when a person says there is no reason why everyone should have the existential fear of dying during a pandemic at the thought of contracting the coronavirus, but they can see why some people might not be able to avoid it.

Working with Psychological Defenses against Emotions

In addition to psychological defenses against emotions, people use physiological as well as energetic defenses against emotions. Physiological defenses against emotions and how to work with them will be covered in the next step of the emotional embodiment process, the expansion, in the next chapter. For now, there are some important things to keep in mind about the relationships among psychological, physiological, and energetic defenses.

Physiological and energetic defenses are often, if not always, the underlying mechanisms of support for what are called psychological defenses. For example, secondary dissociation experiences of numbing out or out-of-body experiences are often driven by defensive biochemical surges in the physiology. It is easier to work with simple physiological defenses—such as holding one's breath, which is used to reduce the intensity of an unpleasant emotion—by just becoming aware of the holding and letting it go. For different reasons, it is harder to work with more complex physiological defenses, such as constriction. Just becoming aware of them with the intention to change them is often not enough to shift them. They might require more active interventions, such as stretching, self-touch, therapist's touch, yoga, bodywork, energy work, or even medication, to shift. Physiological defenses are also often unconscious for both clients and therapists, as opposed to psychological defenses such as denial and displacement, which are easier to observe in clients' behavior.

It is also good to keep in mind that, at times, one might have to work first with complex physiological and energetic defenses to loosen them up before working with emotions, because strong physiological and energetic defenses can make undoing psychological defenses and accessing emotions extremely difficult. That is, one might have to work with the third step, the expansion, first or at the same time as the second step, the emotion, in the emotional embodiment process. Working with more complex physiological defenses to expand the emotional experience in the brain and body physiology is part of the next step, the expansion, the subject matter of chapter 12.

There are many ways of working with psychological as well as physiological defenses. However, the most effective way to work with these defenses is to provide the necessary emotional support to clients to help them access and regulate their emotional experiences so there is no need to defend against them. While providing the necessary emotional support in all the ways we have seen above, we can also point out and work with the specific psychological and physiological defenses as they emerge in the process; educate clients about how the defenses are coming in to protect them from the suffering; and continue to address, support, and regulate the vulnerabilities that are triggering the defenses. This way, clients can become increasingly aware of their defenses so they can even see through them when they are on their own. Different therapy modalities approach working with psychological defenses in different ways, some more complex than others. Specialized information on such complex strategies for working with psychological defenses is beyond the scope of this book.

Simple Self-Inquiry for Self-Help

Some readers who are not mental health professionals might have found the information presented so far on how to find a situation and work with the emotion a bit too theoretical. So, here are some questions you can ask yourself to identify a situation and support an emotion:

- When did I start to suffer from my symptom?

- What was happening in my life around that time? Personally? Professionally?

- What significant changes occurred around that time? Did I move or change jobs? Did I lose a relationship or get into a new one? Did something become more stressful at work or at home?

- What do I notice as a reaction in my brain or body as I run through the situations?

- Which situation appears to elicit more of a reaction?

- Which aspect or details of the chosen situation bring up more charge?

- What do I feel?

- Do I feel more stress thinking about the situation?

- Do I feel bad or awful when I think about the situation?

- Do I recognize the bad feeling as something more specific? As sadness or fear, for example?

- If I feel anger, is it something I have as a typical response to unpleasant, uncomfortable, or frustrating situations? If so, in what ways might I be feeling bad or vulnerable that my anger might be covering up?

- Whom do I go to for emotional support when I am feeling bad?

- What happens when I imagine them here with me with their caring attitude to my suffering?

- What happens when I imagine I am expressing what I am feeling now to them? Does it help me to stay with and deepen into my emotion? Does their imagined support make the emotion more tolerable for me?

- If I cannot get to a specific emotional experience, what else can I do?

- What happens if I imagine my bad feeling about the situation being expressed by a facial expression or vocalization by another person?

- What changes when I try to express this bad feeling, this awful feeling, or this pain, on my face or through a vocalization? In my imagination? Or when I actually do it?

Conclusion

If working with the situation in step 1 and working with the emotion in step 2 yield an emotion to work with, we can go on to the next step of expanding the emotional experience to as much of the brain and body physiology as possible. What if we come up short? Then we can look at the possibility that the situation chosen for the work might not be sufficiently relevant, emotionally charged, or concrete, and try to mend that. We can also look at the possibility that more emotional support and more work on innate and psychological defenses might be needed to get there.

There are also other possibilities. For instance, the physiological defenses against emotions may be too strong for the emotion to come through. In this case, one might have to work with physiological defenses to expand the brain and body physiology, either before or at the same time as working with the emotion.

Another possibility is that there are severe deficits in the person's affect development, limiting their ability to generate, differentiate, identify, or express emotional experiences. In this case, we can proceed as follows: One, educate the person about the different kinds of emotions possible in the situation, especially the simple sensorimotor emotions of just feeling bad or uncomfortable. Two, have the person imagine themselves or another person actually expressing the emotion of feeling bad or awful in the brain or the body physiology through vocalization and facial expression. If necessary, have the person actually do the vocalization and facial expression. Three, proceed to embody the simple sensorimotor emotion of feeling distressed or painful to as much of the brain and body physiology as possible. Four, mirror the person's expressions, resonate with the person's experience, and look for simple, basic, universal emotions such as fear or sadness, and then go from there.

This often works, for two reasons. First, when clients approach us for help, it is because they are suffering, and they can at least identify "feeling bad" in the brain or body physiology. Second, expressing simple sensorimotor emotions through vocalization and facial expression almost always helps in differentiating emotional experiences into basic emotions, because of the multiple roles played by the face and throat physiology in emotional experiences, as seen in earlier chapters.

In chapter 10, we saw how to work with the details of the situation to bring up the relevant emotions. In this chapter, we saw how to support clients' emotions in various ways and how to work with their innate and psychological defenses to help them access their emotions. In the next chapter, we will look at how to work with physiological and energetic defenses against emotions to expand and regulate the brain and body physiology, to expand the experience of emotion to as much of it as possible. The chapter after that will discuss how to manage the intensity of the emotional experience during the expansion process and how to exploit the increased capacity for emotional experience to expedite symptom resolution.

12

The Expansion

Chapter summary: presents different methods for expanding different areas of the body, to expand an emotional experience to as much of the body as possible and thus to make it more tolerable to be with over a longer period.

In chapter 7, we saw the different ways in which defenses can form in the brain and body physiology against overwhelming emotional experiences, and how they can get in the way of accessing and processing unresolved emotional experiences. In chapter 8, we saw how undoing such physiological defenses against emotions can help us in expanding an emotional experience to more of the physiology, and how that can lead to a greater capacity to tolerate, be with, and process the difficult emotional experience. We saw in chapter 6 how creating a greater capacity to be with an emotion by expanding the physiology involved in its experience can improve not only emotional but also cognitive and behavioral outcomes.

As mentioned earlier, we use the phrase "expanding the physiology" to mean "undoing defenses against emotions to involve more of the physiology in the emotional experience." In expanding the physiology to expand an unpleasant emotion, it would be optimal if we could minimize the difficulty in experiencing the unpleasant emotion. In Integral

Somatic Psychology (ISP) professional trainings, we use a model of physiological regulation, a model of energetic regulation, and a number of different strategies and tools to optimize the expansion process, in order to minimize the stress, dysregulation, and distress inherent in the experience of unpleasant emotions. A full discussion of both models of regulation and all strategies and tools used in the expansion process is not possible in this book, to keep its length manageable. In this chapter, we will look at some simple, essential, and effective strategies and tools for undoing defenses in the brain and body physiology, to optimize the expansion process that readers can put into immediate practice for embodying emotions in themselves or their clients.

General Strategies for Expansion

From chapter 5, we know that an emotional experience, especially an overwhelming one, can potentially involve the entire brain and body physiology. In such circumstances, if the emotional experience is limited to one area of the brain and body physiology, we know that physiological defenses are preventing the other areas from fully participating in the emotional experience. When an emotion is present in one area, we can try to expand the emotional experience to the area that immediately adjoins it. We will call this strategy the "local expansion" strategy. Or, we can try to expand it to other areas, which we will call the "area to area" expansion strategy. Both of these are the general strategies for expansion of emotion in the physiology.

The Body in Parts and Layers

For the purpose of having a simple framework for implementing local and area-to-area expansion strategies, we can do a simple division of the brain and body physiology into different areas: the head, the neck, the arms, the thoracic cavity (from the shoulder to the diaphragm muscle), the abdominal and pelvic cavities (from the diaphragm muscle to the pelvic floor), and the legs. We can also do a simple classification of the physiology into three layers. The outer layer consists of the skin, fascia, muscles, membranes, bones, ligaments, and tendons. We consider the muscles, governed by the somatic nervous system, to be the most dynamic component of the outer layer. The middle layer consists of the organs, the glands, and the blood vessels, which are governed by the autonomic nervous system. The third and inner layer consists of the central nervous system areas of the brain and the spinal cord, and the peripheral somatic and autonomic nervous systems.

Simple Tools for Expansion

There are a number of tools we can use to work with physiological and energetic defenses to expand the emotional experience locally or from one area to another. Awareness, intention, visual imagination, detailed tracking of sensations in the brain and body physiology, movement, breath, self-touch, the therapist's imaginal touch, the therapist's actual touch, bodywork, and energy work are all possible tools. In this chapter, we will limit our discussion to the use of simple tools, such as awareness, intention, and self-touch, which can be used more easily for self-help as well as for helping others. I hope that those who touch clients as part of the treatments they offer can translate the information on self-touch presented here into use with their clients through therapeutic touch.

Detailed tracking of body sensations, an effective evidence-based tool that is used widely in psychology these days, is not suggested as a tool here. It is complex to use, and it suffers from its potential to neutralize or regulate away difficult emotional experiences when we are trying to create a greater capacity to tolerate them. If you are interested in reading more on this topic, you can read my paper "How to Avoid Destroying Emotions When Tracking Body Sensations?"[1] Movement and breath, effective tools that can also be in the expansion process, are also excluded from discussion here for the same reasons. Those of you who use the great tools of breath, movement, and detailed tracking of body sensations in your work, please make sure they do not regulate the emotions away when you are using them to embody emotions.

Intention: Intention is an important tool. When we use tools such as awareness or self-touch, the intention with which we apply the tool determines the outcome. In general, a tool can be used with one or more of four intentions:

- A tool can be used in an area to simply calm, soothe, neutralize, and regulate away physiological defenses as well as emotional experiences that the defenses are mobilizing against.

- It can be used to undo the defenses in an area to uncover the emotional experience being defended against.

- It can support an unpleasant experience in an area and make it more tolerable.

- It can support a pleasant experience in the area and make it more durable and enjoyable.

Whenever a tool is used, there is always an intention, be it conscious or unconscious. It is important to make the intention conscious so it is not in opposition to what we are trying to achieve. For example, when inviting a client to use self-touch to undo a defense in an area to uncover the vulnerability it is defending against, if we do not make this intention explicit, the client might just use the self-touch to soothe the area and free it from both the defense and the vulnerability. Intention can be used with a tool to determine the outcome of using the tool as well as to directly expand the emotional experience. For example, we might use self-touch in an area with the intention to undo physiological defenses there, accompanied by a statement such as "Place your hand on the constriction in your chest to soften it to uncover what the constriction is hiding." Or we might use intention to expand the emotional experience locally in an area or from one area to another with a statement such as "As you experience the fear in your chest, please try to expand the fear to more of the chest or to the belly."

Awareness: Awareness is a tool that is always used with an intention. When we are paying attention to an experience mindfully, we are using awareness to pay attention to the experience with the intention of accepting the experience and reacting to it as little as possible. Awareness works in different ways. When we bring our awareness to an area of the body, the brain mobilizes more neurological resources to gather more information on the condition of the area and to send commands to different parts of the brain and body physiology to regulate the area, if the area is dysregulated. Also, when we bring awareness to an area, the energy tends to increase in that area, increasing the possibility of an experience there, according to the first principle of energy psychology, which is: energy follows awareness, and experience follows energy.

The second principle of energy psychology, which will come in handy when our task is to expand an emotional experience from one area to another, is: when two areas in the body are connected through tools such as awareness, self-touch, therapist's touch, or needles, the two areas will get connected energetically. Because experience follows energy, we can expect an emotional experience to expand from one area to the other when those areas are connected energetically. When working to expand an experience from one area of the body to another with awareness, we can hold both areas in our awareness at the same time, or we can go back and forth between the two areas.

These two principles of energy that connect awareness, energy, and experience are easy to verify. Give them a try right away before you read further. For example, if you find yourself feeling an intense emotion in the chest, place one hand on the chest and the second hand on the abdomen, with the intention to connect the two areas in energy and emotion. You can go back and forth between the chest and the abdomen with your awareness, or you can have them both in your awareness. What changes do you notice in your experience of the emotion? Is it less intense in the chest? Do you notice that qualities of the emotion you first noticed in the chest are now in the abdomen? Is the experience of the emotion more or less bearable now?

Self-touch: Different parts of our brain and body physiology, such as our brain and heart, generate fields of bioelectric and biomagnetic energy. These fields of information extend beyond the systems that originate them. They can integrate to become larger fields of energy with greater reach than the individual fields, even beyond the skin boundary. These information fields function as another system of regulation of our brain and body physiology, in addition to the nervous system. They can regulate not only our brain and body physiology but also those of other people they interact with. Our hands are good conduits for these bio-electric and biomagnetic energy fields. They provide a scientific basis for why therapist touch is effective in bodywork and energy work healing modalities.[2] We will look at this topic in greater depth in chapter 14 on interpersonal resonance.

We can use self-touch with one or both hands on different parts of our brain and body physiology, with different intentions, to assist with different steps of the emotional embodiment process. Self-touch can be used in step 2 to support our emotions, in step 3 to expand them, or in step 4 to aid in integration. In general, therapist touch can be expected to be more effective than self-touch because of the involvement of the resources of two systems, the client's and the therapist's, as opposed to one. However, self-touch does have some advantages. It can be used for self-help at home. It can be suggested more freely in different therapy modalities, in different cultures, across genders, for clients who have difficulty being touched, and for therapists who have difficulty touching their clients. It is also quite simple to learn to use. For all these advantageous reasons, self-touch has proved to be an effective workhorse in emotional embodiment work. We will see many examples of the use of self-touch below.

Simple Strategies for Local Expansion

Before we look at area-specific strategies for local expansion of emotion for different parts of the brain and body physiology, let us look at simple strategies we can use to expand emotion locally in any area, using the physical heart as an example. It makes sense to expand the emotional experience to the immediate neighborhood of where it is already present. The emotion's presence in an area signals that the area is either resourced enough to allow it to be experienced there or that the defenses cannot inhibit it out of the area altogether.

Our awareness tends to become dysfunctional in areas where we are struggling with an emotional experience. Either we try to pay less attention to the area, or we concentrate our awareness in the area in hopes that the experience will simply go away. This reduces the support we could provide the experience by using a more functional awareness strategy. When we concentrate our awareness in an area, the energy in the area tends to increase, according to the first principle of energy. As the energy in the area increases, it can energize the emotional experience, the defenses against it, or both. This in turn is likely to increase the level of stress and dysregulation in the area and make the emotional experience even more intolerable than before. People with chronic pain suffer from this dynamic. They cannot help paying attention to pain. The more attention they pay to the pain, the worse it gets, until physiological defenses such as numbing kick in to provide some relief.

In order to facilitate local expansion in an area without such dynamics, we can make the following suggestion to the client: "As you experience the grief in the heart area, please allow your awareness to expand beyond the heart to envelop more of the chest, so that those additional areas in your chest, such as your lungs, can expand physically as well as emotionally with your grief, to reduce the physical and emotional difficulty in the heart area."

Here we are using the tool of awareness with intention to help facilitate the local expansion of emotion in the heart to the chest area, between the shoulders and the diaphragm muscle. Because many people experience difficulty in using awareness as a tool, and awareness alone is often not effective when the defenses are strong, one can bring in the additional tool of self-touch. For example, we could suggest the following: "Place your hand on your heart area to help it expand physically and emotionally in order to expand your experience of grief in the heart, and to areas around the heart, so it can become more tolerable."

We could also make use of the second principle of energy—energy tends to flow between two areas that are connected somehow—and suggest the following: "Place one hand on the heart area, and place the other hand on the lung area, with the intention of helping both areas expand and connect physically and emotionally. Please notice if your experience of grief expands in the heart area, and then from the heart to the lungs. Also, at some point, please notice if there is greater physical ease in the heart area and whether your grief is more tolerable than before." The last statement belongs to the fourth step in the embodiment process, integration, covered in the next chapter. One aspect of integration is paying attention to improvements in physiology, energy, and affect tolerance. Such improvements can be theoretically expected from embodying emotion, as we saw in chapter 8. Integration can be used from time to time as a resource in the expansion process to make the emotional experience more bearable.

Simple Strategies for Area-to-Area Expansion

Sometimes it is difficult to engage in local expansion. It could be that the intensity of emotional experience is simply too much when expanded locally. Perhaps there is simply too much energy or emotion locally causing extreme distress. Or local expansion simply may not work, for one reason or another. In these cases, one has to use strategies to expand the emotion to other areas. Also, it is part of the emotional embodiment process that emotional experience is expanded to more parts of the body.

Let us look at simple strategies we can use to connect any two parts of the body, using the chest and the abdomen as an example. We can use one or more of the following suggestions that use awareness, intention, and self-touch: "As you are aware of the anxiety in your chest, which makes sense given the situation of job loss you find yourself in, please expand your awareness to the abdomen. Hold both your chest and your abdomen in your awareness, or go back and forth between the anxiety in your chest and your abdomen, to see if you can expand the experience of anxiety to the abdomen as well. The experience in the chest might not feel exactly the same as in the abdomen, but search the abdominal area to see if you can find any of the qualities of the anxiety you first felt in the chest. Place one hand on the chest and the other hand on the abdomen, not to regulate your anxiety away but to expand both areas and connect them to each other in the experience of anxiety that is related to your job loss."

When we use awareness and self-touch in two areas at the same time, we are using the second principle of energy: two areas that are connected in any way tend to come together in energy. When we continue to remind the person of the situation and the emotion, and we continue to validate and support the emotional experience as appropriate, the two areas are more likely to come together in the emotional experience as well. These simple strategies for facilitating expansion of emotion from one area to the next can be used with two areas that are next to each other, such as the chest and the abdomen, or distant from each other, such as the head and the legs.

Next, we turn to area-specific self-touch strategies for expanding specific areas (local expansion)—the chest, the abdomen, and so on— and for connecting two parts of the body to each other (area-to-area expansion), especially areas that are adjacent to each other.

Area-Specific Self-Touch Strategies

We begin with the arms, the legs, and the head and neck areas. They are the organs of action in the body with which we take care of ourselves in the world. We express ourselves primarily through the head and neck area and act mainly with our arms and legs to deal with the world. We can form defenses in these areas to hold ourselves back from expressing and doing things, or we can inhibit these areas so as to not feel emotional experiences in these or other areas of the body.

The Legs

The legs can be further divided into three segments: the foot, the lower leg, and the thigh. These segments are joined by the ankle and knee joints. The thigh and the entire leg are connected to the rest of the body by the hip joint. Osteopaths have known for a long time that defenses such as constriction in these three joints can disrupt nervous system, blood, interstitial fluid, lymph, and energy flows across them, which can cause

247

dysfunctions by dysregulating each of the segments locally or the entire leg globally. The connection between the leg and the rest of the body can become compromised at the hip joint, creating problems in the rest of the integrated brain and body physiology. To work with the legs, osteopaths have found it most efficient to work at these three joints.[3,4] They have also found it more effective to do touch work with two of these joints at a time rather than just one joint: with the hip and the knee joint, the knee and the ankle joint, or the hip and the ankle joint.

We can work with the legs to expand them locally, as well as to connect them to the rest of the body, especially with the adjacent abdominal and pelvic areas. We can ask clients sitting in a chair to draw one leg up, support its lower portion on the thigh of the other leg, and use touch to work with two joints at a time. We can touch the joints from above or below. To work with a hip joint, you can place a palm on top of the hip bone with your fingers pointing toward the groin, with the focus of your attention on the hip joint below the tips of your fingers. The choice of the two joints for touch would depend on the leg segments not involved in the emotional experience. We can assume that the leg segments not involved in the experience are defended against the emotional experience. For example, if the lower leg and foot segments appear to be involved, it would make sense to work with the knee and the ankle joints. It is not uncommon to find both legs uninvolved in emotional experiences.

The work with the legs in general and the hip joints in particular is important in emotional embodiment work. One reason is that the defense at the hip joint can disconnect the legs and the rest of the body in emotional experience. Another reason is that most people tend to concentrate their emotional energy above the diaphragm muscle. It is also common for people to concentrate emotional energy in the head. This typical top-heavy concentration makes the experience of emotion more stressful than necessary, due to the defenses formed in the rest of the body to keep it out, and due to the defenses formed in the limited areas emotion is present in to cope with it.

In energy psychology, different types of energies have their grounding in different areas of the legs. Any work at the legs therefore tends to produce a downward flow of energy and emotion and an easier experience of emotion in the body above the diaphragm. Self-touch with one hand on one hip joint and the other hand on the other hip joint, and self-touch with one hand at the hip joint and the other at the ankle joint on the same leg, are two effective strategies for expanding the legs and connecting them to the rest of the body in emotional experience, especially to the adjacent pelvic and abdominal areas.

When the emotion of grief is concentrated in the chest or when there is a great deal of difficulty in the chest in the conflict between grief concentrated there and the defenses to cope with it, we could say things such as "Please place both your hands on the hip joints for a while. Observe how it might help your chest as well as your legs to expand physically and feel at greater ease. Look at whether the grief in your chest is expanding in the chest and whether it is easier now to be with your grief there. See if your grief is expanding downward into your abdominal and pelvic area, and even into the legs." When the emotion of fear is strong in the abdominal or pelvic areas, we could suggest things such as "Please place your right hand on your right hip joint and your left hand on your right ankle joint, after you place your lower right leg on the thigh of the left leg. See what happens. Do you notice the right leg expand physically? Do you observe the expansion of the fear in the abdominal or pelvic area? Do you observe the right leg joining in the experience of fear?"

Please remember that we can also use simple area-to-area expansion strategies to expand the grief in the chest to the legs by placing one hand on the chest and the other hand on any part of a leg, with the intention to connect the two in energy and experience. We could similarly expand the fear in the abdomen to the legs by placing one hand on the abdomen and the other hand on any part of the leg.

We could also just use awareness and intention without self-touch. For example, you could suggest, "As you experience the grief in your chest, please also include your legs in your awareness. You can hold both places in your awareness along with your grief, or you can go back and forth between the two places. Notice what changes happen in your chest and your legs. How does that change the grief in your chest? Does the chest expand physically? Does that grief expand in your chest? Is it easier to be with the grief in your chest now than before? Do you notice whether any of the qualities of the grief you first noticed in your chest are now present in your legs?"

The Arms

The muscles of the arm are capable of a large number of fine and gross motor movements. There are a large number of muscles of varying sizes in the arms to carry them out. The neurophysiology of the arms is appropriately more complex than that of the legs. Given the involvement of the arms in a large number of actions in all kinds of situations starting at birth, especially in psychomotor acts such as pulling someone close and embracing them in close relationships, there are many reasons for defenses to form in them. Physiological defenses in the arms can also form as a defense against emotional experience in adjacent areas of the body, such as the chest cavity.

As with the legs, the three joints in the arms (shoulder, elbow, and wrist) are the most efficient places to work with to expand the arms locally and to connect them to the rest of the body, especially to the adjacent chest cavity between the shoulder and the diaphragm. As for connecting two arm joints at a time, we are more constrained with the arms than with the legs. We can get creative by using one arm to hold one of the three joints on the other arm, and then either move one of the other two joints or bring our awareness to it to connect the two joints. Or we can simply keep the two joints in our awareness so as to connect them. We can also use the knee joint on the leg on the same side as the contact point for the other joint. To do that, pull the same-side leg up, bend it at the knee, and place its lower leg or foot on the thigh of the other leg. One can then place the elbow or the wrist on the knee of the leg on the same side while touching one of the other two joints with the opposite arm. For example, we can touch the left shoulder joint with the right hand and connect the left elbow or wrist joint to the left knee.

As with the legs, the decisions about whether to work with one joint or two joints, and which joint or joints to work with, will be determined based on where the person is experiencing and not experiencing the emotion, and whether adjacent areas could be helped by working with the arms. For example, it is possible for the lower arm segment to be uninvolved in the emotional experience. That would indicate that we need to work with the elbow and wrist joints. It is not uncommon for an entire arm to be uninvolved. Working with the arm is often helpful in expanding the adjacent chest area, connected to the arm at the shoulder joint.

Working with the shoulder joint and the wrist joint is a great way to expand the arm and connect it to the rest of the body, especially to the chest area, provided that there is no major block at the elbow joint. Just working at the shoulder joint with the other hand is enough to help to achieve the same objective in some cases. When one is experiencing a high level of anxiety in the chest area, we can have the client sit in a chair, and then we can make suggestions such as "Please place your right hand on the left shoulder and the left wrist on your left knee after drawing up the left leg and placing the lower left leg on the right thigh. Then, as you stay with your experience of anxiety, which makes sense given the situation you are facing, notice how it might help to expand the left arm and the chest area. Then observe whether your anxiety is expanding more through the chest area, and whether it is also spreading to your arm. And notice whether it is easier to experience the anxiety in the chest now than before."

I have chosen to illustrate working with the arms with the emotion of anxiety as an example because this can be helpful in working with panic attacks, a common symptom. In the formation of panic attacks, there is usually a great deal of fear about something and constriction of the breathing muscles as a defense to cope with the fear, which constrains the fear to the chest area. When the source of the fear continues to be present, the breathing muscles are constricted even more, making breathing increasingly difficult, creating panic in the brain as it is deprived of oxygen. It can be said that a panic attack is an attempt on the part of the brain to release the defenses in the breathing muscles all at once to survive. So when one is working with panic attacks, it is extremely important to quickly expand the adjacent areas of the arms, head, and neck, to expand the experience of anxiety so that the breathing muscles—especially those in the chest—do not constrict too much and scare the brain into a panic attack. (In working with anxiety attacks, it is also important to move the energy and the anxiety downward into the abdomen across the diaphragm.)

We can also use simple area-to-area expansion strategies with just awareness and intention. You could say, "As you feel the anxiety in your chest, please enlarge your awareness to include your arms. You can go back and forth between your chest and your arms in your awareness, or you can hold them both in your awareness at the same time. How does that change your experience of anxiety in your chest? Does the chest feel more expanded or a little less constricted? Does the anxiety expand more in the chest area? Does it feel more tolerable than before? What about your arms? Do they feel more expanded? Do you now feel in your arms any of the qualities of the anxiety you feel in your chest?"

The Head, Face, and Neck

This is an important area in emotional embodiment work for a number of reasons. One, it houses the brain. The brain can generate emotional experiences on its own without involving the rest of the body. Also, the brain can construct emotions from information the body provides on the situation's impact on the person's well-being. Two, the neck musculature, especially its posterior section, is known to mediate the information flow between the head and the body. Blocking the neck area can compromise the flow of information between the two areas. Three, muscles and other structures in the head, face, and neck area (such as the tongue and the larynx) are known to perform a number of important functions in relation to emotions. They play important roles in generating, expressing, regulating, and defending against emotions; in understanding the emotional states of others through mirroring; and in facilitating the processing of emotional experiences in the brain as well as the rest of the body. Defenses against emotions in these areas can therefore significantly compromise the expansion and embodiment of emotional experiences in the brain as well as the rest of the body.

The polyvagal theory of the autonomic nervous system identifies seven muscle groups in the head, face, and neck area as part of what it calls the social engagement system.[5] They are: a) the jaw muscles; b) the eye muscles; c) the inner ear muscles; d) the other facial muscles; e) the muscles of ingestion and expulsion at the throat; f) the muscles of vocalization; and g) the muscles that move the neck and the head. This is one area where we can use movement effectively to undo defenses against emotions and thus to access and expand emotional experiences. In order to work with these muscles through movement, we can open and close our jaws; open and close our eyes; move our eyes around in multiple directions; focus our hearing on faint sounds in the background, moving the focus away from loud sounds in the foreground, to activate the inner ear muscles; contort our facial muscles into different facial expressions; swallow, cough, or simulate throwing up; vocalize different sounds; and engage our head and neck in movements in different directions (forward, backward, and side to side).

In addition to movement, we can also work with these areas to undo defenses in them by just bringing our awareness to them or by gently touching them or massaging them, to expand an emotional experience locally or as preparation for connecting to an emotional experience in the brain or in other parts of the body.

Working with the head, face, and neck area with one or more of the above methods can counteract defenses and help in recruiting the area to participate in generating, experiencing, and expressing emotion. Connecting the brain or other parts of the body to the "bridge" of the head, face, and neck area can allow emotion in those areas to become more expanded throughout the brain and body physiology, more regulated, and more clarified. When the facial muscles are being blocked during emotional experiences, processing of the emotion and the situation in the brain is severely compromised.[6] When the face and throat physiology become involved in emotional experiences in the rest of the body through facial and vocal expression, greater clarity about one's emotional experience is possible. Because vocal and facial expression of emotion are closely linked to nonverbal expression of emotion throughout the body, these expressions can help in further expansion of the emotional experience throughout the body. In addition, when we get the emotion to the face, the likelihood of support for it from other people increases, which would make it easier to tolerate the emotional experience.

To connect this area to the emotional experience in the brain or in other parts of the body, we can make suggestions such as "Imagine someone making a sound or a facial expression that matches the emotional experience in your brain or body." "Imagine yourself making a sound or a facial expression that matches the emotional experience in your brain or body." or "Try to express the emotion you feel in the brain or body as a facial expression or as a sound through vocalization." When there is no clear emotion in the brain or the body, we can work in the same way with the distress that a situation or a psychophysiological symptom is causing in either place, to check if it can be clarified as a possible emotional reaction to the situation. To do that, we can use suggestions such as "As you feel how bad this situation or the abdominal pain or headache is making you feel, please try to express it through a facial expression or vocalization that matches your distress. I will do it with you."

The polyvagal theory of the autonomic nervous system also offers us an understanding of how movement of the seven muscle groups in the head, face, and neck listed earlier can expand the head, face, and neck area and the upper chest area at the same time and help connect the two areas in energy and emotional experience. Evolution has given rise to an extremely fine-tuned coordination between the seven muscle groups and a parasympathetic nerve called the ventral vagal nerve. An intent to move any of the seven groups of muscles immediately triggers the ventral vagal nerve to stimulate the heart and lungs to increase heartbeat and breath rate to increase cardiovascular output, in order to supply the muscle group with the energy needed for the movement. This means that if one wants to expand the emotional experience in the chest to the head, face, and neck area or vice versa by working with the head, face, and neck area, movement of the seven groups of muscles (including muscles of facial expression and vocalization) can be of assistance.

For example, to expand an emotional experience from the chest to the adjacent head and neck area, we can make suggestions such as "As you feel the fear in the chest, open and close your mouth to loosen the jaw muscles, open and close your eyes to expand the muscles of the eyes, turn your head and neck in different directions, or express the fear through facial expression or vocalization. Do one or more of the above actions, and notice what you experience in your chest and in your head and neck as a result. Do you notice physical expansion in either area? How do you experience the fear in the chest now? Is it more expanded? Is it more tolerable than before? Do you experience any fear in your head, face, or neck area?"

To connect the head, face, and neck area to any other area of the body, we can also use the simple area-to-area expansion strategies employing awareness, intention, and self-touch. For example, if we wanted to connect the experience of sadness in the face and throat area to the abdomen, we could make suggestions such as "While paying attention to the sadness in your face and throat, expand your awareness to include the abdomen, hold both areas in your awareness, or go back and forth between the two. See if you can move the sadness down into your abdomen with your intention. What happens in your abdomen? Does it expand? Does it start to experience the qualities of sadness you are experiencing in your face? Do you find your sadness more tolerable than before?"

You can also bring in self-touch to expand the emotion to another area as follows: "As you feel the sadness in your face and throat, place one hand on your face in a comfortable manner and the other hand on the abdomen, with the intention to connect the two areas. Notice whether the sadness or some quality of it in your face and throat is expanding into your abdomen. Is the sadness now more tolerable than before? Do · the face, throat, and abdominal areas feel more expanded now?"

The body psychotherapy system of Bodynamic Analysis has empirically found that the muscles of the neck, especially those in the back of the neck, can form a block to compromise the flow of information between the head and the rest of the body.[7] In addition, the neck muscles have also been found to have the ability to cope with or defend against high levels of energy, stress, fear, and shock. In order to work with the neck to expand the neck area locally as well as to connect the head and the rest of the body in emotional experience, we can just become aware of the neck with the intent to make it more available. We can also move our neck in different directions or touch the back of the neck with one hand with the intent to undo the defenses in the area.

I once asked a woman who suffered from anxiety where she experienced her anxiety when she thought of a situation that triggered it. She said it was all in her brain. I asked her if I had her permission to gently place my hand on the back of her neck, to help connect her anxiety to the body. She said yes. In a dramatic demonstration of how effectively the neck could block the expansion of emotional experience from the brain to the body, within a minute, she reported that her anxiety was all over her body. So I always check on the neck during emotional embodiment sessions, to see whether defenses there are in the way of emotions expanding from the head to the body or vice versa. This holds true for all emotions in general but especially for fear, terror, and grief. Why grief? We often repress our grief by holding back its expression at the throat. Touching the back of the neck seems to help in releasing the inhibition in the throat.

The Chest, Abdominal, and Pelvic Areas

The torso, from the shoulders to the pelvic floor, includes the chest, abdominal, and pelvic areas. The viscera (organs, glands, and blood vessels in the interior of the torso) are protected by muscles, bones, fascia, and skin on the outside. The functioning of the viscera is dependent on the functioning of the torso musculature. For example, the lungs depend on the breathing muscles of the torso for respiration. The viscera constitute the core metabolic machinery of respiration, digestion, and blood circulation through which energy is produced and distributed, to cope with life situations ranging from the ordinary to the extraordinary. The generation of emotional experience, an assessment of how situations affect our well-being, therefore has a lot to do with this core physiology. The torso muscles such as the diaphragm, the intercostals, and the abdominal muscles, identified as the primary breathing muscles, have also been identified as the primary muscles of emotional management in body psychotherapy. We can readily verify this by holding our breath to reduce the intensity of most of our emotional experiences. These connections show how intertwined the viscera and the torso musculature are in their physiological and psychological functioning. In working with ourselves and others, we can also notice how working on one brings about changes in the other.

In emotional embodiment work, we are often interested in expanding the emotional experience locally in the chest cavity between the shoulders and the diaphragm or in the abdominal and pelvic cavities between the diaphragm and the pelvic floor. We are also often interested in integrating the torso area above the diaphragm with the area below it, connecting the chest cavity with the head and neck above, or linking the abdominal and pelvic areas with the legs below. There are many ways to work with the torso in emotional embodiment. As with our work with the arms and legs, we will borrow methods from osteopathy to work with the torso.

Osteopaths have identified three diaphragms within the torso: at the shoulder, at the diaphragm muscle, and at the pelvic floor. A diaphragm is a horizontal structure in the body that, when dysfunctional, can reduce the level of regulation in the body by interfering with vital biological flows, such as blood and intercellular fluid, from one area to another. Osteopaths have found working on the torso's diaphragms to be effective in working with the torso's internal structures, such as organs, and external structures, such as muscles.[8,9]

We can work with the shoulder diaphragm with awareness or with self-touch by placing a hand on the opposite shoulder or at the center of the top of the chest, where the breastbone and collarbones come together. This can be done with the intention to help the chest cavity expand locally in the downward direction or to integrate the chest area with the head and neck area above.

We can work with the diaphragm muscle with awareness or with self-touch with one hand on the middle of the solar plexus just below the breastbone, or with two hands placed on the front of the rib cage, on either side of the one-handed position described immediately above. This can be done with the intention to expand the chest cavity locally in the upward direction, to expand the abdominal and pelvic cavities in the downward direction, or to integrate the chest cavity with the abdominal and pelvic cavities in emotional experience.

We can work with the pelvic diaphragm at the pelvic floor in a number of ways. We can place one hand on the pubic bone or place one hand on the pubic bone and the other on the sacrum. We can also place a hand on either hip bone with the fingers pointing into the groin, as we did for working with the hip joint, with the attention now focused on the pelvic floor instead of the hip joint. We can work with the pelvic diaphragm with self-touch in all of the above ways, with our awareness focused on the pelvic floor to make it more functional, and with our intention to expand the pelvic and abdominal cavities locally in the upward direction, or to integrate them with the legs below in emotional experience.

When we work with two diaphragms at a time, we can expect the area in between to expand and to integrate with the area above the upper diaphragm and with the area below the lower diaphragm. For example, when we work with our awareness or both hands at the shoulder and the diaphragm muscle, we can expect the chest area to expand locally and for it to integrate with the head and neck area above (provided there is no significant blockage at the neck) and with the abdominal and pelvic areas below. When we work with our awareness or both hands at the diaphragm muscle and the pelvic diaphragm, we can expect the abdominal and pelvic areas to expand and to integrate with the chest area above and with the legs below (provided there is no significant problem at the hip joints). We can also work with the shoulder diaphragm and the pelvic diaphragm with awareness or with both hands, to expand the entire torso from the shoulder to the pelvic floor on the inside as well as on the outside (provided there is not a significant blockage in the diaphragm muscle), and to connect it to the legs below and the head and neck area above (provided there is no significant disruption in the neck or at the hip joints).

We can also use simple strategies for local as well as area-to-area expansion, with awareness or self-touch with intention, at other locations on the torso. We have illustrated what that might look like in the earlier sections on simple strategies for local and area-to-area expansion.

The Brain Physiology

In the ISP professional training, trainees also learn how to expand emotional experiences across different layers of the brain and body physiology: the muscular system, the viscera, and the central nervous system areas of the brain and the spinal cord. Detailed discussion of all the strategies that could be used is not feasible here. However, because of the brain's importance, we will learn some ways of working with the brain to regulate and expand emotional experiences in the brain as well as the body, and to expand emotional experiences in the brain to the other layers of the body, the viscera and the muscular system.

The brain regulates the body. Emotional experiences generated in the brain or in the two outer layers of the body can overwhelm the brain and dysregulate it. Defenses can form against this dysregulation in the physiology of the brain and the spinal cord. When the brain is thus overwhelmed, either the emotional experience can disappear all of a sudden, or symptoms such as migraines, confusion, loss of speech, and fainting can form quickly. Working with the brain as well as the viscera just through awareness and intention is not as effective as working with them through self-touch. This is because we cannot sense detailed physiological sensations of what is happening in the brain, the spinal cord, and the viscera through our conscious awareness. We can sense detailed physiological sensations of what is happening in the muscular system and the skin much better.

Two areas of the brain that are involved in emotional overwhelm are the brain stem and the prefrontal cortex. The brain stem manages vital functions, such as breathing and circulation, through the autonomic nervous system, which has its origin in the brain stem. Our survival depends on it. A blunt trauma to the brain stem can result in instant death. The prefrontal cortex—especially the orbito-prefrontal cortex, also called the limbic cortex—is the junction where the higher brain structures that manage emotion come together with the lower brain structures that have to do with generating emotion. In emotional overwhelm that involves the brain, both the brain stem and the prefrontal cortex areas are likely to be overwhelmed. Because some people are more easily overwhelmed than others, and because emotional overwhelm is not an uncommon experience even for those with a great deal of affect tolerance, I have found that knowledge of how to work with the brain directly with self-touch is quite often useful in emotional embodiment work. The self-touch strategies I use to work directly with the brain physiology are inspired by craniosacral therapy.[10]

In order to reach the brain stem with self-touch, one has to place a hand on the occipital bone, the lowest portion of the back of the skull, with the thumb and the forefinger below the bone, on the neck. Then one must set an intention of depth to reach the brain stem, which is located anterior to the occipital lobe and the cerebellum. In order to work with a deeper structure in the brain such as the brain stem, or a deeper structure in the body proper such as the heart, we place our hand on the surface above the deeper structure, with an intent of depth to direct bioelectric, biomagnetic, and quantum energies through our hands to find their target. The prefrontal cortex is easier to locate and work with. We can simply place the palm of one of our hands on our forehead with the intention of depth to regulate the prefrontal cortex.

When we run into a situation where there is overwhelming emotion, or a sudden disappearance of emotion due to the overwhelm, we can make suggestions such as "Please place your hand on your brain stem or forehead, or on both places at the same time, with the intention of depth to reach and regulate the brain structures under your hands. If you can visualize them, that would even be better. If you cannot visualize them, do not worry. Notice what starts to happen in your body. Notice how things start to get more regulated and expanded in the brain and the body. Observe whether emotions that were lost are coming back or whether emotions that were so overwhelming are becoming more manageable or tolerable. See if your brain is getting more regulated, more spacious, calmer, and so on, even though you are processing the fear of dying."

When we worked in Indian villages with survivors of the Indian Ocean tsunami of 2004, simultaneous self-touch at both the brain stem and the prefrontal cortex was quite effective in regulating and expanding the high level of activation. I still remember the women who had just received their treatments showing women who were waiting to receive theirs how to do self-touch at the brain stem and at the prefrontal cortex, which we had taught them as a self-help tool to help themselves as well as others.

Expansion across Layers of the Brain and Body Physiology

We can touch either the brain stem or the prefrontal cortex with one hand and touch another part of the body in the same layer, such as the spinal cord, to expand within the central nervous system area. With one hand on the brain stem or the prefrontal cortex and the other hand on a part of the viscera or the muscular system, we can expand emotional experience across different layers of the physiology. We could, for example, make suggestions such as "As you feel the overwhelming grief in your heart, please place one hand on your brain stem or the prefrontal cortex, and the other hand on your heart to connect the heart and the brain stem with the intention to reach, regulate, and expand the heart. Observe the changes. Does it make the grief more expanded and regulated in your heart or your brain? Does it help to make the grief more present in one place where it was not present before? Does it make your experience of grief overall more tolerable than before?" When the overwhelming grief disappears suddenly, you can suggest, "Please place one hand on the brain stem or the prefrontal cortex and the other hand on your heart. And as you go back to remembering the situation that caused you much grief, please observe whether the grief is beginning to surface in your brain or your heart. Is it more bearable than before?"

We can use simple area-to-area expansion strategies for expanding emotion across the viscera and the muscular system, with awareness, intention, and self-touch. For example, to expand both areas and connect them to each other in emotional experience, we could suggest, "Please place your hand on the large intestine in your abdomen in the area just above your navel. Imagine touching it through your skin and muscle in the area, to undo any defenses there. Place your other hand on your thigh musculature to undo any inhibition there. Now, notice how the two areas might start to connect in energy and in emotion. Is the hint of fear that was present in the large intestine area expanding more throughout the abdomen? Is the fear in the abdomen connecting to the thigh and expanding there? Look for the quality of the fear in the abdomen in the thigh area. Please try to express the fear you feel in the abdomen through a facial expression and a vocalization to help expand it throughout the body. Is your experience of the fear more manageable than before?"

Some Considerations regarding Expansion

When we undo defenses in the brain and body physiology, the physiology tends to get more regulated, especially when we expand it using models of regulation. This could regulate the emotion away if we are not focused on the emotion and the situation causing it. That is okay if that is what our intention is. However, when we wish to increase the capacity to tolerate the emotion, we need to continue to remind the person of the situation, especially those details that are tied to the emotion, such as "You saw your wife alive but not your child when the tsunami retreated." We must also continue to support the person emotionally in all ways possible, with statements such as "Of all the grief I know, the grief of losing a child is the worst. It is the hardest thing in the world to lose a child." Otherwise, the emotion might just disappear, regulated by our singular focus on the expansion that excludes the emotion and the situation.

Questions are often asked about the optimal directions for expanding emotion from one area of the body to another. A good rule of thumb is to expand it to the adjacent areas of the body. For example, if the emotion is present in the chest area, one could expand from the chest to the arms across the shoulder joint, to the abdomen across the diaphragm, to the head and neck area through the shoulder diaphragm, or to the head through the neck. If emotion is initially present in the abdomen, one could expand upward toward the chest through the diaphragm or downward to the legs through the hip joints or the pelvic diaphragm. At times, when the emotional difficulty is too concentrated toward one end of the body, one might have to work at the other end of the body in a nonadjacent area, to pull the energy down and make the emotional experience more bearable. When the difficult emotional experience is too concentrated in the head or the chest, it often helps to work with the legs to expand the emotional experience downward, all the way down into the legs.

Other questions that are often asked about the expansion phase are: How much expansion does one do? Narrow expansion, confined to local expansion in the area or expansion to only one or two other areas? Widespread expansion, involving many other areas? In working on local expansion in an area, does one stay superficial or go deep? And how much time does one spend on the expansion task? The answer to all these questions is a frustrating one: well, it depends. It depends on what is necessary to get the symptom to resolve. It also depends on the capacity of the client, as well as the capacity of the therapist, because what is possible in a session depends on both the client and the therapist.

In general, the lower the client's affect tolerance, the more superficial one needs to stay in expanding an area locally. The longer we stay focused on locally expanding an area, the deeper the opening. The deeper the physiological opening, the more difficult an unpleasant experience becomes, especially when the rest of the body is defended against it. In such circumstances, it is better not to spend a lot of time expanding the emotion locally in the initial area of emotion and instead to recruit another area to expand the emotion into, so that the burden of emotion is shared by both places to make it more bearable.

Sometimes, when affect tolerance levels are really low, the best strategy is to superficially expand the emotional experience to as many places as quickly as possible. We often work with the symptoms of anxiety attacks or migraines caused by emotions this way. There are times when we need to work deeply in one place, such as the heart, in order to resolve a symptom. In such cases, before we get to the deep local work in an area, it is recommended that more parts of the body are first recruited through superficial expansion in earlier cycles of emotional embodiment. Going deep into one place without some support from other areas can make the experience of the emotion more unbearable than it needs to be.

How much expansion one needs to do, how many areas an emotional experience needs to be expanded into, and how deep the expansion needs to be in one place for symptom resolution are all ultimately empirical questions, with answers varying from one client to the next, and from one situation to the next for the same client.

Next, we look at the last step in the emotional embodiment process: integration.

13

The Integration

Chapter summary: shows how improvements in physiological and energetic regulation that continuously accrue from a greater embodiment of emotion can be used to stabilize the practice of embodying emotion, if needed, in different places in a session.

What Is Integration?

Integration usually refers to bringing things together. In general, therapists understand integration as things that happen after a session, on their own, to further the process. For example, integration could occur in the form of a dream that works through another aspect of the problem situation, a change in the person's symptom, or a change in the person's thinking that is helpful for healing. In emotional embodiment work, integration is defined as spontaneous positive developments that occur as a consequence of developing a greater capacity for emotional experience. Such integration can happen even during the session. The creation of a greater capacity for an emotional experience through its expansion can yield tangible improvements in one's physiological and energetic regulation. It can make the brain and body physiology more available for optimal changes in cognition and behavior. It can facilitate greater access to collective resources.

Integration is a continuous process. It can be likened to the process of recovering from an illness such as the flu. As we heal gradually, our body, energy, cognition, behavior, and ability to engage our animate and inanimate environment improve steadily. In the step of integration, we exploit such favorable consequences from embodying emotion as resources for facilitating further embodiment of emotions and resolution of symptoms.

Uses of Integration

When we start to work with a problem situation, we are starting a cycle of embodying emotion. After we have identified an emotion, supported it, and expanded it to the extent possible, we might just end the cycle there, without much attention to integration. A session of emotional embodiment work can have one or many cycles of processing an emotion or different emotions. Integration can be used as the final step in a cycle of processing emotion, or it can come at the end of a session consisting of many cycles, to bring more stability or change at the end of a cycle or a session. However, integration can also be used at other times. It can be used within a cycle to support and stabilize the brain and body physiology. It can also be brought in to keep the emotional experience within a person's window of tolerance.

In embodying an emotion, we might have to take a break from the emotion from time to time so we can process the emotion in many short cycles as opposed to one long cycle, to keep the experience bearable. In such instances, integration can help in breaking up the process into shorter cycles in a stable manner. Please note that conscious use of integration is an optional step in emotional embodiment work. That is, it is not always necessary within a session.

Because integration is always happening, it might become conscious in a client on its own. Here, we are talking about making a conscious use of it. Let us now look at different positive developments that embodying emotion can bring in its wake, how they come about, how they appear, how to look for them, and different ways in which they can be used as resources for improving embodiment of emotions and resolution of symptoms.

Positive Developments from Embodying Emotion

Improvement in physiological and energetic regulation: An unpleasant emotional experience is a state of stress and dysregulation. As we saw in chapter 8 on affect tolerance, the level of stress and dysregulation in the body during an unpleasant emotional experience increases with the engagement of physiological and energetic defenses when we are actively trying to access the emotional experience to resolve it. A pleasant emotional experience is a state characterized by increasing regulation and decreasing stress. If the pleasant emotional experience, such as sexuality, is inhibited through physiological and energetic defenses, the level of stress and dysregulation in the body also increases. When we ease physiological and energetic defenses against the emotional experience to expand an emotional experience and support the person to experience more of the emotion, our body and energy move in the direction of greater regulation or lesser dysregulation, even as we are experiencing unpleasant emotions. In fact, it is this relative improvement in the regulation of body and energy in the process of embodying emotion that plays a major role in making us experience the unpleasant emotion as less painful or more tolerable.

As physical and energetic defenses are undone to expand the brain and body physiology to expand the emotional experience, blood, nervous system, interstitial, lymphatic, and energy flows that regulate the body improve, increasing regulation and well-being in the physiology, even as we are processing an unpleasant emotional experience. In general, in integration we are looking for shifts in the body and energy experienced as increases in well-being or decreases in stress and distress.

One can experience this aspect of integration in the body in many ways: less inhibition, less constriction, more freedom, more space, more comfort, less discomfort, less pain, easier breath, relief, ease, and so on, even as one might be processing a terrible emotion such as the fear of dying. In terms of energy, one might experience integration as reduction in unease or discomfort in one's experience of energy, more positive energy, less energy with greater comfort, more flow, expansion, balance in the distribution of energy in the body, and so on.

Paying attention to shifts in the underlying body and energy experience toward less discomfort or more comfort can be helpful in making the emotional experience more regulated, stable, and tolerable during a cycle, at the end of a cycle, or at the end of a session. One can go back and forth in one's attention from improvements in the body and energy experience to the emotional experience, or one can hold them both in the awareness at the same time.

The increase in stability, regulation, and tolerance of the emotional experience can come about in at least three ways. One, sensing the increase of regulation beneath the unpleasant emotion can make the unpleasant emotion more tolerable, as the swallowing of bitter medicine is made easier with a bit of sugar mixed in. Two, paying attention to regulation supports its growth. When we do that in the same physiology in which we are working with an unpleasant emotional experience, it can counter the unpleasant experience and reduce the level and intensity of it, making it more stable and bearable. Three, the more attention we pay to an experience, the more intense it can get, as we are adding more energy to the experience by paying attention to it, in accordance with the first principle of energy. So when we split the brain's attention between the unpleasant emotional experience and the underlying improvement in body and energy, we dilute the attention we are paying to the unpleasant emotional experience, distracting ourselves from it, and that can reduce the suffering from it, making it more stable and bearable.

Potential for improvement in cognition and behavior: As we saw in chapter 6, cognition, emotion, and behavior depend not only on the brain but also on the body and the environment. And as we saw in chapter 8, defenses formed to cope with overwhelming emotions render our body less available for cognition and behavior, compromising both in a situation and hampering our ability to cope with the situation effectively. When we create a greater capacity to tolerate emotions by expanding the body, both the body and its connection to the environment are more available for optimal cognitive and behavioral shifts. As cognition and behavior become more optimal in relation to a situation, our ability to cope with the situation through cognition and behavior improves.

There are situations where changes in cognition or behavior can lead to the resolution of an emotional difficulty. For example, while processing the hurt I felt from an instance when I felt rejected by my wife and the subsequent difficulty I have had in reaching out to her when I am in need, both my hurt and my disconnection from my wife could be resolved by realizing that the hurt I feel around my wife might have to do with my mother (cognition); or it could be resolved by feeling an impulse to reach out to my wife again (behavior). There are also situations where changes in cognition or behavior can help in tolerating the emotion. For example, realizing that the hurt I feel might have more to do with my mother than with my wife (cognition) can help in making the hurt more tolerable to process. As another example, the recognition that the fear of dying from a childhood trauma is mixed up with the fear of dying during the pandemic can render both fears more tolerable to process to completion. Just naming a feeling (cognition) can sometimes help make the experience more tolerable. Realizing that one has more options for responding to a situation (behavior) can make one's emotions in the situation, such as fear and frustration, more tolerable to process.

In integration, we can look for helpful cognitive and behavioral shifts that happen during emotional embodiment work—whether during a cycle, at the end of a cycle, at the end of a session of many cycles, or between sessions—that can make the emotional experience more tolerable, stable, and resolvable. These shifts often emerge on their own as part of the process. If not, we can facilitate them by asking questions such as "What do you think about the situation now?" or "What do you think you can do differently in the situation?" Engaging a person in cognitive and behavioral aspects of the experience in the midst of an overwhelming emotional experience by splitting the person's attention among the different aspects of experience can help to reduce the intensity of the emotional aspect of the experience, making the emotional experience more tolerable and stable in the middle or at the end of a cycle.

You can ask, "Now that you have developed some ability to tolerate, regulate, and be with your emotions, I wonder how your thinking about the situation, your memory of the details of the situation, and your ideas about what you can and cannot do (or what you could have done and what you could not have done) in this situation may have shifted." You can ask them to engage in such a process with you during the session, or you can have them do such self-inquiry in between sessions.

Integration of the work of emotional embodiment, like any other psychological work, is likely to continue in waking life as well as in dream states. Keeping this in mind, we can also suggest the following to our clients: "You have done an important and hard piece of work successfully. The process is likely to continue for some time when you are awake as well as when you are asleep. Please keep track of changes in your thinking and your memory of the situation; your emotions about the situation, including the ones we worked on today; and what you think you can or cannot do about the situation. Please also keep track of your dreams, and reflect on how your dreams in the aftermath of the session might reflect changes in your cognition, emotion, and behavior in relation to the situation you worked with."

Improvement in collective resources: When a greater capacity for an unbearable emotion is generated, the mind and the body can be more open to the environment, which allows them to be better connected with the collective energies of the universe. For example, when I am able to connect more with people in my environment after working with my fear of making eye contact with others, a fear that goes back to my childhood, the extra support I can now take in from others in my collective can help me process deeper levels of my fear of making contact, with greater affect tolerance. We can use this interpersonal resource during a cycle, or at the end of a cycle or a session, to make the emotional experience more stable, regulated, and tolerable, and to resolve symptoms.

Paying attention to positive shifts in energy (whether from the inside or the outside, because we cannot always distinguish between the two in the body) at any stage during emotional embodiment work—but especially at the end of a session, when we can expect the collective energies to be more available after several cycles of embodying emotion—can help in making the emotional experience more stable, regulated, and tolerable, and in reorganizing persistent long-term body and energy patterns to resolve symptoms. I remember sitting with a woman after she had worked with embodying her sadness in her chest, resonating with the swirls of energy that came into her lungs, and expanding them in slow motion from the inside, the kind of deep integration that I have seen precede symptom resolution. That particular client reported that soon afterward she gained major relief from her long-term symptom of frequent episodes of breathing difficulty.

Integration in Different Stages of Emotional Embodiment

Within a cycle: A cycle of embodying emotion consists of the four steps of situation, emotion, expansion, and integration. At any point in the cycle, especially in the first three steps, there are times when emotion can become too much to bear, and defenses become stronger. There can be an increase in stress, dysregulation, and instability in body and energy. One can then use physiological and energetic phenomena of integration to manage the process to keep the experience within the window of tolerance.

You can do this by making statements such as "You are really doing a great job, working hard to embody your grief. It looks like it is becoming too much for you, for now. Grief is hard. I know from my own experience how hard it can be. Shift your awareness a bit to notice how your body and energy might feel a bit better than before, from the hard work you did to expand your grief. Specifically, your breath might be just a little bit easier. The body might feel less constricted somewhere, especially in places you have expanded the grief to. You might even feel more energized in a good way in some places or throughout your body. Your brain might feel less stressed. Please place your awareness on such tiny improvements in your body and energy, for a little while, from time to time, as you continue to pay attention to your expanding grief. You can go back and forth between your grief and the small improvements in your body and energy, or you can hold them both in your awareness at the same time. Notice how that makes you feel better in being with your grief, and continue expanding it further in your body."

When things get hard within the cycle, we can also bring in cognitive and behavioral aspects of integration to ease the suffering and decrease stress, dysregulation, and instability. As we saw earlier, it might make it easier to be with the grief because one's attention is taken away from emotional experience or divided between emotional experience and cognitive and behavioral aspects of the experience. Or we might be able to tap into the potential for improvement in cognition and behavior, to help ease the pain and reduce the instability in the process.

We can make statements such as "It is great that you have managed to grasp your grief to this extent. It is not the easiest thing in the world to do, to be with an emotion as difficult as grief. When we develop a greater capacity to tolerate an emotion by expanding it in the body, research shows that it can change what we think about the situation and what we can do in the situation, for the better. Let us now take a moment to assess how the work you have done so far might have changed what you think or recall about the situation—and your ideas about what you can or could have done differently in the situation—for the better. For example, you could have said or not said something. You could have done or not done something, things that are more feasible to you now than before. Also, does the grief you are feeling now in this situation remind you of other situations in your life, especially from your childhood?" The last sentence taps into the possibility that cognitive insight about the influence of the past on the present can be helpful in tolerating the emotion in the present.

During the cycle, we can also use an increase in a person's ability to make contact and take in support from you or from the group if you happen to be working with the person in a group, to help bring more stability, containment, and capacity to the emotional experience. You can facilitate such contact by saying, "Please look at me or the group, and see if you notice a difference in your ability to make contact with me or the group, and take in my or the group's support. It is okay if you can do that only to a limited extent. Even a little can go a long way. Take in as much support as you can. Does it help you become more stable, your physiology or energy get more regulated, and your grief feel more tolerable?"

At the end of a cycle: A person can be with a difficult emotion only for so long. Either the cycle leads to the resolution of the emotion, or of the physical, energetic, cognitive, emotional, behavioral, or relational symptoms; or, more likely, the emotion goes away because the person can no longer stand it or has done enough for now, and needs a break before engaging the emotion again in another cycle. It is also possible that the psyche is pausing to integrate the cognitive and behavioral implications of embodying an emotion.

In such instances, we can shift to the integration mode and bring in physiological, energetic, cognitive, behavioral, and environmental aspects of integration with statements similar to the ones we saw earlier in this chapter, in the section about integration within a cycle, with one difference. The opening statement could be, "Now that you have successfully completed one cycle of processing a difficult emotion, let us turn to the benefits you have accrued from the hard work you did. Please do not think of it as failure if you could not hold onto the emotion longer. It is natural for emotion to come and go. We can stay with an emotion for only so long. Your body, your energy, how you look at the situation, and your perception of what you can do or could have done in the situation are all likely to be different, if not better."

When we are trying to integrate the benefits or stabilize the process at the end of a cycle, it would not generally be productive to continue reminding the person of the details of the situation that evoked the emotion or to continue to refer to the emotion and support it. For example, we would not go back and forth between the emotion and the physiological and energetic improvements from embodying emotion. We might, however, hold both at the same time, to stabilize the person in the emotion before shifting to the cognitive and behavioral aspects of integration. The end of a cycle is also a good place to bring in the potential improvement in a person's ability to connect with others and take in their support, using statements we have mentioned earlier, as a resource for consolidating the work done and for the work ahead.

For shortening or ending cycles: There are times when we need to keep the cycles short because the affect tolerance level is so low that a person might not be able to handle longer cycles. There are other times when the emotional experience is simply so overwhelming, the stress, dysregulation, and distress so high, the process so unstable, that we need to end a cycle as an emergency measure. In such instances, we can use integration deliberately to shorten or end the cycle. To do this, we as therapists need to shift our focus away from the situation and the emotion for the time being and toward physiological and energetic benefits that have accrued from whatever emotion has been embodied. Integration of cognitive and behavioral shifts is less likely to be beneficial after a short cycle; it is likely to be more beneficial after a number of short cycles or after a long cycle or at the end of a session, but it should not be ruled out altogether. Having the client make contact with you or the group in ways we have seen earlier can be helpful in distracting them from their process so you can end a cycle. This can also be helpful for obtaining support from others for stabilizing the process if the cycle ended on shaky ground, or for use as a resource for the next cycle.

Managing extreme emotional states: When an emotional experience becomes too dysregulated, or when it regresses into unbearable childhood states, integration as we have suggested so far might be inadequate to end the cycle, manage the emotion, and stabilize the physiology. In such instances, we need measures for managing such overwhelm to bring a cycle to an end. Let us look at some simple things we can do to manage extreme activation. As therapists, we need to stop referring to the situation and supporting the emotion, as that can continue to fuel the emotion. We also need not to show excess concern; instead, we need to reassure the client that the overwhelming experience can be managed. We can make statements such as "You have really gotten into the emotion, and it appears that your brain and body are having a hard time dealing with it. It would be good to get out of it altogether now, for the time being. We can go back to it later. This happens to everyone from time to time, especially to those who are really willing to dig deeper into their suffering for healing.

"Please open your eyes [if the client's eyes are closed] and put all of your attention on the outside, or as much attention on the outside as you need to make your experience more manageable. Please move your head and neck in different directions to help you orient to the present. Please let go of thinking about the situation and what you did or could not do in the situation. Please stop paying attention to the emotion now. We will get back to it later. To help yourself orient more to the present, please pay attention to the environment through your five senses. What do you see? What colors do you see? What do you smell here? What do you hear? Do you hear the wind in the trees or the traffic? What taste do you have on your tongue? How does your clothing feel on your skin now? If it is helpful to stand up from sitting in the chair, please do.

"Please move your body. Please move your arms, legs, torso, head, and neck, so you start to feel them more. Coming more into your muscles through awareness and movement can help you combat excess emotion, especially in child ego states. Please hold back the crying, because it can keep you regressed in child ego states and leave you helpless. Please look at me. See if that contact helps you contain your emotional experience and make it more manageable.

"There are specific things we can do together to make the emotional experience more manageable. While sitting in a chair, bring your legs together, put your hands on the sides of your knees, and then try to open your thighs while resisting that action by pressing your knees together with your hands. This will activate the fascia on the outsides of the thighs, which has the function of containing one's experiences, especially difficult ones. You can also do this in the standing position. Please stand up and try to imagine lifting both legs to the side while at the same time resisting the movement of the legs by pressing your feet into the ground. This will activate the fascia on the sides of your thighs, to contain your experience. Do you feel more together and less helpless when you do that? Lift your chest by pushing from the middle of your back to experience more containment. Play with pulling your chest in or lifting it in the opposite direction to get a sense that you can open and close your chest to manage vulnerable emotions there. Raise your arms to the sides, and bring them together over your head. Please do that a few times to see if you feel that you have more space around you that feels protective, and observe how that might make your experience easier to be with."

At the end of a session: The end of a session of one or more cycles of embodying emotion is a really good time for integration. It can help in stabilizing the process and the client's physiology before they go out into the world. It can also help in making the emotional experience more contained and tolerable if the client is still in the thick of the emotional experience at the end of the session. And it can help in exploiting the gains of various forms of integration from many cycles of embodying emotions (increase in physiological and energetic regulation, greater potential for cognitive and emotional change, and increase in access to collective resources) for resolving symptoms. Many of the statements we have offered earlier for use in integration at the end of the cycle can also be used at the end of a session.

In addition, when exploiting physiological, energetic, and collective aspects of integration at the end of the session, one can encourage a person to pay more attention to global or overall improvements in their body, energy, and collective resources, as opposed to local or specific improvements. Paying attention to global changes in body, energy, and collective resources has the advantage of bringing more stability to the process before the session ends. It can also offer more support and deeper resources for quicker symptom resolution. We can make statements such as "Now that we have done some really hard work, let us pay attention to how your whole body and energy might feel better, as opposed to paying attention to improvements in specific locations such as arms or legs. Notice how your whole body or energy might feel more regulated, changed for the better, freer, more pleasurable, less pained, and so on. If you are still with the emotion we worked with, please notice whether it is easier to be with the emotion now than it was before, as you notice these global shifts in your body and energy."

To exploit improved connection to the collective, which can be expected to be there to a greater extent in a more noticeable way after several cycles of emotion, we can make statements such as "Now that you have worked very hard with the really difficult emotion of shame, let us see how it might have helped you to connect more to the world.

Please look at me or the group [if you happen to be working in front of a group] and see whether it is easier to make contact with others. Do you feel more connected and supported than before? Do the fear and shame that inhibit you from making contact have the same grip on you?"

We can also say, "When it is tolerable to be with a difficult emotion such as fear or shame connected with making contact, the body does not have to defend against it. The body is then more connected to the environment and to the primal energies of creation. When your body and energy are more open to the collective energies of the environment and the primal energies of creation, they can come in and work on your body and energy to change your long-term patterns and symptoms. These energies are experienced in the body in different ways. They can feel like some new energy is coming in. They can feel like they are filling up parts of the body or the whole body. They can feel like they are expanding parts of the body or the whole body. Their flow can be experienced in different ways. They can be moving from the top to the bottom or from the bottom to the top. They can appear in spiral patterns, with the spirals going from the left to the right or from the right to the left, or spiraling from the top to the bottom or from the bottom to the top. They can feel like they have qualities and dynamics of movement of air or water. It is important that we support these healing energies with our awareness so they can transform us. We do not have to do anything other than to observe them and support them in doing their work."

Between sessions: After the session, the psyche will continue to heal. All aspects of integration will continue. It is said that when we take one conscious step on the path of healing, the unconscious will help us by taking several more steps toward our goal. A number of elements can come up to be processed between sessions in both waking states and dream states, such as other aspects of the situation, other emotions that have to do with them, deeper levels of the same emotion, other situations that are related to the situation worked with, and emotions that have to do with them. All aspects of integration we have discussed (physiological, energetic, cognitive, behavioral, and collective) can be expected to continue as well. And symptoms can resolve.

Most systems of psychotherapy understand all of the above phenomena as integration, as opposed to our more limited definition of it. It is a good practice to educate clients to expect all of these possibilities between sessions and teach them how to work with these occurrences on their own, to the extent that they are able. In Integral Somatic Psychology, we expect clients to learn the skills of embodying emotions so that they can use them throughout their lives, to help themselves and others. It is always good to review the session with clients at the end so they can remember the attitudes, self-touch positions, and other skills, including how to notice and use different aspects of integration—all the things that worked well for them in the session. This way, they will remember to use them to the extent that they are able, to work with themselves between sessions. It is also a good practice at the beginning of the next session to ask them about things that have happened since the last session, to quickly orient to the work to be done and to gather the new resources that have accrued from integration since the last session.

Use and misuse of integration: Working with integration is an optional step in a cycle of embodying emotion. Cognitive and behavioral aspects of integration usually happen naturally during the session or afterward to stabilize the process, contribute to the healing, or bring up new situations to work on for symptom resolution. However, one might have to work on generating cognitive and behavioral aspects of integration deliberately if they do not occur on their own and if they appear to be necessary for stabilizing the process and making the experience tolerable, or for ideas for further work to be done for symptom resolution. Conscious work with other aspects of integration, such as improvements in body, energy, and access to collective resources, might not be always necessary. These aspects of integration usually happen in the background, stabilizing the process, making the experience bearable, and contributing to symptom resolution. We do not have to make them conscious and use them as long as the emotional experience continues to be stable and the experience tolerable.

As we have seen, conscious use of all aspects of integration can be of considerable help in regulating overwhelming experiences during emotional embodiment work. However, caution is in order, especially in relation to the use of positive developments in body, energy, and access to collective resources. Because these aspects of integration tend to counteract the stress and dysregulation that are inherent in unpleasant emotional experiences, excess attention to them at the expense of the emotion could regulate the emotion away. It could become a learned defense against the experience of unpleasant emotions because of the brain's innate resistance to pain and suffering. So we should be careful in using positive developments to manage overwhelming unpleasant emotional experiences. It would be better to manage the intensity of the emotional experience by manipulating the level of emotional support, the level of emotion, the depth and width of body expansion, and the length of the cycle. If we fail, we can always fall back on integration to save the day. However, it is important to remember an exception to the general rule that the use of integration, especially with respect to improvements in access to collective resources, can contribute significantly to symptom resolution at the end of the session.

A Seven-Step Protocol for Embodying Emotion That Includes Integration

People like step-by step protocols. Here is one for one cycle of embodying emotion in seven steps, with integration included. It is especially useful for working with those who have very low levels of affect tolerance because it limits the time a person spends with an unpleasant experience between periods of integration.

1. Work with a situation and find an emotion to work with and support it to the extent necessary.

2. Locate the emotion in one place in the brain and body physiology. Locally expand it, but not for long. Please remember that the longer you stay in one place, the deeper you will go into it. The level as well as the intensity of the emotional experience there could become too high to tolerate.

3. Locate the emotion in another place. Again, locally expand it, but not for too long.

4. Pivot to paying attention to physiological and energetic aspects of integration. Let go of your attention to the situation and support for the emotion. Let the emotion remain in the background.

5. Locate physiological or energetic ease of integration in one place in the brain and body physiology, especially in one of the places where emotion was present. Expand it locally, but not for long. If you do, the physiology will deepen in the area, which might make the experience of the unpleasant emotion in the next cycle more difficult to manage.

6. Locate physiological or energetic ease of integration in another place, especially in one of the places where emotion was present. Expand, but not for long.

7. Expand your awareness to the whole of your body or energy and pay attention to the overall improvement in your body and energy, especially energy. Stay here a bit longer than in other steps.

Ordering of the Four Steps

People often ask in which order one should conduct the process of emotional embodiment. Because an emotion is always tied to a situation, it is best to start with the first step of finding the situation to work with. Most of the time, people come to us to sort out difficulties in specific situations. Therefore, it is relatively easy to zero in on a specific situation to focus on. However, there are times when the situation might not be clear. People might come in with a physical or energy symptom they are suffering from even though they are more likely to see a medical or bodywork practitioner than a psychotherapist first when they suffer from physical or energy symptoms. Or they might come with an emotional symptom, such as depression or anxiety, with no idea of what situations are causing it. When people come in with an emotional symptom, one can help them to explore what situations might be causing their emotional suffering. One can also work with the emotion to expand and support it, with the expectation that the situation will reveal itself if necessary as their capacity for suffering is enhanced.

The four steps of emotional embodiment are ordered in a logical sequence. However, the order should not be viewed as a rigid component of the protocol. One does not move from one step to the next while leaving the previous steps behind. In order to keep the emotion alive and relevant to the situation, one has to cycle back to the details of the situation as often as necessary to keep the fire of emotion burning. Also, in order to keep the emotion alive, one has to continually provide the necessary support for it and work with the innate and psychological defenses as they crop up. As we saw earlier, the optional fourth step of integration—in its physical, energetic, and collective aspects, as well as its cognitive and behavioral dimensions—can be done during a cycle, at the end of a cycle or session, or between sessions. There are times when, even as the situation and the emotion are clear and there is adequate support for the emotion and for dismantling the innate and psychological defenses against emotion, the unconscious physical and energetic defenses are so strong that it is hard to access the emotion, let alone expand its capacity in the body. In such situations, a therapist might work with a client's physical and energetic defenses for a while, first in a session or for a whole session, to loosen them as a preparation before focusing on a specific situation.

So, the four steps should be viewed more as different sets of tools or ingredients that the therapist can draw upon throughout a session of emotional embodiment work, rather than as a rigid sequence to be followed in every session. Often, the therapist engages the client with more than one step at the same time. The therapist has to continually support the client through empathy and other forms of emotional support; refer to the situation that the emotion has to do with often enough to keep the emotion alive and relevant; work with the innate, psychological, physical, and energetic defenses as and when they show up; and bring in the step of integration in its physical, energetic, collective, cognitive, or behavioral aspects when necessary for the different purposes for which they can be used.

Therapists who have conducted a detailed intake of a client might have strong hypotheses about past situations that might be contributing to the present emotional difficulty and might wish to focus on a past situation. A question that is often asked in supervision is whether one should work with the emotion in relation to the original situation or in relation to the current situation to which the emotion has been transferred. My preference is to work with the current situation that has triggered the old emotional response, with the thinking that creating a greater capacity for the emotion through its embodiment will eventually evoke the cognition that the emotion has to do with a past situation, if such a cognition is necessary for therapeutic change. This works most of the time. One then works with the past situation, if it is necessary to resolve the symptom.

But the spontaneous connection to a past situation that is necessary for healing does not always show up, for the following reasons. One, even though the creation of greater capacity for the emotion through its embodiment in relation to the current situation theoretically increases the possibility of cognitive grasp of its link to a relevant past situation, psychological defenses might still remain strong enough to prevent the cognitive insight from emerging. Two, some people might have an undeveloped capacity for psychological insight in relation to the past that might get in the way of the resolution to their suffering. Three, the memory of the relevant past situation might be from an early stage of childhood for which explicit memory is not available for recall. Four, when we build capacity for the emotion in relation to the present situation without an accompanying link to the past, due to strong psychological defenses, undeveloped capacity for psychological insight, or lack of explicit memory, we might erroneously and convincingly fix the blame for the emotional suffering on the present situation. This conclusion can get in the way of resolution of the present situation.

In each of these situations, it might be better for the therapist to work with a past situation than with the present situation, even if the client is insistent that their suffering has to do with the current situation. After all, interpreting the unconscious roots of a conscious problem with the help of known but not personally remembered history is one of the most important elements of the practice of psychotherapy.

14

Interpersonal Resonance

Chapter summary: discusses the scientific basis of interpersonal resonance, through which our bodies can exchange information with each other and regulate each other, over short and long distances; and how to use it to attune to emotional states in others and regulate them, in the process of helping them embody their emotions.

Helping others embody their emotions involves getting them to consciously experience their emotions in more places in their brain and body physiology than they have previously. But more often than not, people have difficulty accessing and expressing their emotional experiences for a variety of reasons. For example, strong psychological and physiological defenses might be in the way. But the most likely reason is that they grew up with little or no support for generating, experiencing, identifying, symbolizing, and expressing their emotions.[1] This means that, in working with emotions in others, our ability to support their emotional experiences is the most important ability we bring to the therapeutic setting.

In chapter 11, we discussed a number of concrete ways to support emotions in others. In this chapter, we will see yet another way of supporting and regulating others' emotional experiences: through the innate ability we all have to resonate physiologically with each other. This ability is poorly understood and underutilized in therapy. We will call it "interpersonal resonance," or simply resonance. This chapter will discuss what resonance is, what its mechanisms are, and how to use it consciously to access and regulate emotional experiences in others as well as in ourselves.

According to findings in attachment theory,[2] a mother's capacity to feel her child's emotional states in her own body, which we shall call the capacity for "embodied emotional attunement," is the best predictor of her ability to regulate her child emotionally.[3] In order to support emotions in others, we need to know what their emotional experience is by "tuning in" or "attuning" to their emotional experiences. The term "emotional attunement" can be thought of broadly as the understanding of what another person is experiencing emotionally. We can arrive at this understanding in a number of ways. We can simply ask the other person what they are experiencing; we can put ourselves in others' shoes and imagine what we might have felt in their place in the situation they are describing; we can use what we have observed others go through in similar situations in life, literature, and movies. We might also use psychological theories to deduce others' emotional states. We can use all of these usual methods for understanding where others are emotionally and then attempt to feel it in our own bodies as much as possible to arrive at an embodied emotional attunement to another's emotional state.

In addition, we can mirror the vocal, facial, and body expressions of others to experience and support what they might be experiencing emotionally in their bodies, as is often the practice in body psychotherapy approaches. We can use what neuroscientists call "mirror neurons" in our brains, which can mimic the movements of others to simulate their emotional experiences in our brain, if not in our body physiology.[4] Together, all of these methods might be sufficient for experiencing another's emotional responses in our bodies. In cases when all such methods prove to be inadequate, or in addition to these methods, we can use our innate ability for interpersonal resonance to sense the emotional experience of others in our bodies.

Let us now look at what interpersonal resonance is, the scientific evidence for it, and the differences between interpersonal resonance and countertransference. Then we will explore how we might use interpersonal resonance to help others and ourselves to embody emotions.

Interpersonal Resonance:
An Alternative Method of Information Exchange

In psychology, all information exchanges between two bodies are generally assumed to happen through our five senses of sight, smell, hearing, taste, and touch. Simulating the experiences of other bodies in ours through mirror neurons or mirroring others' facial, vocal, and body expressions can be understood within this framework of information exchange through the five senses. Interpersonal resonance has to do with the possibility that our brain and body physiologies can directly exchange emotional and other information with each other without involving the five senses. Our ability to "feel" on the back of the neck that someone behind us might be staring at us indicates that the physiology of our five senses might also be involved in such information exchanges in ways we do not fully understand. Our experience that resonance can happen not only over short distances involved in a typical consulting room but also over greater distances involved in online video sessions or audio phone sessions implies that we have other physiological mechanisms for resonance, over and above the five senses.

What are the implications of such resonant possibilities for exchanging information with each other? Our attunement and empathy can become embodied. We can use our bodies to find out what others are experiencing in theirs. Then we can help others in understanding, conceptualizing, naming, and expressing their emotional experiences. We can also communicate directly with the bodies of others to regulate them. When we can sense what others are experiencing in their bodies and can regulate their experiences in our bodies, we can then share that regulatory information with others through resonance, or we can simply communicate regulatory information upon just sensing what others might need. For example, if we sense another person's anxiety in our body, we can send regulatory information to calm them immediately upon sensing their anxiety or after calming their anxiety within our bodies.

Kleinian psychoanalyst Wilfred Bion imagined such a process happening between mothers and their babies all the time.[5] An anxious baby is ill equipped physiologically to handle such distress, so it sends or "projects" its unbearable experience into the receptive mother. The mother, with a more developed and capable physiology, receives or "projectively identifies" with the child's anxiety. Externally, she engages in soothing behaviors to help regulate the child's anxiety. Internally, she assimilates and transforms the anxiety into calm and projects the calm state back to the desperate baby. The baby projectively identifies with the mother's calm and is soothed by it. Bion likens this process to that of a mother bird feeding a baby bird predigested food that the baby bird's physiology cannot yet handle due to its immaturity. Bion, however, did not specify the mechanisms through which projection and projective identification took place. As we shall see, the dynamics of interpersonal resonance could offer a physiological basis for Bion's theory.

The Scientific Basis of Interpersonal Resonance

Cellular biologist James Oschman became interested in bioenergy fields, such as bioelectric and biomagnetic fields generated by different systems in our brain and body physiology, how they are generated, how far they travel, what functions they serve, and so on. Oschman's findings from his survey of research across multiple disciplines are published in two volumes, *Energy Medicine: The Scientific Basis*[6] and *Energy Medicine in Therapeutics and Human Performance*.[7] Bioelectric and biomagnetic energy fields are generated by different systems in our body. All of our organs, including the brain and the heart, generate such bioenergy fields. These bioenergy fields can be measured in the form of frequencies along the electromagnetic spectrum. The specific bioenergy fields generated by individual organs such as the brain and the heart become integrated bioenergy fields through the connective tissue fabric that is woven into every part of our brain and body physiology.

Bioenergy fields capture and transmit information on the state of the local physiology. Electrocardiograms and electroencephalograms capture important information on the state of the heart and the brain physiology, respectively. Internally, different parts of the brain and body physiology communicate status and regulatory information to each other through nerves as well as blood. They also send and receive status and regulatory information through local as well as global, or more integrated, bioenergy fields. The connective tissue matrix that is woven into every structure in the physiology is ideal for rapidly transmitting physiological information from one part of the body to another, earning the privilege of being studied as an extra nervous system outside the central and peripheral autonomic and somatic nervous systems.

The bioenergy fields generated by the brain and body physiology are capable of expanding beyond the skin into the environment. The bioenergy field of the heart is one hundred times more powerful than that of the brain, and it can be detected several feet from the body.[8] When our bioenergy fields extend beyond the body, as in figure 14.1, they can interact with other people's bioenergy fields as well as with

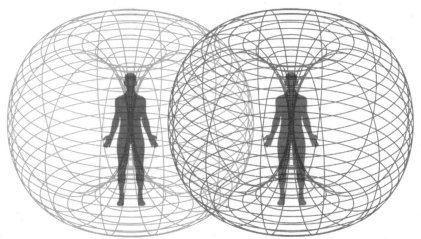

FIGURE 14.1 Interacting Human Bioenergy Fields

structures in others' brain and body physiologies. In this way, bodies can inform, influence, and regulate each other, like birds in synchronized flight patterns; or dysregulate each other, as in a mob frenzy. Bioenergy fields from the hands of healers can reach deep into the brain and body physiology of others to initiate transformation, even when the hands are at a distance from their bodies.

The fasciae in different parts of the body interweave with each other to create a continuous fabric. This connective tissue matrix, with its crystalline structure, functions as radar for information reaching the body in the form of bioenergy fields from the outside. Deep within our cells, tiny antennae-like filaments on our genes, known to have the capacity to alter gene expression, vibrate with information from bioenergy fields inside and outside our brain and body physiology.[9]

So there appears to be adequate scientific evidence that we have structures in place to inform, influence, regulate, and dysregulate each other through interpersonal resonance. I am no longer astonished by instances that demonstrate the phenomenon of resonance, as when a horse grazing in a field comes straight up to me and puts its nose against my heart on a day when my heart is extraordinarily wide open with love. As when my wife comes down from the third floor to the kitchen on the ground floor and kisses me and says she loves me, immediately after my heart is moved to tears from reading a moving newspaper story about reconnection. As when my wife, who is sleeping next to me but not touching me, drops deeper and deeper into her sleep and breath as I hold my head in my hands to regulate myself down from a nightmare.

So far, we have only seen physiological evidence for interpersonal resonance across short distances, as between client and therapist in the same room, involving measurable frequencies of the electromagnetic spectrum. This book is being written during the coronavirus pandemic, when therapy has moved increasingly online. Concerns abound regarding whether therapists can provide as much support and connection online as they can in person; as does pleasant surprise about how much connection and support both clients and therapists experience in online sessions. Given this unique situation, it makes sense to explore the evidence for interpersonal resonance over longer distances. We will see that some of the possible dynamics involved in long-range interpersonal resonance, such as quantum entanglement, could also contribute to the strength of interpersonal resonance over short distances.

Interpersonal Resonance over Longer Distances

Around four a.m. one morning in Los Angeles, I woke up from an awful dream. A man had died in India, and his coffin was being lowered into the ground; and it was expected that his wife would be buried alive with him. I wrote the dream down on a notepad on the night table to get it out of my system, and I went back to sleep. Around six a.m., the phone rang. One of my maternal uncles was calling to tell me that my forty-nine-year-old brother-in-law had died of a heart attack, and that they had been trying to contact me for a while. The dream had brought me information about what had just happened. Years later, I would realize that the dream had also brought me information from or about the future. It foretold the very difficult times my sister would undergo for many years after her husband's death. When I share the dream with students around the world as an example of interpersonal resonance, I often hear similar personal stories, reinforcing my impression that such experiences are not extraordinary and that there must be a scientific explanation for them.

A less dramatic and more frequent experience that occurs is just thinking of calling or writing someone, only for that person to contact us first, a phenomenon that Rupert Sheldrake calls "telepathic telephone calls." In a study to investigate the extent of this phenomenon, Sheldrake and David Jay Brown found that 78 percent of two hundred respondents reported that they have had the experience of telephoning someone who said that they were just thinking about calling them.[10] It turns out that there are scientific explanations for such long-range information exchanges or resonance, in the discipline of quantum physics.

Quantum physics is concerned with the world of subatomic particles, the tiny particles that everything in the universe would break down into if we were to keep breaking things down to get at the stuff that the universe is made of. In the strange behavior of these very tiny things, we might find an explanation for long-range resonance. Two subatomic particles are said to be "entangled" when a change in one cannot happen without effecting simultaneous changes in the other, with no time lag whatsoever, even when they are great distances from each other. This behavior among entangled particles, which Albert Einstein called "spooky action at a distance," has been experimentally validated many times.[11]

Does this mean that the information on the change in one particle travels to the other particle faster than the speed of light (186,000 miles per second)? Some scientists have theorized that speeds faster than the speed of light are indeed possible in the world of subatomic particles. According to one theory, there are hidden variables of subatomic particles that are capable of traveling faster than light—variables we cannot measure because, as you may have guessed already, they are hidden.[12] According to another controversial theory, subatomic particles are able to achieve speeds faster than light through a behavior called "quantum tunneling."[13]

The standard explanation for quantum entanglement is nonlocality. We live in a world characterized by space and distance, but there is no space or distance in the world of subatomic particles.[14] So when something changes in one particle, it leads to changes in the other particles that are entangled with it. In the world we know, defined by space and time, the speed of our communications with each other can be measured in time. It is difficult for us to grasp a world without space and time. But we do also exist at the quantum level, where we can communicate with each other instantaneously, according to quantum physics. So nonlocality is another feasible scientific explanation for interpersonal resonance at a distance, in addition to communication at faster-than-light speeds.

If all of this is making your head spin, please do not worry. The key is that it is possible for information to travel great distances between two entangled particles instantaneously or at speeds greater than the speed of light; and that we exist, as all things in the universe do, at both quantum and nonquantum levels of reality. At the subatomic level, some of us are perhaps more entangled than others because we belong to the same species, ethnicity, family, or close relationship. Quantum entanglement may be the mechanism through which I learned of my brother-in-law's death in a dream.

Larry Dossey, MD, offers many more examples of information exchange over long distances through interpersonal resonance in his book *One Mind: How Our Individual Mind Is Part of a Larger Consciousness and Why It Matters,* a required reading in Integral Somatic Psychology professional training.[15] This is a very interesting read for anyone who wants to learn what is behind our ordinary knowledge of who we are and what reality is. I have the trainees read it for one reason: to overcome their bias against long-range information exchange through interpersonal resonance so they can at least allow it as a possibility in their minds and explore it in their awareness, which is very important, because quantum phenomena are known to be affected by our awareness and intention.

Countertransference and Resonance

Countertransference is a serious concern among therapists across the board, for good reason. When a therapist has a reaction to a client that has very little to do with the client, but the therapist incorrectly interprets the reaction as having to do with the client, it can compromise the quality of the therapy and even bring harm to the client. For example, if a therapist is triggered unconsciously into his unresolved anger toward his mother because the client subliminally reminds him of his mother, the therapist could insist that the anger he is feeling toward the client is actually the client's unconscious anger toward the therapist.

Earlier Freudian psychoanalysts wrongly believed that therapists could eliminate countertransference reactions altogether and become "abstinent" by undergoing therapy themselves. Even though our understanding of countertransference has evolved to include the possibility that it could be useful in understanding and helping the client, the concern about harming the client through countertransference persists, as therapists in country after country have told me when I suggest that they start to examine their inner reactions for clues to their clients' conscious and unconscious experiences.

Initially, transference was understood as a client's reaction to a therapist that had nothing to do with the therapist, and countertransference was a therapist's reaction to a client that had nothing to do with the client. Later, the understanding of countertransference evolved to include the possibility that a therapist's experience in relationship to a client might be useful in understanding and regulating the client. A type of countertransference called "concordant" or "mirror" countertransference allows for the possibility that sometimes the therapist can experience what the client is experiencing. Another type of countertransference called "complementary" countertransference allows for the possibility that the therapist's experience in relation to a client can be exactly the opposite of the client's experience in relation to the therapist.

For example, in mirror countertransference a therapist might feel anxiety in the presence of an anxious client whose anxiety might even be unconscious to the client. In complementary countertransference the therapist might start to feel extremely calm in the presence of an anxious client so as to help the client manage their anxiety. When a therapist experiences a sudden urge to hit their client when the client is afraid, that is another example of complementary countertransference where the client is communicating to the therapist the abuse they experienced. Mirror and complementary countertransference experiences are possible through the information from the five senses, in all the ways we have seen. They are also possible through interpersonal resonance, based on the ability our physiologies have to share physiological information directly with each other.

Transference and countertransference are real. They can be harmful or beneficial, depending on how they are handled. A therapist with an ego that believes countertransference is a sign of imperfection on their part and does not admit to it might be a danger to their clients and themselves. As we have seen, the capacity for interpersonal resonance is also real. It offers therapists a profound additional tool for joining, understanding, and regulating the experience of their clients. But experiences of countertransference and resonance can be confounded. As much discrimination as one might bring to a situation, it might still be insufficient to untangle the two, in part because all that we can make conscious in terms of the dynamics in any situation is limited relative to what is there in the unconscious, and in part because it might be impossible to separate one's experience from that of another in relationship. Intersubjective psychoanalysts such as Robert Stolorow, one of my teachers, dispute the very idea that one's experience can be clearly separated from that of another in a relationship.[16] So the use of resonance requires humility in addition to discrimination—the humility to acknowledge that one can be just as incorrect as correct. Resonance also requires the ability to let it go if its use does not lead to anything.

Resonance in Mutually Regulating Systems

In his book *The Developing Mind: How Relationships and the Brain Interact to Shape Who We Are,* Daniel Siegel states that when two human beings come into any cooperative relationship, the two systems come together to form a supersystem.[17] A supersystem has a greater capacity to regulate both systems than the sum of its constituent individual capacities. In such a supersystem, the individual systems might be involved in different activities at different times. At times, they might be synchronous in their activity; at times, they might be complementary; at times, their activities might appear to have nothing to do with each other. In mutually regulating systems, one system might lead at times and follow at other times. At still other times, the systems may appear to be in no apparent relationship to each other, doing their own things, but still be in a mutually regulating relationship.

What does this mean for our experiences in resonance—for what we sense in our brain and body physiology when we are working with another? Let us look at it through an example. We are sitting with a client and we suddenly feel a surge of energy in our legs. Does this mean it is happening in the client at the same time? That is one possibility. It is equally possible that it is happening in us first so as to regulate the client, whose energy is becoming too top-heavy for their own good. Their system, in resonating with the downward shift of energy in us, might move toward more balance. It is also possible that a third factor, the psyche at large, could be triggering simultaneous movement of energy in the legs of both therapist and client, as in Jungian psychology. It is also possible that one cannot find a reason for it in the client's process. But that does not mean it is not helpful to us or the client in some way that we cannot understand. In a way, it is not unlike a conversation between friends. One says something, and the other says something else, and so on, until both end up feeling better and clearer about the situation they have been discussing.

The Practice of Interpersonal Resonance in Three Steps

Let us now see how we might go about using resonance to sense, interpret, and regulate emotional experiences in others as well as in ourselves.

1. Allow for the possibility for the direct exchange of information between one brain and body physiology and another through bioenergy fields or quantum fields, and set an intention to allow it to happen.

Intention is important, especially for quantum phenomena, because they are subject to awareness and intention. Observe your brain and body physiology from time to time—your body sensations, changes in energy states, and emotions. Look out for sudden shifts in your experience such as pain in the heart, loss of energy in the legs, or anxiety. Simply accept your experience, and if it is unpleasant, try not to change it in any way to feel better. Please remind yourself that you could be resonating with the client's process and feeling its impact on you. Being mindful of it, not reacting to it but supporting it with your awareness and intention, can help to regulate the client's experience in the resonance.

2. Regulate yourself, in whatever way you know how, if your experience becomes too much for you to bear.

This turn of events might mean the client is struggling with how overwhelming the experience is for them. It might also mean that the experience is simply too much for your system. We often work with experiences in others for which we do not have the capacity or personal reference, such as those who have been through war or specific forms of physical or sexual abuse.

In these instances, regulate yourself so as to make the experience more bearable, but please take care not to regulate yourself away from it and compromise the resonant relationship you have with your client through sharing their experience. Sharing another person's experience, especially with one's body, is extremely important in helping another person process their emotional experiences. It is akin to one person helping another person lift a heavy load, or lending a hand to support another person as they walk. The emotional load is shared and supported in the resonance. This is why sometimes the best thing we can do for a person who is grieving is to simply sit with the person, sharing their grief in as much of our body as possible. I remember sitting with a distant cousin whom I had just met as she was grieving the loss of her father. Six months earlier, she had also lost her mother. As I sat with her for nearly an hour, I felt her trembling, grieving, and despairing, often in silence. A few months later she wrote to me and said that, even though she had just met me for the first time in her life that day, and we hardly talked to each other in the brief time we spent together, she felt something really had happened between us to establish a strong bond. I felt that way too, and I still feel it.

There are several ways in which we can regulate ourselves when we are struggling with another's experience in resonance or in reaction to their experience, without losing contact with the person. We can place a hand gently on the part of our brain and body physiology where the discomfort is most difficult, to help ease it. We can take a deep breath to make it more bearable. We can place one hand on that spot and the other hand on another part of the body to help distribute the energy between the two spots to reduce the pain in the initial spot. We can sense our legs to ground ourselves or sense the lower abdomen to center ourselves to withstand the experience. With our awareness and intention, we can expand the difficult emotional experience to more areas of the body so as to create a greater capacity to be with it. We can place a hand on our brain stem (the lowest part of the back of the skull) or on the prefrontal cortex (the forehead) in a casual way to help regulate ourselves while we stay focused on the other's suffering.

When we regulate ourselves this way in the resonance, we mobilize its powers to help others regulate their experience and work through it, without even drawing their attention to it. This way of working within the resonance is particularly helpful when we are working with children or those who have much difficulty working consciously with their experiences, especially in the body.

3. Make further use of the information we gather in the resonance by sharing it with the client.

We saw in chapter 5 how conscious awareness of an emotional experience can be of extra help in regulating the experience and can inform the person more fully of the impact of the situation. If we were to feel sadness in our chest in the course of working with the client, we could bring it to the person's attention by asking, for example, "What do you experience in your chest now?" "What emotion do you feel in your chest now?" "Do you feel sadness or happiness in your chest?" "Do you feel sadness anywhere in your body?" We could also say, "I feel sadness in my chest now. I do not know what it is about. Do you feel sadness too? If so, where in your body do you experience sadness?" And so on. In these instances, there would seem to be an assumption that we are picking up the emotion that the client is also consciously experiencing at the moment. However, it could be that the emotion is unconscious and needs the mirroring and support of the therapist to become conscious and bearable. It is also possible that the client is projecting the unpleasant or unacceptable emotion outward and that the therapist is projectively identifying with it in order to understand the client's condition.

It is also possible that the sadness is the therapist's own, in reaction to the client's situation; or the therapist could be having a countertransference reaction that has nothing to do with the client. Therefore, it is important not to press the issue if the intervention does not lead to anything, unless of course the therapist is absolutely sure from knowing the client that the intervention is being defended against, and pursuing it is in the client's best interest. When nothing comes of an intervention based on information from resonance or other means, it does not mean that the intervention might not somehow be helpful to the client. It is possible that the client is not ready to deal with it. The intervention might, however, seed the client's psyche and lead to its emergence in the future. The therapist might be modeling the experience and expression of emotion for the client. The client might also receive the information that the therapist is experiencing sadness in response to their situation as empathic support, which could lead to the client sharing not only sadness but also other vulnerable emotions with the therapist.

Issues in Working in Resonance

Too much resonance: Therapists often complain about suffering from resonating too much with their clients. Some report that they have no choice but to resonate a lot and suffer. Embodying the unpleasant emotions of others in oneself does involve suffering. Resonating with emotions of others, however, does not mean therapists need to suffer as much as their clients. The pattern of resonating too much might go back to one's childhood. One might have learned it from one's caregivers, or one might have had to do it to maintain connection with caregivers. This might have been reinforced in therapy, as the pattern of resonating too much can be of significant help to clients. Therapists who do this might have even become identified with it as a characteristic of a really good therapist—something I had to unlearn myself.

The first thing to do to correct the pattern of resonating too much is to understand that one has a choice regarding how much to resonate with someone and whether to resonate with someone in the first place. We do not resonate with everyone we run into in our life, just as we do not try to relate to everyone we run into in the same way. So the first thing we can do is to set conscious intentions to not resonate with someone or to limit the extent to which we resonate with someone. These intentions work to some extent. Setting such intentions is likely to bring into consciousness unconscious intentions from childhood or later in life that contribute to the problem of resonating indiscriminately and without limit. We can then work with those intentions to change them.

In addition, we can adjust certain behaviors to manage the extent to which we engage others in resonance. Doing less mirroring of tone of voice, facial expression, and body expressions such as posture, movement, and gesture, along with reducing eye contact, are some of the simple things we can do to reduce the extent and intensity of resonance. If the problem of resonating too much continues across the board or persists in relation to some clients, one can seek personal therapy to uncover and work through unconscious attitudes, experiences, and vulnerabilities that resist change, in order not to suffer more than necessary in working with others in resonance.

Too little resonance: Some therapists have the opposite problem. They have a hard time engaging their clients in resonance in general. If they have difficulties with resonating with specific clients, the problem could be with the client or the therapist. In either case, they could try all the methods that were suggested for reducing the extent of resonance, but in the opposite direction. For example, one could set the intent to resonate more or to do more mirroring of tone of voice, facial expression, and body posture. If these methods do not work, the therapist who has difficulty resonating in general or with specific clients could do personal therapy to uncover and resolve what is in the way. One important reason why people find it difficult to resonate with others is that they do not have the capacity to tolerate the suffering that resonance could bring.

Also, resonating is a two-way street. It is something a person can control consciously or unconsciously. This was the case with a dear friend of mine who was Jewish. Toward the end of World War II, when he was a four-month-old baby in France, his young parents left him in the care of a priest and fled to the hills with the French Resistance. The priest hid him in a dark cellar two levels below the ground and cared for him until his parents returned. When his parents came to get him four or five months later, he was so emaciated that they thought he could have died.

I could never get a sense of my friend through resonance, despite my skill in resonating with people. It is as though he instinctively learned very early in life that it was not safe to be detected in the resonance. However, when he was diagnosed with terminal cancer, I could not stand to be around him. It was simply too much stress for my body to handle. His ex-wife and son reported the same experience. It was as though the wall he had put up during the war and maintained ever since broke down when he was faced with certain death, and all the stress and vulnerabilities he had managed to hold at a distance came flooding back, overwhelming him and those who cared for him very much.

Attitudes that therapists develop during their training also get in the way of their ability to help their clients through resonance. Therapists who believe that they can become free of countertransference, who do not know they have the ability to help their clients through resonance despite possible countertransference reactions, or who hold the view that their inner experiences are of no value in understanding clients' experiences are likely to have difficulty in resonating with their clients. Similarly, therapists who are afraid they could do harm to their clients by making suggestions based on their experiences; who are trained in therapy modalities that emphasize that awareness of client's experiences should come from clients, and the role of the therapist is to follow them and validate them; or who do not pay attention to their body experiences are also likely to have difficulty with resonance. Therapists across therapy modalities often bring up the fear of causing harm by imposing one's countertransference reactions on clients as a major concern about trusting their resonance.

In body-oriented and energy-oriented psychologies, there is at times excess concern about "merging" with clients. It appears that "not merging" is sometimes understood as "not exchanging energies at all." Merging could also mean identifying oneself with another's experience so completely as to give up one's own experience. That is of course not desirable if it is a default mode for interacting with others, or if it is a defense, called the "confluence" defense in gestalt therapy. If not merging is understood as not exchanging energies at all, or if identifying completely with another person's experience even for a short time is always regarded as pathological, those attitudes can become an impediment for engaging others in resonance. This is because in the exchange of information involved in resonance, there is always an exchanging or mixing of energies to a greater or lesser extent. And putting oneself in another's shoes completely for a short period of time might be at times necessary to help the other in resonance.

Stuck in resonance: When we resonate with clients during sessions, a number of things could happen that might leave us stuck with the client's experiences or our reactions to them, compromising our well-being and our availability for resonating with other clients. Let us look at some of these possibilities with one or two examples. When we resonate with a client's experience, the experience could just be too much for our system. We might not have the capacity to tolerate the experience, either because it is unfamiliar or just too intense, or it could trigger unbearable and unresolved experiences of ours. In such instances, physiological defenses could kick in to maintain our system's functionality to help the client. This is analogous to a person who grabs another person to prevent them from falling over a cliff, and not noticing that an arm muscle was torn in the process due to the instinctual physiological defense of numbing, until after the rescuer successfully gets the other person to safety. In the same way, therapists might not notice until after the session (sometimes hours after the session) that their system is left holding incomplete and unresolved experiences, sometimes with symptoms.

Once in a training in Europe, I worked with a Jewish woman who felt terror in large groups. The only daughter of two Holocaust survivors who lost all of their family members in the concentration camps during World War II, she still had difficulty revealing her Jewish identity to her neighbors in the small village where she lived. At some point when she was an adult, her father took his own life by hanging himself. In a session in front of a class, we used the presence of the group to trigger the terror she lives with so we could use her body to embody and tolerate the terror of being killed, which she had probably inherited from her parents as well as from the collective Jewish experience. At the end of the session and during the rest of the training, she reported that she felt more present and at ease in making contact with others in the group. I said to her that I felt more present and connected to others as well, adding that it was an illustration of the wisdom of Swiss psychologist Carl Jung, who said every therapy session has the potential to change both the therapist and the client.

However, during the session I felt a slight constriction in the back of my neck on the left side. The next morning, I woke up with pain in the same spot. I did not think much of it because it is a familiar symptom of mine. I knew that the posterior neck muscles have many psychological functions, including the management of high energy, stress, fear, and shock or traumatic stress. I also knew that the familiar constriction pattern with pain in my neck might have to do with what remained unresolved from the trauma of my birth, in which my mother and I both came very close to death. Based on past experiences, I thought I could resolve the pain with yoga and, if necessary, by working with the terror by myself or with my therapist. As time went on, I grew increasingly concerned when neither method worked; nor did the subsequent body-work sessions I received. In fact, the constriction and the pain spread from one side of the neck to the other and started to recruit the shoulders in what appeared to be a complex regional pain syndrome. I started to look for simple medical reasons for the pain: perhaps I had injured my neck during a yoga posture.

It was in this state of distress that I arrived in India for my annual visit with my mother on her farm, at the beginning of a new year. With the stress of being back in the family of origin, my neck condition worsened, and I felt helplessness and despair. Out of the blue, my wife suggested that I contact a local energy healer who had helped her with a chronic hip pain symptom some years ago. I called him reluctantly. He is a bit of an odd fellow, even to his family. The first time I met him, he said, "I prefer the company of plants and trees in the forests near where I live. They taught me about energy and how to do energy healing." Also, in contrast to most energy healers, who normally exude calm and solemnity, he was a nervous wreck, talking ceaselessly about random

301

things while he "worked." He worked on my neck for a short time, his fingers moving at my neck as though they were trying to catch a butterfly very delicately so as not to injure it, while I looked on with my usual skepticism and ego. I wondered what he could accomplish that I could not with all the work I had done to fix the problem.

I did not have to wait long to find out. That night, as my neck relaxed and with it my entire body, high levels of energy started to course all over my body. With the energy came high levels of terror, helplessness, and despair, but mostly terror—the terror of dying—that in repeated cycles exhausted me but also managed to dissolve my regional pain syndrome around my neck for good. The next morning I felt like a new person. I wondered to what extent the emotions I had felt the previous night had to do with my own near-death trauma around my birth; to what extent it had to do with the Jewish woman I had worked with; and to what extent it had to do with the terror of all of her ancestors. I would never know for sure. But what I do know for sure is that the session healed me and made me more capable of being there for others in resonance. The whole several-month episode also taught me that, in order to work efficiently at undoing physiological defenses to help people access and embody their emotions, I need to also learn how to work with physiological defenses at the energetic, subtle, or quantum level as well, the level that seems to be more involved in coping with unbearable experiences and the physiological defenses against them, the more traumatic the situations become.

Resonance and vicarious traumatization: When therapists are stuck with experiences they encounter while working in resonance with their clients, cannot resolve the experiences, and develop symptoms from them, therapists are said to be vicariously traumatized by other people's traumas. There is much discussion among trauma therapists about how to avoid vicarious traumatization. Suggestions usually involve better self-care: keeping a manageable caseload, not working with too many challenging clients, having enough downtime, exercise, sleep, peer support, supervision, and so on. They also usually involve better management of one's physical and energetic boundaries. At times, concern with vicarious

traumatization and maintaining boundaries to avoid it—such as visual-
izations that imagine a white light protecting oneself—can undermine
the therapy by compromising the deep relationships therapists could have
with their clients in the resonance. In my view, the best protection that
therapists can have to minimize vicarious traumatization, in addition to
making sure one is not resonating too much in all the ways discussed
above, is to develop a greater capacity for tolerating a range of difficult
experiences, using such instances as opportunities for personal work and
as gateways to further personal and professional development.

Learning and resonance: Children can also learn about the world
and how to respond to it by resonating with the brain and body physiologies of the adults around them. Children have this capacity from
very early on, as far back as their life in the womb. They resonate with
adults' vulnerabilities as well as their defenses against them. This is one
way in which children can be vicariously traumatized, and the effects of
collective and individual traumas in a family's history can be passed on
from one generation to the next.

As we saw in chapter 5, resonance might also have a role to play in
learning about emotions. When adults pick up children's physiological patterns through resonance and name them as this emotion or that
emotion, children learn to identify different physiological patterns that
they are experiencing as different emotions through words that adults
use to describe them. Because it is possible to resonate with both brain
and body physiologies, it is possible for one to resonate not only with
patterns of sensations in the body but also with the abstract patterns
that the brain might form from them prior to their being attached to
linguistic concepts to become communicable emotional experiences.

Touch and resonance: Our hands are powerful tools through which
we are able to sense and transmit bioelectric and biomagnetic energies
for regulating and healing others as well as ourselves.[18] Our hands can
serve these functions even at a distance from the body because our bioenergy fields extend beyond the skin boundary. But when our hands are
in contact with the skin, their effects are even more pronounced, making
touch and self-touch effective healing tools. Because touch combines

information from resonance with input from one of the five senses, the experiences a therapist has in resonance with a client when there is touch might differ from when there is no touch.

The Archetypal Basis of Resonance?

We have tried to understand the phenomenon of interpersonal resonance as a manifestation of the intricate mechanisms laid down by evolution to maximize our survival by increasing the possibilities of interactive regulation among members of our species. We have tried to understand its structural specifics in terms of short-range bioelectric and biomagnetic fields and short- and long-range quantum fields. Does interpersonal resonance have deeper sources in our psyche? Mara Sidoli, a Jungian analyst with a developmental focus, characterizes the spontaneous rocking behavior babies in distress use to soothe themselves along the following lines, which I find quite moving: when personal mothers disappear, archetypal mothers rock the baby from the inside.[19]

In Jungian psychology, the individual psyche is conceptualized as a unique combination of energy patterns, such as the good mother and the bad mother, that are common to all of us.[20] These common energy patterns, called archetypes, are seen as guides for our development in different stages of our lives, and as playing a role in our wellness as well as illness. Every archetype, such as the good mother, appears in different cultures as different symbols, such as the Virgin Mary in the West and the goddess Shakti in the East. On closer examination, archetypal symbols from different cultures reveal themselves as having core qualities in common, such as good mothering or bad mothering. The good mother and the bad mother archetypes interact with us through individuals around us to mother us and impart the qualities of mothering to us, which we use to mother others in turn.

I think the following story is a fitting end to this chapter on the fascinating subject of interpersonal resonance. Once I went to see a close friend who had just given birth to her first child, a girl. The baby was about four to six weeks old. The mother looked exhausted. The baby was hard to regulate and kept my friend up all night long. While she ate the Chinese meal I had brought her, I held the baby in my arms and talked with my friend, catching up with a lot of stuff that had happened in both our lives since the last time we had met.

I started to notice that the baby was settling into my body and making strange sounds that my body seemed to be responding to with sounds of its own. She dropped deeper and deeper into sleep while I carried on a conversation with her mother through the haze of a trance that seemed to be enveloping me and the baby. At some point, I bid my friend goodbye, handed her the baby, and drove back to my apartment.

It was around four p.m. when I got back to my apartment. I felt exhausted—more exhausted than I could ever remember being. I wondered if that was what it took to mother a child, day after day. I had a plan to go to a seven p.m. movie, and I thought I would take a long nap to recover and then go to the movie as planned. I lay down for my nap and woke up to the sound of my telephone ringing at seven a.m. the next morning. My friend was calling to say she had not had such a good night of sleep in a very long time. The baby had slept through the night too, she added. She asked me what I had done, and she ended our conversation by saying, "You should visit more often!"

My instinctual body reaction to her suggestion was a strong *no,* which was understandable given what it had felt the evening before upon returning to the apartment. My ever-insecure ego, always on the lookout for something to take credit for to feel inflated, imagined that it might even be a better emotional coregulator (borrowing a term from attachment theory) of the child than the mother was.[21]

The psyche at large does not brook such inflation. The compensation came swiftly, the very next morning, just before I woke up. In a dream, I was visited by my paternal grandmother, a matriarch, an archetype of the unconditional mother, by whom I felt more unconditionally loved than by anyone else growing up. In the dream, I was asleep or unconscious. She woke me up and had the following message to deliver: "Raja, it is time for you to do a ceremony for all the mother goddesses of the world. Go to our village, where you will find a young mother with a newborn. I mothered her when she was a child. Tell her that I sent you, and ask her baby for the ceremony. She will give you the baby. Take the baby and go up in the sky to where all the mother goddesses abide. Do not forget Mary and her infant son. Lay the baby at their feet and pray to them in all humility."

I woke up from this dream quite humbled, all right, with chills going up and down my spine. To me, the message was loud and clear. Whatever mothering I had brought to my friend's baby, it had ultimately come from the archetypal mother goddesses of the world. The young mother in the village represented my mothering ability that my grandmother had nurtured in me by channeling all the mother goddesses of the world in her interactions with me. The baby from the village that I had laid at the feet of the goddesses in the dream, I interpreted as the further fruition of my mothering ability I had gained from regulating my friend's child—a gift from the goddesses, no less, a gift for both the mothering and the mothered. When I tell my students this story of the divine or archetypal source of our ability to resonate in the collective psyche of all human beings, to reassure those who are unsure of their ability to resonate and regulate, I often see awe on their faces, the same awe I felt after the humility the dream brought me.

Conclusion: The Future

Writing this book has only deepened my interest in emotion as a subject of study. It has connected me to a worldwide community dedicated to the pursuit of the complexity that emotion is. It has inspired me. It has also left me feeling deeply humble. For as much knowledge as our species has collectively accumulated on emotion over its span of existence, it appears that there is so much more we do not know as yet. The span of an individual life and its contribution is even more limited. Therefore, for further inquiry, one can only focus on a limited number of topics of utmost personal interest.

I will focus this chapter on two subjects for further exploration, both for myself and for others who might feel similarly inclined:

- How does one explain, with more theory and evidence than this book presents, that it is possible for a person to "experience" an emotion such as sadness throughout one's brain and body physiology? If this question puzzles you, please note that the evidence we have seen so far—showing that the entirety of the brain and body physiology could be involved in the generation of an emotional experience such as love—does not necessarily imply that it is possible to consciously experience it throughout the brain and body physiology.

- With advances in quantum physics and that discipline's insight into deeper structures and processes within us, what can we gain from exploring how such quantum or subatomic levels of our physiology contribute to our emotional experiences, for understanding emotions as well as for working with our physiology at the quantum level, to improve emotional, cognitive, and behavioral outcomes?

Generation versus Experience of Emotion

My interest in emotion started with the observation that my clients and I had considerable difficulty with accessing emotions as well as with tolerating them long enough to process them through. I had already learned from intersubjective psychoanalysis, Jungian psychology, alchemy, and Advaita Vedanta that affect tolerance—the capacity to tolerate opposites in emotional experience—is important for psychological as well as spiritual growth, so building capacity for greater affect tolerance became a focus of my personal and professional work from very early on in my career in psychology. Just staying with the emotional experience wherever it appeared in the brain and body physiology did not always help; in fact, it often made symptoms worse. Therefore, I started to look for better methods for increasing affect tolerance in my clients and myself, especially in the body, because that is where the difficulty in tolerating an emotional experience often showed up.

I also got into the habit of asking my clients where in the body they felt the emotional experiences they were reporting, in part because I was oriented to the body from the very beginning of my career, and in part because I needed to get back into the body. From my early reading on emotion and the body, I was particularly influenced by learning that the generation of an emotion as well as its experience could potentially involve the entirety of the brain and body physiology, and that basic emotions might have distinct patterns in the brain and the body physiology. So I was naturally curious to check whether there were any patterns in the emotional experiences my clients and I had. That is, did all of us feel a basic emotion such as fear or sadness in the same places in the body?

It turned out that, consistent with findings from the early research on emotions and the autonomic nervous system, there was no pattern such as people always feeling anger in one place and sadness in another. Different people reported experiencing an emotion such as fear in different places—the brain, the eyes, the chest, the abdomen, and so on. Some places, such as the heart and the chest, showed up often, but not always. When I started posing this question to large groups of people in my classes, the sum total of all the areas reported in the experience of an emotion such as fear often ended up covering the entire brain and body physiology.

There was, however, one pattern I did observe. When people were able to tolerate being with an emotion for longer periods of time without falling apart or forming symptoms, they started reporting that they could feel their emotional experience as being more spread out in the body than before. These observations led me to believe that not only is it possible to expand the experience of emotions to more places in the body, but it might also lead to a greater capacity for tolerating the emotional experience. So I started to make interventions such as "As you experience the emotion in the chest, please expand your awareness to more of your chest, with the intention to expand your emotional experience to more of your chest." "Where else do you experience the emotion in the body?" "Are there other places in the body where you experience this emotion or some qualities of this emotion?" And so on, to good effect, which increased my confidence in the fledgling approach of embodying emotion.

As I continued to develop the practice of embodying emotion in my clients and myself in the above manner, I also continued to read on the subject for ideas about how to enrich the practice and ground it in hard science. From the literature on the physiology of emotions, I learned more about how the generation of emotion could involve the entirety of the brain and body physiology. From the body psychotherapy approaches I gathered that people tend to form strong physiological defenses in the body to minimize emotional experiences (especially unpleasant ones). I inferred that physiological defenses could compromise vital physiological flows such as blood and increase the level of stress in the physiology, thereby making emotional experiences in the body potentially more difficult to tolerate than if the emotional experiences were allowed to involve more of the body.

Putting this all together with my observation that an emotion could be potentially experienced throughout the brain and body physiology, I theorized that undoing physiological defenses against emotion to decrease the level of stress and increase the body areas involved in generating emotion could expand the experience of emotion in the body and increase a person's capacity to tolerate an unpleasant emotion for a longer period. This turned out to be a productive path, one that led eventually to the maturation of the method of embodying emotion, and to this book, at the end of which I am left wondering how much I really know about emotion!

I was fortunate enough to discover the idea that an emotion could be experienced throughout the brain and body physiology—the idea that inspired me to observe where we experience different emotions in the body in the first place—early in my reading of the literature on emotions. Candace Pert attributes this idea to Paul Ekman, and she paraphrases Ekman's understanding as follows: "Each emotion is experienced throughout the organism and not in just the head or body, and has a corresponding facial expression."[1] I say I was fortunate because I have not been able to find another scientific source supporting the idea that an emotion could be potentially experienced throughout the brain and body physiology, even though emotion is now generally understood as an assessment of the situation's impact on the well-being of the whole organism. Ekman believes, with some evidence, that every emotion such as fear is generated by a unique physiological pattern in the brain as well as the body. It therefore makes sense that he would state that the experience of it could involve the whole organism.

Ekman's theory that an emotion is a product of simultaneous activity in both the brain and the body has support in the more recently formulated enactive approach to emotion.[2] This is a dynamic systems approach which theorizes that emotion is a product of simultaneous—not sequential—activity across the brain and body physiology. In contrast, in the sequential or hierarchical model of Damasio[3] and Craig[4] that we saw in chapter 5, for example, a situation happens that impacts the body, and the brain then makes emotion from the information it gathers from the body about the impact. In Ekman's model, something happens, and there is a simultaneous brain and body instinctual reaction to it that is emotion.[5] In the dynamic systems perspective of enactive emotion, all experiences—cognition (including perception), emotion, and behavior—are constantly, continuously, and concurrently happening, simultaneously involving the brain, the body, and the environment. The contrast between Ekman's theory and the enactive emotion approach is that in the latter, there is no immediate implication that there are different physiological patterns for different emotions in the brain and the body, as in Ekman's model.

I wondered why the scientific literature on emotions contains hardly any statements on how emotions are experienced in the body. One possible reason is scientists' skepticism toward using self-reports of subjective experience as evidence in research studies. Another possible reason is that emotion researchers have been focused more on the mechanisms of how emotions are generated in the brain and the body, and whether they are generated more in the brain or the body, than on where and how they are experienced. Because the basic premise behind the practice of embodying emotion is that an emotion could potentially be experienced throughout the brain and body physiology, I think an analysis of different evidence-based theories of emotion, to determine the extent to which they imply that emotions could be experienced throughout the brain and body physiology, is in order.

Theories that limit generation of emotion to the brain imply that the experience of emotion is limited to the brain as well, because they do not allow the body a role even in the generation of emotion. Theories other than those of Ekman and his followers that allow a role for the body in the generation of emotion differ with respect to how they see the body's involvement in the generation of emotion. In the theories of Damasio and Craig, in the tradition of William James, the brain processes detailed information from the body on the impact of the situation to generate higher-order body maps (or abstractions of the more detailed body information, akin to seeing a face in a cloud) that are then somehow recognized as emotions. In Barrett's constructive theory of emotion, very general information on the situation's impact on the body, such as valence (good or bad) and arousal (low or high), is combined with learned linguistic concepts to arrive at emotional experiences.[6] In all three theories, emotions are constructed in the brain. There is no implication that such brain-constructed emotions such as sadness could potentially be experienced throughout the body.

So if an emotional experience such as sadness is a construction in the brain, even though it might be based on body information, how does one account for observations that emotions such as sadness are experienced throughout the body—something we can easily verify personally with a little bit of effort? Either these evidence-based theories offer limited explanations of the ways in which emotions are generated and experienced in the brain and the body; or there are brain and body mechanisms we do not yet know about that would make it possible for emotions constructed in the brain to be experienced throughout the body.

The Projection Hypothesis and the Information Transfer Hypothesis

Theories that say emotions are generated in the brain, through instinctual brain circuits or through abstraction of information from the body, need to add mechanisms through which such emotional experiences could be experienced in the rest of the body. Two possible avenues for exploration are projection and transfer of information. Let us explore each in turn.

The brain is known to have the capacity to project an experience on the body and experience it as though it were the actual first-hand experience of the body. For example, according to Damasio, even our very basic experiences of body sensations such as heartbeat are projections on the body of abstractions of more detailed body sensations from the area. If this is the case with even simple body sensations, then one can well imagine that the brain indeed does have the capacity to project emotions such as sadness onto different places in the body. Another example of the brain's ability to project an experience on the body is the phantom limb phenomenon, in which the brain is capable of experiencing the pain in an amputated leg. We shall call this the projection hypothesis.

It is also possible for information on emotion generated in the brain to be transferred to the body through deeper physiological structures and processes, such as through information molecules in interstitial fluids in the way Pert theorizes;[7] or through subatomic particles at the quantum level, even involving instantaneous information exchange through quantum entanglement. We shall call this the information transfer hypothesis.

In emotional embodiment work, when we are working with an emotion such as fear and we work with physiological defenses in an area of the body in which we do not experience the emotion, it becomes possible to experience the emotion in that area. This has been my experience, both in my work with clients and in my own life. Some might argue that this empirical phenomenon tends to support the information transfer hypothesis more than the projection hypothesis as an explanation for how emotions generated in the brain could be experienced throughout the body. One could argue that removal of physical defenses against regulatory flows such as blood to an area allows for the transfer of information on the emotional experience generated in the brain to that part of the body.

But one could also argue that our experience of being able to expand an emotional experience to a part of the body after working with physiological defenses that limit vital regulatory flows such as blood to the area can also support the projection hypothesis. In order to project an emotional experience generated in the brain onto a part of the body through interoception, that part of the body has to be available for interoception. The work with the physiological defenses that limit the regulatory flows to that area, through which we also become aware of that part of the body, makes the sensing of that area through interoception more possible. So the empirical phenomenon that an emotion can potentially be experienced throughout the body could support both hypotheses. It remains for science to verify which dynamic is more likely and whether both dynamics could be in play.

Quantum Physics, Quantum Psychology, and Energy Psychology in the West

Current research on the physiology of psychological processes such as emotions is done at the level of relatively large objects such as muscles, organs, neurons, hormones, and so on—objects large enough to be measured. These objects are made of different types of molecules, such as water and nitrogen molecules. A molecule is made of two or more atoms. For example, water is made of two atoms of hydrogen and one atom of oxygen. An atom can be broken down into subatomic particles. The three major subatomic particles are protons, electrons, and neutrons. These subatomic particles break down further into a larger number of even smaller subatomic particles. Quantum physics is the study of such small or fine or subtle subatomic particles of matter, which are hard if not impossible to observe and measure. Scientists at the European Center for Nuclear Research on the French-Swiss border use a huge subterranean particle collider to accelerate larger subatomic particles such as protons close to the speed of light and crash them against each other or against barriers. This impact breaks them down into finer subatomic particles, allowing researchers to detect more of them and study how they interact with each other at the quantum level of our existence.[8]

Given the expense and effort required to study subatomic particles in the optimal environment of a particle collider, it makes sense that little is known about how quantum mechanics operating within our physiology at the subatomic level might contribute to generating and regulating our psychological experiences of cognition, emotion, and behavior. There have been attempts in the West to formulate a quantum psychology on the basis of methods and findings from quantum physics, to add to our understanding of how the deeper level of our physiology affects our psychological experience.[9,10] These attempts appear to be having a limited effect on the field of psychology.

Eastern Psychology

Eastern psychological approaches, which date back centuries, have a two-level model of human physiology that can accommodate the world of subatomic particles. The level of physiology that is relatively easy to observe and measure, from the atomic scale and upward, is called the gross layer (or gross body), with reference to the relatively larger size of the objects involved, such as muscles, organs, and neurons. The level of physiology that is relatively harder to measure if not observe, the world of subatomic particles, is called the subtle layer (or subtle body), with reference to the relatively smaller, finer, or "subtler" sizes of the objects involved. The subtle layer is theorized as the deeper layer of our physiology. Changes in the subtle layer affect the gross layer, and vice versa, in the process of generating and regulating our physiological and psychological experiences.

These Eastern psychological approaches present theories of structures and processes of the subtle body and how they affect structures and processes in the gross body, physiologically and psychologically, as well as methods for working with both layers to facilitate physiological and psychological well-being. These theories, which date back thousands of years, were developed primarily through well-developed introspection and self-observation of one's physiology and psyche, and they were tested based on the effectiveness of the methods derived from the theories. In case you think this is all too subjective, please note that the use of introspection—self-observation of one's own processes—to build psychological theories is not uncommon in Western psychology, even today. In addition, physiological measurement of structures and processes (and even outcomes) of Western psychological theories remains limited by our ability to measure psychological structures, processes, and outcomes or to afford the measurements, even at the gross level of neurons and biochemicals, not to mention the subtle level of fermions and bosons, as subatomic particles of matter and energy particles are categorized.

Before we proceed further, it is important to clarify that the equivalence between the Eastern concept of the subtle body and the body layer of subatomic particles from quantum physics, which was arrived at through introspection, cannot be exact. The Easterners differentiated the gross body and the subtle body thousands of years ago in terms of how difficult their components were to perceive and measure through the five senses as well as by introspection, according to the standards of what they could measure in those days. Clearly, science is still constrained in its measurements of many things at the gross level of atoms and their combinations that make up the larger objects and energies in the world. So the many things at the gross level that are hard for us to observe through the five senses or through sophisticated instruments that can be thought of as extensions of the five senses these days could also be included in the Eastern concept of the subtle body.

It is understandable that there are a number of models of the subtle layer of the body and its relationship with its gross layer, given that they are products of introspection, however refined it might have been. One of these models is the meridian system, which is the basis for the evidence-based practice of acupuncture.[11] Even though the effectiveness of acupuncture is now studied and explained in the West in terms of its demonstrated ability to bring about nervous system, biochemical, and bioelectrical changes in the gross body, the original theory, which is still taught in acupuncture schools, involves a subtle substance called *chi* that can be felt but not measured. The chi in the individual is connected to the chi of the universe. The universal chi differentiates itself into different types of chi and is distributed along the different meridians that are distributed in the gross body to maintain physiological and psychological well-being in an individual. The meridians can be thought of as channels for chi in the body. When there are blocks to the flow of chi along the meridians, physiological and psychological dysfunction can result, depending on the meridians along which the chi is blocked or excessive. Acupuncture practice unblocks the obstructions to the chi along the meridians, balances the chi in different parts of the body, and connects the chi in the individual to the universal chi.

In 2012, the American Psychological Association (APA) approved Thought Field Therapy (TFT)[12] and Emotional Freedom Technique (EFT),[13] two similar evidence-based energy psychology approaches, for meeting the continuing education requirements of licensed psychologists. Both methods involve simple routines of self-tapping with one's fingers along certain easily located meridian points in the body. More than thirty randomized controlled studies have been done on these approaches—more than the total number of studies of all body psychotherapy approaches—for the treatment of posttraumatic stress in a number of populations.[14] A significant advantage of these methods is that they can be easily taught to clients as tools for self-help practice at home.

I became curious about what these techniques could add to trauma treatment, so I took a course in EFT. When I listened to the two facilitators and practiced the method with other participants, I realized that I was quite skeptical—as skeptical as the mental health professional audiences I used to experience in the 1990s when I tried to persuade them about the importance of working with the body for treating trauma. I thought about why I was so skeptical. It may have had to do with the labeling of these methods as energy psychology techniques, and the reflexive rejection of anything that has to do with "energy" as New Age psychology with no scientific basis, not only among mental health professionals but also in the general population.

It may have also had to do with instances when I heard some energy psychology practitioners claim that these techniques could resolve all kinds of problems, at times even cancer. When we have known for a long time that energy and matter are equivalent through Einstein's famous equation ($E = mc^2$), it is perhaps a bad idea to label a psychology as an energy psychology given the deep prejudice against the word "energy." "Quantum psychology" would be a far better classification. It would run into less resistance, given that findings in quantum physics provide a scientific basis for these and other methods that have been traditionally described as having to do with energy.

What was my experience with EFT? In the course itself, I was eventually impressed with how it could regulate unpleasant emotional states quickly. At the end of the course, I was still not sure how it could be used as a tool in the practice of embodying emotion. I thought perhaps it could be used to regulate extremely dysregulated emotional experiences to make them more tolerable for their embodiment. I never followed it up. However, I encountered its power to regulate extreme distress soon afterward. Two friends, both therapists, were diagnosed with cancer within a short period. One underwent a complicated surgery and a series of treatments, and he was suffering from a great deal of anxiety about how it would turn out for him. The other was awaiting surgery shortly after his diagnosis.

He and his wife were naturally quite anxious. In both instances, I was so grateful that I knew EFT to help them manage their anxiety relatively quickly and leave them with a self-help tool that they said worked better than anything else they had tried to help keep their anxiety down.

Physiological and psychological models that include the subtle layer of energy are not exclusive to the West. In both the East and the West, there are many different treatment models of physical and mental health, from the simple to the complex, that incorporate energy into their mix. (Here I am excluding methods that manipulate the energies produced by the gross body, such as electromagnetic waves emanating from the brain or the heart). As varied as these treatment models appear to be, they have some features in common:

- All physiological and psychological experiences are theorized to originate as impulses from the subtle level.

- Disturbances in the flow or balance in the energies at the subtle level are often coping mechanisms in the face of difficult experiences.

- The disruption in the flow or balance of subtle energies contributes to physiological and psychological symptoms at the gross level.

- Working to balance energies and restore their flow at the subtle level is one way of treating difficulties at the gross level.

When I went to Russia to teach Integral Somatic Psychology (ISP) and the practice of embodying emotion in 2011, I did not know that Russians (even Russian physicians) were quite open to alternative medicine,[15] especially traditional Chinese medicine, of which acupuncture is often a key component.[16] The Russians wanted to know if I could enrich the method of embodying emotion by adding an energy component to it. They were particularly interested in what I, a person from India who had spent the first twenty-six years of his life there, could offer them with regard to the use of energy in psychological work.

The potential benefits of working with the subtle body for the practice of embodying emotion were in my peripheral vision, given the attention TFT and EFT were getting in the field after their accreditation by the APA and because of an experience I had in treating trauma symptoms among tsunami survivors in India, which I will share in a moment. However, I was quite reluctant to jump in with both feet. I shared the collective resistance (or prejudice) of my colleagues and the population at large about anything that had to do with energy. I was quite concerned that the use of energy could damage the professional reputation of the science-based practice of embodying emotion. But I could not overcome the enthusiastic demands of the Russians and finally yielded.

Fortunately, I did not have to look far for an energy psychology model to experiment with in the practice of embodying emotion. In 2001, after I had completed three years of heady coursework for my doctoral studies in clinical psychology, to get back into my body I signed up for a two-year training in Biodynamic Craniosacral Therapy, an approach that works with both the gross and the subtle layers of the body, with an emphasis on connecting the subtle energies of the individual to those of the universe to bring about healing.

During that training I started to refine my interoceptive ability to start to differentiate the gross from the subtle in my awareness. Franklyn Sills, an American who lives in the bucolic, windswept county of Devon in the United Kingdom, is a well-known writer in the field. I relied a lot on his book on Biodynamic Craniosacral Therapy during my training.[17] Prior to his incarnation as a Biodynamic Craniosacral Therapist, he was a practitioner of Polarity Therapy. I had encountered this modality a few times, both as a client for a few free sessions from a friend in Los Angeles, and through classmates who were also Polarity Therapists in the Somatic Experiencing trauma training. Franklyn had written a book on Polarity Therapy titled *The Polarity Process*, which immediately grabbed my attention because it appeared to have an Eastern energy approach incorporated into it, based on the cover design.[18] I bought it on impulse, put in on my bookshelves with hundreds of other books, and forgot all about it. When I returned from Moscow, it was there where I had put it many years ago, waiting for me.

Polarity Therapy is an East-West bodywork/energywork modality developed by an Austrian osteopath after he moved to Chicago and changed his name to Randolph Stone. Driven by an intuition that healing involved more than changes in the muscles, organs, nerves, and brain, Stone had an epiphany while reading an old Indian text on energy or the subtle body. Reading further, and combining elements of Indian and Chinese subtle body theories with his understanding of the gross body from Western osteopathy, he developed what eventually became known as Polarity Therapy.

In Dr. Stone's Polarity Therapy, our body has a gross level and a subtle level. Our physical and mental experience and health depend on interactions between the two as well as their interactions with the environment. In case this sounds familiar, it is because we have seen earlier in this book that modern neuroscience is almost exactly in this place these days: the proposition that our physiological and psychological well-being depends on our brain, our body, and our environment, in equal measure. The only difference is that in Polarity Therapy, the body is explicitly modeled as having two levels. Defenses can form on both levels and disrupt the connection between the individual body and its environment.

In Polarity Therapy the subtle body is modeled as having five layers, and subtle defenses are theorized to take the form of disruptions to the flow of the energies of the subtle body in the gross body. There is a map of the distribution of the subtle body energies in the gross body, which Dr. Stone often called the map of the "wireless anatomy of man." Polarity Therapy has methods for working with both the gross and the subtle levels of the body and for restoring the connection between them and the environment. In addition to hands-on manipulation of the gross and subtle levels of the body, which we have translated into self-touch positions for use in psychotherapy settings that do not involve therapist touch, the integral approach of Polarity Therapy also includes nutrition, exercise, and psychological processing.

In Polarity Therapy, as in most other models of the subtle body, the subtle body is theorized as the source of stimulation of all physiological and psychological experiences, health, and illness in the gross body. There is no measurement-based verification of this theory, of course, given the generally hard-to-measure nature of the subtle body. However, there are reports of some very preliminary but controversial and much discounted research done in Russia based on measurements of the energy field around the human body that has found that changes in the energy field occur at the same time as or prior to the changes in brain activity associated with a decision-making task, implying that subtle body activity precedes activity in the gross body.[19]

As we have seen, in models of the subtle body (including Polarity Therapy), the inadequate supply or imbalances in the distribution of subtle body energies in the gross body are theorized to lead to physical and mental suffering by stimulating the gross body unevenly, excessively in some places and sparsely in others. Treatment then involves working to increase the supply of subtle body energies and balance their distribution in the gross body. We know from chapter 8 what happens when the emotional experience is too concentrated in one area of the brain and body physiology: it becomes difficult to tolerate and process, with attendant problems.

Just to ensure you are not left with the impression that incorporating the subtle body into your treatment modalities is too "subtle" to implement, let me give you an example of how easy it would be to implement it in clinical settings, even by those who cannot track subtle body dynamics in awareness or through touch. Acupuncturists do not need to see the energy along clients' meridians or be able to sense the energy flow in their own meridians to treat clients or themselves with needles. People who live in remote villages in Africa do not have to sense energy flow in their bodies to treat themselves by tapping on certain points on their body identified by EFT or TFT, to relieve themselves of posttraumatic stress.[20]

In the Polarity Therapy model, a subtle body energy called the air element, which is associated with the heart, can form a defense of imbalance in its distribution in the gross body toward the head. This has the effect of making emotional experiences too intense in the chest area, inviting gross body defenses such as muscular constriction to kick in to further the difficulty and dysfunction. Each type of subtle energy has three areas in the gross body that are important for its even distribution throughout the gross body. In the case of the subtle energy of air, the three areas are the chest, the kidneys and large intestine, and the lower legs. This subtle body energy can be redistributed in the gross body toward a more even and tolerable experience of the emotion by connecting two of these three areas at a time with both our hands, based on the second principle of energy we have seen before, which is that energy will flow between any two areas that are connected by awareness, needles, or touch.

I started using Polarity Therapy as the primary model and Biodynamic Craniosacral Therapy as the secondary model for working with subtle body defenses against emotions in the practice of embodying emotions. I did this in as simple a manner as possible so people who had no background in energy work could implement these techniques—a task that TFT and EFT have succeeded in, with great results. I tried it first in Russia and then in India, two places where there is less resistance to the concept of subtle energy and more willingness to experiment with it, to see if it helped to improve outcomes. Due to encouraging outcomes and increasing interest, working with the subtle body is now a smaller part of the practice of embodying emotion in ISP professional training. Even though working with the subtle body in the practice of embodying emotion appears to yield incremental outcomes in emotional regulation at times over and above working solely at the level of the gross body, I must add that the experiment with the subtle body is still ongoing as far as I am concerned. I invite like-minded clinicians to join this experiment, to add yet another dimension of embodiment to psychotherapy—a dimension that has the potential to further improve cognitive, behavioral, and emotional outcomes.

When I invite my classes to experiment with applying the methods of energy psychology in the practice of embodying emotions, I motivate them by telling them there are a large number of therapy modalities out there; estimates range from two hundred to four hundred. Most modalities that have remained viable because of the outcomes they deliver do not have hard scientific evidence for their theories in terms of physiological measurements. A theory is formulated on the basis of introspection, observation, or inference. Methods are developed on the basis of the theory. When methods deliver good outcomes, the theory is held as not falsified unless another theory can better explain the outcomes. As therapists, we use such methods all the time. So as you implement the science-based practice of embodying emotion at the level of the gross body, why not experiment with adding some work with the subtle body from time to time, to see for yourself if your outcomes are better with it than without it? If you get better results, does it matter whether the theory is not verified by rigorous scientific evidence with physiological measurements, when most of the methods we use are equally unverified?

In 2005, after the Indian Ocean tsunami, when we worked with tsunami survivors in Indian fishing villages to treat them for symptoms of posttraumatic stress, one therapist refused to follow my instructions not to use an energy work method she was trained in, in addition to the gross body method we were all using. This therapist ended up with results so much better than the rest of the team that we had to exclude her data when we published the very good outcomes of our study.[21] We had to do this so we could claim that the significant differences were due to the common method we were using and not because of differences among the therapists. That was my earliest impression of the power of adding subtle body techniques to standard gross body methods for treating trauma symptoms.

TFT and EFT have since developed a body of evidence.[22] A recent pilot study comparing EFT and cognitive behavioral therapy (CBT) in the treatment of depression shows that EFT might be better than CBT in maintaining therapeutic gain at three and six months after treatment.[23] If it is possible to further improve outcomes by adding subtle body methods such as EFT to gross body methods such as CBT in treatment, why deprive ourselves and our clients of better outcomes, just because we have a collective resistance to the word "energy"?

Some of you are probably working with an energy psychology modality already. Good for you! You are probably a pioneer in the field, advancing the embodiment project in psychology by adding yet another dimension to the body in psychology. You might wonder, as many in my classes do when I introduce the subtle body, which level—gross or subtle—to work with, and when, in the practice of embodying emotion.

The subtle body, the brain physiology, and the body physiology can be thought of as three systems constantly interacting with each other to generate and regulate our experiences. Changes in one lead to changes in others. Therefore, we need to be ready and able to shift our work from level to level depending on need. But that answer might be too complex for a beginner, so my usual answer is to remind my students that our interest is in building a greater capacity to tolerate emotions in the gross body of the brain and body physiology; so work on that first. Within the brain and body physiology, work on the body physiology first, unless it is necessary to work with the brain physiology because the work with the body physiology does not result in access to or regulation of emotion. If the work with neither the brain nor the body physiology leads to access to or regulation of emotion, then work with the subtle body, with the ultimate goal of creating a greater capacity for emotion in the gross body.

Good luck to all of you! And thank you for reading this book! I hope you find it of value to you in both your personal and professional lives.

A

Two Lists of Emotions

The following list of 149 emotions from around the world was compiled by Tiffany Watt Smith.[1] Please note that foreign words (in italics) on this list do not translate precisely into English.

A

Abhiman

Acedia

Amae

Ambiguphobia

Anger

Anticipation

Anxiety

Apathy

L'appel du vide

Awumbuk

B

Bafflement

Basorexia

Befuddlement

Bewilderment

Boredom

Brabant

Broodiness

C

Calm

Carefree

Cheerfulness

Cheesed (off)

Claustrophobia

Collywobbles, the

Comfort

Compassion

Compersion

Confidence

Contempt

Contentment

Courage

Curiosity

Cyberchondria

D

Delight

Dépaysement

Desire

Despair

Disappear, the desire to

Disappointment

Disgruntlement

Disgust

Dismay

Dolce far niente

Dread

E

Ecstasy

Embarrassment

Empathy

Envy

Euphoria

Exasperation

Excitement

F

Fear

Feeling good (about yourself)

Formal feeling, a

Fraud, feeling like a

Frustration

G

Gezelligheid

Gladsomeness

Glee

Gratitude

Greng jai

Grief

Guilt

H

Han

Happiness

Hatred

Heebie-jeebies, the

Hiraeth

Hoard, the urge to

Homefulness

Homesickness

Hopefulness

Huff, in a

Humble, feeling

Humiliation

Hunger	Miffed, a bit
Hwyl	*Mono no aware*
I	Morbid curiosity
Ijirashi	**N**
Ilinx	*Nakhes*
Impatience	*Nginyiwarrarringu*
Indignation	Nostalgia
Inhabitiveness	**O**
Insulted, feeling	*Oime*
Irritation	Overwhelmed, feeling
J	**P**
Jealousy	Panic
Joy	Paranoia
K	Perversity
Kaukokaipuu	*Peur des espaces*
L	Philoprogenitiveness
Liget	Pique, a fit of
Litost	Pity
Loneliness	Postal, going
Love	Pride
M	Pronoia
Malu	**R**
Man	Rage
Matutolypea	Regret
Mehameha	Relief
Melancholy	Reluctance

Remorse

Reproachfulness

Resentment

Ringxiety

Rivalry

Road rage

Ruinenlust

S

Sadness

Satisfaction

Saudade

Schadenfreude

Self-pity

Shame

Shock

Smugness

Song

Surprise

Suspicion

T

Technostress

Terror

Torschlusspanik

Toska

Triumph

V

Vengefulness

Vergüenza ajena

Viraha

Vulnerability

W

Wanderlust

Warm glow

Wonder

Worry

Z

Żal

The Human-Machine Interaction Network on Emotion has proposed an Emotion Annotation and Representation Language that classifies the following forty-nine emotions.[2]

NEGATIVE AND FORCEFUL

Anger

Annoyance

Contempt

Disgust

Irritation

NEGATIVE AND NOT IN CONTROL

Anxiety

Embarrassment

Fear

Helplessness

Powerlessness

Worry

NEGATIVE THOUGHTS

Doubt

Envy

Frustration

Guilt

Pride

Shame

NEGATIVE AND PASSIVE

Boredom

Despair

Disappointment

Hurt

Sadness

AGITATION

Shock

Stress

Tension

POSITIVE AND LIVELY

Amusement

Delight

Elation

Excitement

Happiness

Joy

Pleasure

CARING

Affection

Empathy

Friendliness

Love

POSITIVE THOUGHTS

Courage

Hope

Humility

Satisfaction

Trust

QUIET POSITIVE

Calmness

Contentment

Relaxation

Relief

Serenity

REACTIVE

Interest

Politeness

Surprise

References

Introduction

1 Stolorow, R. D., & Atwood, G. E. (1993). *Faces in a cloud: Intersubjectivity in personality theory.* Lanham, MD: Jason Aronson.

2 Marcher, L., & Fich, S. (2010). *Body encyclopedia: A guide to the psychological functions of the muscular system.* Berkeley, CA: North Atlantic Books.

3 Levine, P. A., & Frederick, A. (1997). *Waking the tiger: Healing trauma.* Berkeley, CA: North Atlantic Books.

4 Shea, M. J. (2007). *Biodynamic Craniosacral Therapy, volume one.* New York: Random House USA.

5 Damasio, A. R. (2005). *Descartes' error: Emotion, reason, and the human brain.* New York: Penguin Books.

6 Damasio, A. R. (2004). *Looking for Spinoza: Joy, sorrow and the feeling brain.* New York: Vintage.

7 Pert, C. (1999). *Molecules of emotion: The science behind mind-body medicine.* New York: Simon & Schuster.

8 Gendlin, E. T. (1981). *Focusing.* New York: Bantam Books.

9 Johnson, M. (2017). *Embodied mind, meaning, and reason: How our bodies give rise to understanding.* Chicago: The University of Chicago Press.

10 Barrett, L. F. (2018). *How emotions are made: The secret life of the brain.* Boston: Mariner Books.

11 Beilock, S. (2017). *How the body knows its mind: The surprising power of the physical environment to influence how you think and feel.* New York: Atria Books.

12 Colombetti, G. (2014). *The feeling body: Affective science meets the enactive mind.* Cambridge, MA: MIT Press.

13 Colombetti, G., & Thompson, E. (2008). The feeling body: Towards an enactive approach to emotion. In W. F. Overton, U. Muller, & J. L. Newman (Eds.), *Developmental perspectives on embodiment and consciousness* (pp. 45–68). Hillsdale, NJ: Lawrence Erlbaum Associates.

14 Niedenthal, P. (2007). Embodying emotion. *Science, 316,* 1002–1005.

15 Hufendiek, R. (2016). *Embodied emotions: A naturalistic approach to a normative phenomenon.* London: Routledge Taylor & Francis Group.

16 Swami, D. (1998). *Introduction to Vedanta.* New Delhi, India: Orient Paperbacks.

17 Sills, F. (2002). *The polarity process: Energy as a healing art.* Berkeley, CA: North Atlantic Books.

18 Sills, F. (2011). *Foundations in craniosacral biodynamics.* Berkeley, CA: North Atlantic Books.

1. The Beginning

1 Parker, C., Doctor, R. M., & Selvam, R. (2008). Somatic therapy treatment effects with tsunami survivors. *Traumatology, 14*(3), 103–109.

2 Barrett, L. F. (2018). *How emotions are made: The secret life of the brain* (chapter 6). Boston: Mariner Books.

3 Damasio, A. R. (2004). *Looking for Spinoza: Joy, sorrow and the feeling brain* (chapter 3). New York: Vintage.

4 Craig, A. D. (2015). *How do you feel? An interoceptive moment with your neurobiological self* (chapter 2). Princeton, NJ: Princeton University Press.

5 Barrett, *How emotions are made.*

6 Dossey, L. (1997). *Healing words: The power of prayer and the practice of medicine.* New York: Harper Paperbacks.

7 Selvam, R. (2017, July). *How to avoid destroying emotions when tracking body sensations.* Integral Somatic Psychology. https://integralsomaticpsychology .com/how-to-avoid-destroying-emotions-when-tracking-body-sensations/

8 Niedenthal, P. (2007). Embodying emotion. *Science, 316,* 1002–1005.

9 Oschman, J. L. (2015). *Energy medicine: The scientific basis.* London: Elsevier.

10 Foa, E. B., Hembree, E. A., & Rothbaum, B. O. (2007). *Prolonged exposure therapy for PTSD: Emotional processing of traumatic experiences.* New York: Oxford University Press.

2. Variations in Emotional Embodiment Work

1 Porges, S. W. (2011). *The polyvagal theory: Neurophysiological foundations of emotions, attachment, communication, and self-regulation.* New York: W. W. Norton.

2 Okon-Singer, H., Hendler, T., Pessoa, L., & Shackman, A. J. (2015). The neurobiology of emotion-cognition interactions: Fundamental questions and strategies for future research. *Frontiers in Human Neuroscience, 9.* https:// doi.org/10.3389/fnhum.2015.00058

3 Burghardt, G. M. (2019). A place for emotions in behavior systems research. *Behavioural Processes, 166,* 103881.https://doi.org/10.1016/j.beproc.2019.06.004

4 Tyng, C. M., Amin, H. U., Saad, M., & Malik, A. S. (2017). The influences of emotion on learning and memory. *Frontiers in Psychology, 8,* 1454.

5 Damasio, A. R. (2005). *Descartes' error: Emotion, reason, and the human brain.* New York: Penguin Books.

6 Damasio, A. R. (2004). *Looking for Spinoza: Joy, sorrow and the feeling brain.* New York: Vintage.

7 Pert, C. (1999). *Molecules of emotion: The science behind mind-body medicine.* New York: Simon & Schuster.

8 Harrsion, A. M. (1993). Affective interactions in families with young children. In Ablon, S. L., Brown, D., Khantzian, E. J., & Mack, J. E. (Eds.), *Human feelings: Explorations in affect development and meaning* (pp. 145–160). Hillsdale, NJ: Analytic Press.

9 Siegel, D. (2012). *The developing mind: How relationships and the brain interact to shape who we are* (p. 222). New York: Guilford Press.

10 Landa, A., Peterson, B. S., & Fallon, B. A. (2012). Somatoform pain: A developmental theory and translational research review. *Psychosomatic Medicine, 74,* 717–727.

11 Haller, H., Cramer, H., Lauche, R., & Dobos, G. (2015). Somatoform disorders and medically unexplained symptoms in primary care: A systematic review and meta-analysis of prevalence. *Deutsches Ärzteblatt International, 112*(16), 279–287.

3. The Contribution of Emotional Embodiment to Working with Individual, Collective, and Intergenerational Traumas

1 van der Kolk, Bessel A. (1996). The body keeps the score: Approaches to the psychophysiology of posttraumatic stress disorder. In Bessel A. van der Kolk, A. C. McFarlane, & L. Weisaeth, (Eds.), *Traumatic stress: The impact of overwhelming experience on mind, body, and society* (pp. 214–241). New York: Guilford Press.

2 Levine, P. (1997). *Waking the tiger: Healing trauma.* Berkeley, CA: North Atlantic Books.

3 Kabat-Zinn, J. (2013). *Full catastrophe living: How to cope with stress, pain, and illness using mindfulness meditation.* New York: Little Brown Book Group.

4 Wallen, D. J. (2007). *Attachment in psychotherapy.* New York: Guilford Press.

5 Oschman, J. L. (2015). *Energy medicine: The scientific basis.* London: Elsevier.

6 Widom, C. S., Czaja, S. J., & Dumont, K. A. (2015). Intergenerational transmission of child abuse and neglect: Real or detection bias? *Science, 347*(6229), 1480–1485. https://doi.org/10.1126/science.1259917

7 Sandler, J. (Ed.). (2019). *Projection, identification, and projective identification.* London: Routledge.

8 Oschman, J. L. (2015). *Energy medicine: The scientific basis.* London: Elsevier.

9 Dossey, L. (2014). *One mind: How our individual mind is part of a greater consciousness and why it matters.* Carlsbad, CA: Hay House.

4. Diverse Benefits of Emotional Embodiment in Various Clinical Settings

1 Siegel, D. J. (2010). *The mindful therapist: A clinician's guide to mindsight and neural integration.* New York: W. W. Norton.

2 Barrett, L. F. (2018). *How emotions are made: The secret life of the brain* (p. 182). Boston: Mariner Books.

3 Salzman, C. D., & Fusi, S. (2010). Emotion, cognition, and mental state representation in amygdala and prefrontal cortex. *Annual Review of Neuroscience, 33,* 173–202. https://doi.org/10.1146/annurev.neuro.051508.135256

4 Beilock, S. (2017). *How the body knows its mind: The surprising power of the physical environment to influence how you think and feel.* New York: Atria Paperback.

5 Damasio, A. R. (2005). *Descartes' error: Emotion, reason, and the human brain.* New York: Penguin Books.

6 Niedenthal, P. (2007). Embodying emotion. *Science (316),* 1002–1005.

7 Tyng, C. M., Amin, H. U., Saad, M., & Malik, A. S. (2017). The influences of emotion on learning and memory. *Frontiers in Psychology, 8,* 1454. https://doi.org/10.3389/fpsyg.201

8 Dolan, R. J. (2002). Emotion, cognition, and behavior. *Science, 298*(5596), 1191–1194. https://doi.org/10.1126/science.1076358

9 Nakazawa, D. J. (2015). *Childhood disrupted: How your biography becomes your biology, and how you can heal.* New York: Atria Books.

10 Scaer, R. C. (2014). *The body bears the burden: Trauma, dissociation, and disease.* London: Routledge.

11 Psychophysiologic Disorders Association. (n.d.). https://ppdassociation.org/

12 Landa, A., Peterson, B. S., & Fallon, B. A. (2012). Somatoform pain: A developmental theory and translational research review. *Psychosomatic Medicine, 74,* 717–727.

13 Wallen, D. J. (2007). *Attachment in psychotherapy.* New York: Guilford Press.

14 Stern, D. N. (2000). *The interpersonal world of the infant: A view from psycho-analysis and developmental psychology.* New York: Basic Books.

15 Oschman, J. L. (2015). *Energy medicine: The scientific basis.* London: Elsevier.

16 Dossey, L. (2014). *One mind: How our individual mind is part of a greater consciousness and why it matters.* Carlsbad, CA: Hay House.

17 Howard, K. I., Kopta, S. M., Krause, M. S., & Orlinsky, D. E. (1986). The dose–effect relationship in psychotherapy [Review]. *American Psychologist, 41,* 159–164. https://doi.org/10.1037/0003-066X.41.2.159

5. The Physiology of Emotion

1 Fox, A. S., Lapate, R. C., Shackman, A. J., & Davidson, R. J. (2018). *The nature of emotion: Fundamental questions.* New York: Oxford University Press.

2 Johnston, E., & Olson, L. (2015). *The feeling brain: The biology and psychology of emotions.* New York: W. W. Norton.

3 Damasio, A. (2003). *Looking for Spinoza: Joy, sorrow, and the feeling brain* (p. 37). New York: Harcourt.

4 James, W. (1884). What is an emotion? *Mind, 9*(34), 188–205.

5 Lange, C. (1885). Om Sindsbevægelser. Et Psyko-Fysiologisk Studie [On emotions. A psycho-physiological study]. Copenhagen: Lund. Also published in German (1887, 1910), French (1895, 1902), and English (1922).

6 Friedman, B. H. (2010). Feelings and the body: The Jamesian perspective on autonomic specificity of emotion. *Biological Psychology, 84*(3), 383–393. https://doi.org/10.1016/j.biopsycho.2009.10.00

7 Laird, J. D. (2007). *Feelings: The perception of self.* New York: Oxford University Press.

8 Levenson, R. W., Ekman, P., & Friesen, W. V. (1990). Voluntary facial action generates emotion-specific nervous system activity. *Psychophysiology, 27,* 363–384.

9 Cannon, W. B. (1932). *The wisdom of the body* (177–201). New York: W. W. Norton.

10 Dror, O. E. (2014). The Cannon-Bard thalamic theory of emotions: A brief genealogy and reappraisal. *Emotion Review, 6*(1), 13–20.

11 Craig, A. D. (2015). *How do you feel: An interoceptive moment with your neurological self* (chapter 2). Princeton, NJ: Princeton University Press.

12 Damasio, *Looking for Spinoza* (chapter 3).

13 Kreibig, S. D. (2010). Autonomic nervous system activity in emotion: A review. *Biological Psychology, 84*(3), 394–421. https://doi.org/10.1016/j.biopsycho .2010.03.010

14 Barrett, L. F. (2017). *How emotions are made: The secret life of the brain* (chapter 5). Boston: Mariner Books.

15 Ekman, P., Levenson, R. W., & Friesen, W. V. (1983). Autonomic nervous system activity distinguishes among emotions. *Science, 221*(4616), 1208–1210. https://doi.org/10.1126/science.6612338

16 Philippot, P. Chapelle, G., & Blairy, S. (2002). Respiratory feedback in the generation of emotion. *Cognition & Emotion, 16*(5), 605–627. https://doi.org/10.1080/02699930143000392

17 Rainville, P., Bechara, A., Naqvi, N., & Damasio, A. R. (2006). Basic emotions are associated with distinct patterns of cardiorespiratory activity. *International Journal of Psychophysiology, 61*(1), 5–18. https://doi.org/10.1016/j.ijpsycho.2005.10.024

18 Nummenmaa, L., Glerean, E., Hari, R., & Hietanen, J. K. (2013). Bodily maps of emotions. *Proceedings of the National Academy of Sciences,111*(2), 646–651. https://doi.org/10.1073/pnas.1321664111

19 Nummenmaa, L., Hari, R., Hietanen, J. K., & Glerean, E. (2018). Maps of subjective feelings. *PNAS Proceedings of the National Academy of Sciences of the United States of America, 115*(37), 9198–9203. https://doi.org/10.1073/pnas.1807390115

20 Damasio, *Looking for Spinoza* (chapter 3).

21 Barrett, *How emotions are made* (p. 119).

22 Damasio, *Looking for Spinoza* (chapter 2).

23 Damasio, *Looking for Spinoza* (chapter 3).

24 Damasio, *Looking for Spinoza* (chapter 3).

25 Barrett, *How emotions are made* (chapter 6).

26 Picard, F., & Friston, K. (2014). Predictions, perception, and a sense of self. *Neurology, 83*(12), 1112–1118. https://doi.org/10.1212/WNL.0000000000000798

27 Barrett, *How emotions are made* (chapter 5).

28 Häusser, L. F. (2012). Empathie und Spiegelneurone. Ein Blick auf die gegenwärtige neuropsychologische Empathieforschung [Empathy and mirror neurons. A view on contemporary neuropsychological empathy research]. *Praxis der Kinderpsychologie und Kinderpsychiatrie, 61*(5), 322–335. https://doi.org/10.13109/prkk.2012.61.5.322

29 Oschman, J. L. (2015). *Energy medicine: The scientific basis.* London: Elsevier.

30 Lipton, B. H. (2016). *The biology of belief: Unleashing the power of consciousness, matter and miracles.* Carlsbad, CA: Hay House.

31 Damasio, *Looking for Spinoza* (p. 96).

32 Damasio, A., Grabowski, T., Bechara, A., Damasio, H., Ponto, L., Parvizi, J., et al. (2000). Subcortical and cortical brain activity during the feeling of self-generated emotions. *Nature Neuroscience 3*, 1049–1056. https://doi.org /10.1038/79871

33 Critchley, H. D., & Nagai, Y. (2012). How emotions are shaped by bodily states. *Emotion Review, 4*(2), 163–168. https://doi.org/10.1177/1754073911430132

34 Craig, *How do you feel* (p. 6).

35 Tsakiris, M., & Preester, H. D. (2019). *The interoceptive mind from homeostasis to awareness*. New York: Oxford University Press.

36 Ekman, P. (2009). Darwin's contributions to our understanding of emotional expressions. *Philosophical Transactions of the Royal Society B: Biological Sciences, 364*(1535), 3449–3451. https://doi.org/10.1098/rstb.2009.0189

37 Ekman, P. (2004). *Emotions revealed: Understanding faces and feelings to improve communication and emotional life*. New York: Henry Holt and Company, LLC.

38 Davidson, R. J., Ekman, P., Saron, C., Senulis, J., & Friesen, W. V. (1990). Emotional expression and brain physiology I: Approach/withdrawal and cerebral asymmetry. *Journal of Personality and Social Psychology, 58*, 330–341. https://doi.org/10.1037/0022-3514.58.2.330

39 Cannon, W. B. (1927). The James-Lange theory of emotions: A critical examination and an alternative theory. *American Journal of Psychology, 39*, 106–124.

40 Bard, P. (1928). A diencephalic mechanism for the expression of rage with special reference to the sympathetic nervous system. *American Journal of Psychology, 84*, 490–516.

41 Papez, J. W. (1937). A proposed mechanism of emotion. *Archives of Neurology and Psychiatry, 79*, 725–743.

42 MacLean, P. D. (1964). Man and his animal brains. *Modern Medicine, 12*, 95–106.

43 Panksepp, J. (1998). *Affective neuroscience: The foundations of animal and human emotions*. New York: Oxford University Press.

44 LeDoux, J. (1998). *The emotional brain: The mysterious underpinnings of emotional life*. New York: Simon & Schuster.

45 Pert, C. (1999). *Molecules of emotion: The science behind mind-body medicine* (p. 137). New York: Simon & Schuster.

6. Cognition, Emotion, and Behavior

1 Fincher-Kiefer, R. (2019). *How the body shapes knowledge: Empirical support for embodied cognition*. Washington, DC: American Psychological Association.

2 Beilock, S. (2017). *How the body knows its mind: The surprising power of the physical environment to influence how you think and feel.* New York: Atria Books.

3 Colombetti, G. (2017). *The feeling body: Affective science meets the enactive mind.* Cambridge: MIT Press.

4 James, K. H. (2010). Sensori-motor experience leads to changes in visual processing in the developing brain. *Developmental Science, 13*(2), 279–288. https://doi.org/10.1111/j.1467-7687.2009.00883.x

5 Beilock. *How the body knows its mind* (p. 61–65).

6 Marcher, L., & Fich, S. (2010). *Body encyclopedia: A guide to the psychological functions of the muscular system.* Berkeley, CA: North Atlantic Books.

7 van den Bergh, B., Schmidt, J., & Warlop, L. (2011). Embodied myopia. *Journal of Marketing Research, 48*(6), 1033–1044.

8 Beilock. *How the body knows its mind* (chapter 9).

9 Muehlhan, M., Marxen, M., Landsiedel, J., Malberg, H., & Zaunseder, S. (2014). The effect of body posture on cognitive performance: A question of sleep quality. *Frontiers in Human Neuroscience, 8,* 171. https://doi.org/10.3389/fnhum.2014.00171

10 Peper, E., Lin, I., Harvey, R., & Perez, J. (2017). How posture affects memory recall and mood. *Biofeedback, 45*(2), 36–41. https://doi.org/10.5298/1081-5937-45.2.01

11 Winkielman, P., Niedenthal, P., Wielgosz, J., Eelen, J., & Kavanagh, L. C. (2015). Embodiment of cognition and emotion. In M. Mikulincer, P. R. Shaver, E. Borgida, & J. A. Bargh (Eds.), *APA handbook of personality and social psychology, vol. 1. Attitudes and social cognition* (pp. 151–175). Washington, DC: American Psychological Association. https://doi.org/10.1037/14341-004

12 Niedenthal, P. (2007). Embodying emotion. *Science (316),* 1002–1005.

13 Peper et al., How posture affects memory recall and mood.

14 Damasio, A. (2005). *Descartes' error: Emotion, reason, and the human brain.* New York: Penguin Books.

15 LeDoux, J. (1998). *The emotional brain: The mysterious underpinnings of emotional life.* New York: Simon & Schuster.

16 Kahn, J. (2013, September 11). Can emotional intelligence be taught? *New York Times Magazine.* https://www.nytimes.com/2013/09/15/magazine/can-emotional-intelligence-be-taught.html

17 Dolan, R. J. (2002). Emotion, cognition, and behavior. *Science, 298*(5596), 1191–1194. https://doi.org/10.1126/science.1076358

18 Tyng, C. M., Amin, H. U., Saad, M., & Malik, A. S. (2017). The influences of emotion on learning and memory. *Frontiers in Psychology, 8,* 1454.

19 Laird, J. D. (2007). *Feelings: The perception of self.* New York: Oxford University Press.

20 Storbeck, J., & Clore, G. L. (2007). On the interdependence of cognition and emotion. *Cognition & Emotion, 21*(6), 1212–1237. https://doi.org /10.1080/02699930701438020

21 Salzman, C. D., & Fusi, S. (2010). Emotion, cognition, and mental state representation in amygdala and prefrontal cortex. *Annual Review of Neuroscience, 33*, 173–202. https://doi.org/10.1146/annurev.neuro.051508.135256

22 Okon-Singer, H., Hendler, T., Pessoa, L. & Shackman, A. J. (2015). The neurobiology of emotion and cognition interactions: Fundamental questions and strategies for future research. *Frontiers in Human Neuroscience, 9.* https:// doi.org/10.3389/fnhum.2015.00058

23 Duncan, S., & Barrett, L. F. (2007). Affect is a form of cognition: A neurobiological analysis. *Cognition & Emotion, 21*(6), 1184–1211. https://doi.org /10.1080/02699930701437931

7. Physiological Dynamics Involved in Generating and Defending against Emotional Experiences

1 Reich, W. (1990). *Character analysis.* New York: Noonday Press.

2 Lowen, A. (1994). *Bioenergetics.* New York: Penguin/Arkana.

3 Marcher, L., & Fich, S. (2010). *Body encyclopedia: A guide to the psychological functions of the muscular system.* Berkeley, CA: North Atlantic Books.

4 Marcher, *Body encyclopedia* (p. 255).

5 Marcher, *Body encyclopedia* (p. 171).

6 Porges, S. W. (2011). *The polyvagal theory: Neurophysiological foundations of emotions, attachment, communication, and self-regulation.* New York: W. W. Norton.

7 Marcher, *Body encyclopedia* (p. 503).

8 Lowen, A. (1979). *The language of the body* (chapter 17). New York: Collier Macmillan.

9 Reich, *Character analysis.*

10 Lowen, *Bioenergetics.*

11 Ekman, P. (2004). *Emotions revealed: Understanding faces and feelings to improve communication and emotional life.* New York: Henry Holt and Company, LLC.

12 Marcher, *Body encyclopedia.*

13 Niedenthal, P. (2007). Embodying emotion. *Science (316)*, 1002–1005.

14 Faulkner, G. E. (2010). *Exercise, health and mental health: Emerging relationships.* London: Routledge.

15 Grof, S., & Grof, C. (2010). *Holotropic breathwork: A new approach to self-exploration and therapy.* Albany: State University of New York Press.

16 Craig, A. D. (2015). *How do you feel: An interoceptive moment with your neurological self* (p. 6). Princeton, NJ: Princeton University Press.

17 Keleman, S. (1987). *Embodying experience: Forming a personal life.* Berkeley, CA: Center Press.

18 Reich, *Character analysis.*

19 Keleman, *Embodying experience.*

20 Peper, E., Lin, I., Harvey, R., & Perez, J. (2017). How posture affects memory recall and mood. *Biofeedback, 45*(2), 36–41. https://doi.org/10.5298 /1081-5937-45.2.01

21 Slattery, D. P. (2000). *The wounded body: Remembering the markings of flesh.* Albany: State University of New York Press.

22 Darwin, C., & Ekman, P. (2009). *The expression of the emotions in man and animals.* New York: Oxford University Press.

23 Ekman, *Emotions revealed.*

24 Niedenthal, Embodying emotion.

25 Ablon, S. L., & Brown, D. P. (2015). *Human feelings: Explorations in affect development and meaning* (chapter 1). London: Routledge.

26 Fogel, A., & Reimers, M. (1989). On the psychobiology of emotions and their development. *Monographs of the Society for Research in Child Development, 54*(1–2), 105–113.

27 Porges, S. W. (2011). *The polyvagal theory: Neurophysiological foundations of emotions, attachment, communication, and self-regulation* (chapter 10). New York: W. W. Norton.

28 Finzi, E. (2014). *The face of emotion: How Botox affects our moods and relationships.* London: Palgrave Macmillan.

29 Porges, *The polyvagal theory.*

30 Rossi, M., Bruno, G., Chiusalupi, M., & Ciaramella, A. (2018). Relationship between pain, somatisation, and emotional awareness in primary school children. *Pain Research and Treatment,* 1–12. https://doi.org/10.1155/2018/4316234

31 Cloitre, M., Khan, C., Mackintosh, M., Garvert, D. W., Henn-Haase, C. M., Falvey, E. C., et al. (2019). Emotion regulation mediates the relationship between ACES and physical and mental health. *Psychological Trauma: Theory, Research, Practice, and Policy, 11*(1), 82–89. https://doi.org/10.1037/tra0000374

32 Fisher, H. E. (2017). *Anatomy of love: A natural history of mating, marriage, and why we stray.* New York: W. W. Norton.

33 Oschman, J. L. (2015). *Energy medicine: The scientific basis.* London: Elsevier.

34 Lipton, B. H. (2015). *The biology of belief: Unleashing the power of consciousness, matter and miracles.* Carlsbad, CA: Hay House.

35 Basford, J. R. (2001). A historical perspective of the popular use of electric and magnetic therapy. *Archives of Physical Medicine and Rehabilitation, 82*(9), 1261–1269. https://doi.org/10.1053/apmr.2001.25905

36 Sills, F. (1989). The polarity process. *Self & Society, 17*(6), 23–28. https://doi.org/10.1080/03060497.1989.1108502

37 Sills, F. (2011). Craniosacral biodynamics. *Energy Medicine East and West,* 249–258. https://doi.org/10.1016/b978-0-7020-3571-5.00019-6

8. Emotional Embodiment and Affect Tolerance

1 Gonzalez, M. J., Sutherland, E., & Olalde, J. (2019). Quantum functional energy medicine: The next frontier of restorative medicine. *Journal of Restorative Medicine, 9*(1), 1–7. https://doi.org/10.14200/jrm.2019.0114

2 Ross, C. L. (2019). Energy medicine: Current status and future perspectives. *Global Advances in Health and Medicine, 8,* 216495611983122. https://doi.org/10.1177/2164956119831221

3 Madrid, A. (2005). Helping children with asthma by repairing maternal-infant bonding problems. *American Journal of Clinical Hypnosis, 48*(2–3), 199–211. https://doi.org/10.1080/00029157.2005.1040151

4 Sills, F. (2002). *The polarity process: Energy as a healing art.* Berkeley, CA: North Atlantic Books.

5 Turculeţ, A., & Tulbure, C. (2014). The relation between the emotional intelligence of parents and children. *Procedia—Social and Behavioral Sciences, 142,* 592–596. https://doi.org/10.1016/j.sbspro.2014.07.671

6 Ablon, S. L., & Brown, D. P. (2015). *Human feelings: Explorations in affect development and meaning* (chapter 1). London: Routledge.

7 Madrid, Helping children with asthma.

8 Sills, *The polarity process.*

9 Turculeţ, The relation between the emotional intelligence of parents and children.

10 Ablon, *Human feelings* (chapter 1).

9. Different Types of Emotions

1 Barrett, L. F. (2018). *How emotions are made: The secret life of the brain* (p. 182). Boston: Mariner Books.

2 Suvak, M. K., Litz, B. T., Sloan, D. M., Zanarini, M. C., Barrett, L. F., & Hofmann, S. G. (2011). Emotional granularity and borderline personality disorder. *Journal of Abnormal Psychology, 120*(2), 414–426. https://doi .org/10.1037/a0021808

3 Damasio, A. (2003). *Looking for Spinoza: Joy, sorrow, and the feeling brain* (p. 29). New York: Harcourt.

4 Pert, C. (1999). *Molecules of emotion: The science behind mind-body medicine* (p. 131). New York: Simon & Schuster.

5 Shiota, M. N. (2016). Ekman's theory of basic emotions. In H. L. Miller (Ed.), *The Sage encyclopedia of theory in psychology* (pp. 248–250). Thousand Oaks, CA: Sage Publications. https://doi.org/10.4135/9781483346274.n85

6 Ekman, P., & Cordaro, D. (2011). What is meant by calling emotions basic. *Emotion Review, 3*(4), 364–370. https://doi.org/10.1177/1754073911410740

7 Johnston, E., & Olson, L. (2015). *The feeling brain: The biology and psychology of emotions* (p. 50). New York: W. W. Norton.

8 Ekman, P. (1994). All emotions are basic. In P. Ekman & R. J. Davidson (Eds.), *The nature of emotion: Fundamental questions* (pp. 15–19). New York: Oxford University Press.

9 Lazarus, R. S., & Lazarus, B. N. (1996). *Passion and reason: Making sense of our emotions.* New York: Oxford University Press.

10 Cowen, A. S., & Keltner, D. (2017). Self-report captures 27 distinct categories of emotion bridged by continuous gradients. *Proceedings of the National Academy of Sciences, 114*(38). https://doi.org/10.1073/pnas.1702247114

11 James, B. G. (2016). HUMAINE emotion annotation and representation language (EARL): Proposal. https://pdfcoffee.com/humaine-emotion-annotation -and-representation-language-earl-proposal-emotion-research-pdf -free.html

12 Smith, T. W. (2016). *The book of human emotions: An encyclopedia of feeling from anger to wanderlust.* London: Profile Books.

13 Beaumont, L. R. (n.d.). Learn to recognize these emotions in yourself and others. *Emotional competency.* http://www.emotionalcompetency.com /recognizing.htm

14 Plutchik, R. (2000). *Emotions in the practice of psychotherapy: Clinical implications of affect theories.* Washington, DC: American Psychological Association. https://doi.org/10.1037/10366-000

15 Johnston, E., & Olson, L. (2015). *The feeling brain: The biology and psychology of emotions* (pp. 46–48). New York: W. W. Norton.

16 Barrett, *How emotions are made* (pp. 32–39).

17 Sullivan, M. W., & Lewis, M. (2003). Emotional expressions of young infants and children: A practitioner's primer. *Infants and Young Children, 16*(2), 120–142.

18 Grossmann, T. (2010). The development of emotion perception in face and voice during infancy. *Restorative Neurology and Neuroscience, 28*(2), 219–236. https://doi.org/10.3233/rnn-2010-0499

19 Ablon, S. L., & Brown, D. P. (2015). *Human feelings: Explorations in affect development and meaning* (pp. 346-403, Kindle edition). London: Routledge.

20 Méndez-Bértolo C., Moratti S., Toledano R., Lopez-Sosa F., Martínez-Alvarez R., Mah Y. H., et al. (2016). A fast pathway for fear in human amygdala. *Nature Neuroscience, 19,* 1041–1049. https://doi.org/10.1038/nn.4324

21 Parrott, W. (2001). *Emotions in social psychology.* Philadelphia: Psychology Press.

22 Niedenthal, P. (2007). Embodying emotion. *Science (316),* 1002–1005.

23 Ablon, *Human feelings* (pp. 587–596, Kindle edition).

24 Pert, C. (1999). *Molecules of emotion: The science behind mind-body medicine* (chapters 7 and 9). New York: Simon & Schuster.

25 Shaver, P., Schwartz, J., Kirson, D., & O'Connor, C. (1987). Emotion knowledge: Further exploration of a prototype approach. *Journal of Personality and Social Psychology, 52*(6), 1061–1086. https://doi.org/10.1037/0022-3514.52.6.1061

10. The Situation

1 Barrett, L. F. (2018). *How emotions are made: The secret life of the brain* (p. 78). Boston: Mariner Books.

2 Greenberg, L. S., & Goldman, R. N. (2019). *Clinical handbook of emotion-focused therapy* (chapter 1). Washington, DC: American Psychological Association.

11. The Emotion

1 Turculeț, A., & Tulbure, C. (2014). The relation between the emotional intelligence of parents and children. *Procedia—Social and Behavioral Sciences, 142,* 592–596. https://doi.org/10.1016/j.sbspro.2014.07.671

2 Shai, D., & Meins, E. (2018). Parental embodied mentalizing and its relation to mind-mindedness, sensitivity, and attachment security. *Infancy, 23*(6), 857–872. https://doi.org/10.1111/infa.12244

3 van der Kolk, B. A., McFarlane, A. C., & Weisaeth, L. (Eds.) (1996). *Traumatic stress: The impact of overwhelming experience on mind, body, and society* (pp. 306–308). New York: Guilford Press.

12. The Expansion

1 Selvam, R. (2017, July 25). How to avoid destroying emotions when tracking body sensations? Integral Somatic Psychology. https://integralsomaticpsychology .com/how-to-avoid-destroying-emotions-when-tracking-body-sensations/

2 Oschman, J. L. (2015). *Energy medicine: The scientific basis* (chapter 12). London: Elsevier.

3 Nicholas, A. S., & Nicholas, E. A. (2015). *Atlas of osteopathic techniques.* Philadelphia: Lippincott Williams and Wilkins.

4 Gyer, G., & Michael, J. (2020). *Advanced osteopathic and chiropractic techniques for manual therapists: Adaptive clinical skills for peripheral and extremity manipulation.* London: Singing Dragon.

5 Porges, S. W. (2011). *The polyvagal theory: Neurophysiological foundations of emotions, attachment, communication, and self-regulation* (chapter 10). New York: W. W. Norton.

6 Niedenthal, P. (2007). Embodying emotion. *Science (316),* 1002–1005.

7 Marcher, L., & Fich, S. (2010). *Body encyclopedia: A guide to the psychological functions of the muscular system.* Berkeley, CA: North Atlantic Books.

8 Bordoni, B. (2020). The five diaphragms in osteopathic manipulative medicine: Myofascial relationships, part 1. *Cureus.* https://doi.org/10.7759/cureus.7794

9 Bordoni, B. (2020). The five diaphragms in osteopathic manipulative medicine: Myofascial relationships, part 2. *Cureus.* https://doi.org/10.7759/cureus.7795

10 Agustoni, D. (2011). *Harmonizing your craniosacral system: Self-treatments for improving your health.* Berkeley, CA: North Atlantic Books.

14. Interpersonal Resonance

1 Turculeț, A., & Tulbure, C. (2014). The relation between the emotional intelligence of parents and children. *Procedia—Social and Behavioral Sciences, 142,* 592–596. https://doi.org/10.1016/j.sbspro.2014.07.671

2 Wallen, D. J. (2007). *Attachment in psychotherapy* (p. 48). New York: Guilford Press.

3 Turculeț, The relation between the emotional intelligence of parents and children.

4 Häusser, L. F. (2012). Empathie und Spiegelneurone. Ein Blick auf die gegenwärtige neuropsychologische Empathieforschung [Empathy and mirror neurons. A view on contemporary neuropsychological empathy research]. *Praxis der Kinderpsychologie und Kinderpsychiatrie, 61*(5), 322–335. https://doi.org/10.13109/prkk.2012.61.5.322

5 Sandler, J. (Ed.). (2019). *Projection, identification, and projective identification.* London: Routledge.

6 Oschman, J. L. (2015). *Energy medicine: The scientific basis.* London: Elsevier.

7 Oschman, J. L. (2003). *Energy medicine in therapeutics and human performance.* Burlington, MA: Butterworth-Heinemann.

8 McCraty, R. (2015). *Science of the heart: Exploring the role of the heart in human performance, vol. 2* (p. 36). Boulder Creek, CA: HeartMath Institute. https:// doi.org/10.13140/RG.2.1.3873.5128

9 Lipton, B. H. (2016). *The biology of belief: Unleashing the power of consciousness, matter and miracles.* Carlsbad, CA: Hay House.

10 Sheldrake, R., & Brown, D. J. (2001). The anticipation of telephone calls: A survey in California. *Journal of Parapsychology, 65*(2), 145–146.

11 Jennifer, C. (2018, August 19). Light from ancient quasars helps confirm quantum entanglement. *MIT News Office.* https://news.mit.edu/2018 /light-ancient-quasars-helps-confirm-quantum-entanglement-0820

12 Quantum "spooky action at a distance" travels at least 10,000 times faster than light. (2013, March 10). *New Atlas.* https://newatlas.com/quantum -entanglement-speed-10000-faster-light/26587/

13 Wolchover, N. (2020, October 20). Quantum tunnels show how particles can break the speed of light. *Quanta Magazine.* https://www.quantamagazine .org/quantum-tunnel-shows-particles-can-break-the-speed-of-light -20201020/

14 Musser, G. (2016). *Spooky action at a distance: The phenomenon that reimagines space and time—and what it means for black holes, the big bang, and theories of everything* (chapter 6). New York: Scientific American/Farrar, Straus and Giroux.

15 Dossey, L. (2014). *One mind: How our individual mind is part of a greater consciousness and why it matters.* Carlsbad, CA: Hay House.

16 Stolorow, R. D., & Atwood, G. E. (1996). The intersubjective perspective. *Psychoanalytic Review, 83,* 181–194.

17 Siegel, D. J. (1999). *The developing mind: How relationships and the brain interact to shape who we are* (p. 232). New York: Guilford Press.

18 Oschman, J. L. (2015). *Energy medicine: The scientific basis* (chapter 8). London: Elsevier.

19 Sidoli, M., & Blakemore, P. (2000). *When the body speaks: The archetypes in the body* (chapter 7). London: Routledge.

20 Butler, E. A., & Randall, A. K. (2012). Emotional coregulation in close relationships. *Emotion Review, 5*(2), 202–210. https://doi.org/10.1177 /1754073912451630

21 Jung, C. (2014). *The archetypes and the collective unconscious.* London: Routledge. https://doi.org/10.4324/9781315725642

Conclusion: The Future

1 Pert, C. (1999). *Molecules of emotion: The science behind mind-body medicine* (p. 145). New York: Simon & Schuster.

2 Colombetti, G., & Thompson, E. (2008). The feeling body: Towards an enactive approach to emotion. In W. F. Overton, U. Müller, and J. L. Newman (Eds.), *Developmental perspectives on embodiment and consciousness* (pp. 45–68). Hillsdale, NJ: Erlbaum.

3 Damasio, A. (2003). *Looking for Spinoza: Joy, sorrow, and the feeling brain.* New York: Harcourt.

4 Craig, A. D. (2015). *How do you feel: An interoceptive moment with your neurological self.* Princeton, NJ: Princeton University Press.

5 Barrett, L. F. (2018). *How emotions are made: The secret life of the brain.* Boston: Mariner Books.

6 Ekman, P. (1999). Basic emotions. In T. Dalgleish & M. Power (Eds.), *Handbook of cognition and emotion* (pp. 45–60). Hoboken, NJ: Wiley.

7 Pert, *Molecules of emotion* (chapter 7).

8 *CERN accelerating science.* (n.d.). https://home.cern/about

9 Bohm, D. (2008). *Wholeness and the implicate order.* London: Routledge.

10 Schwartz, J. M., Stapp, H. P., & Beauregard, M. (2005). Quantum physics in neuroscience and psychology: A neurophysical model of mind–brain interaction. *Philosophical Transactions of the Royal Society B: Biological Sciences, 360*(1458), 1309–1327. https://doi.org/10.1098/rstb.2004.1598

11 Ning, Z., & Lao, L. (2015). Acupuncture for pain management in evidence-based medicine. *Journal of Acupuncture and Meridian Studies, 8*(5), 270–273. https://doi.org/10.1016/j.jams.2015.07.012

12 Connolly, S. M. (2004). *Thought field therapy: Clinical applications.* Sedona, AZ: George Tyrrell Press.

13 Church, D. (2018). *The EFT manual.* Fulton, CA: Energy Psychology Press.

14 *Meta analyses, reviews, and theoretical articles on energy psychology* (revised August 2020). Bryn Mawr, PA: Association for Comprehensive Energy Psychology. https://cdn.ymaws.com/www.energypsych.org/resource/resmgr/research/Theoretical_Articles_Reviews.pdf

15 Brown, S. (2008). Use of complementary and alternative medicine by physicians in St. Petersburg, Russia. *Journal of Alternative and Complementary Medicine, 14*(3), 315–319. https://doi.org/10.1089/acm.2007.7126

16 Zhu, B. (Ed.) (2011). *Basic theories of traditional Chinese medicine.* London: Singing Dragon.

17 Sills, F. (2011). *Foundations in craniosacral biodynamics.* Berkeley, CA: North Atlantic Books.

18 Sills, F. (2002). *The polarity process: Energy as a healing art.* Berkeley, CA: North Atlantic Books.

19 Kirlian effect—scientific tool to study mind body functions by reading aura. (n.d.). Thiaoouba. https://www.thiaoouba.com/kir.htm

20 Feinstein, D. (2008). Energy psychology in disaster relief. *Traumatology, 14*(1), 127–139. https://doi.org/10.1177/1534765608315636

21 Parker, C., Doctor, R. M., & Selvam, R. (2008). Somatic therapy treatment effects with tsunami survivors. *Traumatology, 14*(3), 103–109. https://doi.org/10.1177/1534765608319080

22 *Meta analyses,* Association for Comprehensive Energy Psychology.

23 Hannah, C., Stapleton, P., Porter, B., Devine, S., & Sheldon, T. (2016). The effectiveness of cognitive behavioral therapy and emotional freedom techniques in reducing depression and anxiety among adults: A pilot study. *Integrative Medicine, 15*(2), 27–34.

Appendix A: Two Lists of Emotions

1 Emotion classification. (n.d.). In *Wikipedia.* https://en.wikipedia.org/wiki/Emotion_classification

2 Emotion classification, *Wikipedia.*

Index

attachment theory, 82, 284
  emotional coregulator, 305
Auger, Richard, 4, 184
autonomic nervous system
  expansion, 241
  polyvagal theory, 155, 253–254
awareness, and expansion, 242–243

B

"bad feelings" and "good feelings", 29, 42, 88, 192–193, 198–199, 237
Baird, Larry D., 98
Bard, Philip, 98, 109, 114
Barrett, Lisa Feldman, 8, 105, 190, 210, 311
basic emotions approach, 186–189, *188*, 192–197
  vs. constructionist approach, 191–192
  Parrott's model, 194–197
behavior, 1–2. *See also* triad of cognition, emotion, and behavior
  emotion and, 130–132
  impact of lack of emotional capacity, 127–128
  improvement in cognition and behavior, 268–270
  improvement in collective resources, 270–271
behavioral outcomes, 75–81
Beilock, Sian, 8–9
between-session integration, 277–278
biceps, 121, 123
biochemical and bioelectrical dynamics, 157–158
Biodynamic Craniosacral Therapy, 6–7, 9, 319, 322
bioelectric and biomagnetic energy fields, *287*
  self-touch, 243–244
Bioenergetic Analysis, 5
  breaking down constricted muscles, 145
  role of voluntary muscular system, 145
Bioenergetics, 5, 7
  breathing patterns, 151
bioenergy fields, 286, *287*
  interpersonal resonance, 286–289
biological functions, 151, 152
  breathing, 151
  heart rate, 152
Bion, Wilfred, 286

birth trauma, 4, 78–79, 169, 175, 215, 301, 302
blood flow, 165
body
  availability of body for cognition, 125–127
  brain gathers information from body, 102–103
  brain generates emotions from body experience, 103–104
  cognition, emotion, and behavior. *See* triad of cognition, emotion, and behavior
  emotions are constructed from body experience, 104, 105
  flow of information between brain body, 165
  impact of lack of emotional capacity, 127–128
  physiology of emotion. *See* physiology of emotion
  posture, 124
  recent neuroscience research, 100–102
  role in cognition, 118–119, 122–125
  role in learning, 119–122
  science of role of body in emotional experience, 109–112
body maps, 102–103, 311
body physiology, 179, 185, 324
  bioenergy fields, 287
  division into areas for expansion, 240–241
  electromagnetic and quantum mechanical energy, 161
  emotion patterns, 308–309
  expansion, 261–262. *See also* expansion
  experience of emotions, 94–95
  facial expressions and vocalizations, 199
  usage of term in this text, 163
body psychotherapy, 5, 7, 78
  focus on muscular system, 146
  postural analysis, 153
Bodynamic Analysis, 5, 7, 119, 121
  neck muscles, 255–256
  role of voluntary muscular system, 145–146
Bodynamic Institute in Copenhagen, 121
Bodynamic Somatic Developmental Psychology. *See* Bodynamic Analysis
borderline personality disorder, 41–45

About the Author

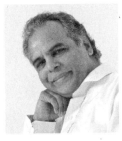

RAJA SELVAM, PhD, a licensed clinical psychologist, is the developer of Integral Somatic Psychology, a therapeutic approach based on emerging scientific paradigms of embodied cognition, emotion, and behavior in cognitive psychology and affective neuroscience as well as on multiple Western and Eastern psychological, somatic, energetic, and spiritual approaches. Dr. Selvam is also a senior trainer in Dr. Peter Levine's Somatic Experiencing Trauma Professional Training Program. He has taught for twenty-five years in twenty-one countries in North and South America, Europe, Asia, the Middle East, and the Far East. His work is informed by the older body psychotherapy systems of Reichian Therapy and Bioenergetic Analysis, the newer body psychotherapy systems of Bodynamic Analysis and Somatic Experiencing®, and the bodywork systems of Postural Integration and Biodynamic Craniosacral Therapy. His work is also inspired by Jungian and archetypal psychologies, the Kleinian and intersubjective schools of psychoanalysis, affective neuroscience, quantum physics, yoga, Polarity Therapy, and Advaita Vedanta (a spiritual psychology from India).

In addition, his work draws upon his clinical psychology PhD dissertation work on Advaita Vedanta and Jungian psychology. Dr. Selvam wrote an article based on his dissertation, titled "Jung and Consciousness," which was published in the international analytical psychology journal *Spring* in 2013. He did outreach work in India in 2005–2006 with survivors of the 2004 Indian Ocean tsunami, and an article detailing an outcome study based on this work, titled "Somatic Therapy Treatment Effects with Tsunami Survivors," was published in the journal *Traumatology* in 2008. Dr. Selvam's current work is also inspired by work he did in Sri Lanka in 2012-2014 with survivors of war, violence, loss, and displacement, and the work he did with mental health professionals working with these survivors, after that country's thirty-year civil war ended in 2009.

About North Atlantic Books

North Atlantic Books (NAB) is a 501(c)(3) nonprofit publisher committed to a bold exploration of the relationships between mind, body, spirit, culture, and nature. Founded in 1974, NAB aims to nurture a holistic view of the arts, sciences, humanities, and healing. To make a donation or to learn more about our books, authors, events, and newsletter, please visit www.northatlanticbooks.com.